Anti-Angiogenesis Drug Discovery and Development

(Volume 4)

Edited by

Atta-ur-Rahman, *FRS*

Honorary Life Fellow,
Kings College, University of Cambridge, Cambridge, UK

&

M. Iqbal Choudhary

H.E.J. Research Institute of Chemistry, International Center for Chemical
and Biological Sciences, University of Karachi, Karachi, Pakistan

Anti-Angiogenesis Drug Discovery and Development

Volume # 4

Anti-Angiogenesis Drug Discovery and Development

Editors: Atta-ur-Rahman and M. Iqbal Choudhary

ISSN (Online): 2210-268X

ISSN (Print): 2452-3240

ISBN (Online): 978-1-68108-397-1

ISBN (Print): 978-1-68108-398-8

need for a court order if at any point you breach any terms of this License Agreement. In no event will any delay or failure by Bentham Science Publishers in enforcing your compliance with this License Agreement constitute a waiver of any of its rights.

3. You acknowledge that you have read this License Agreement, and agree to be bound by its terms and conditions. To the extent that any other terms and conditions presented on any website of Bentham Science Publishers conflict with, or are inconsistent with, the terms and conditions set out in this License Agreement, you acknowledge that the terms and conditions set out in this License Agreement shall prevail.

Bentham Science Publishers Ltd.
Executive Suite Y - 2
PO Box 7917, Saif Zone
Sharjah, U.A.E.
Email: subscriptions@benthamscience.net

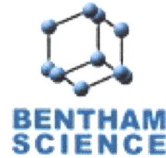

BENTHAM SCIENCE

CONTENTS

PREFACE

Angiogenesis, the process of new blood vessel formation, is both physiological and pathological in nature. A better understanding of the role of angiogenesis in disease process has already helped in the development of several classes of anti-angiogenic agents against various diseases. Inhibition of pathological angiogenesis can help in slowing down the progression of numerous diseases, such as retinopathies, benign and malignant angiogenic tumors, progression of malignant tumors, cardiovascular and CNS disorders. Extensive research in this field is yielding an exponentially growing number of research publications, focusing on various aspects, such as characterization of new pro- and anti-angiogenic factors, their role in various diseases, and identification of natural and synthetic molecules with antiangiogenic properties. This book series entitled, **"Anti-Angiogenesis Drug Discovery and Development"** is an attempt to highlight the major developments in this dynamic interdisciplinary field of research.

Volume 4 of the book series is a compilation of seven scholarly written reviews, focusing on the molecular basis of angiogenesis in various diseases and on the development of anti-angiogenic drugs for therapeutic purposes. Rachel Knott's article is focused on retinal angiogenesis in diabetes, and other macular degeneration conditions, covering molecular initiators of angiogenesis and development of specific pharmacological inhibitors. The review by Ivan Cameron is largely based on his own studies on decline of hypoxia-driven angiogenesis in cancer through short electromagnetic field exposure, in combination with infra-red. Rathinavelu *et al.* have comprehensively reviewed the success and failures, as well as lessons learned in anti-angiogenic drug discovery and development in the last six decades. The chapter by Latrakis focused on various classes of angiogenesis regulators, both positive and negative, and their merits as well as demerits, in his review. Retinal diseases and their treatment through anti-angiogenic/anti-VEGF therapies including clinical outcomes, comprise the theme of the article by Soriano *et al.* The role of angiogenesis in multiple sclerosis (MS) has been a topic of extensive research in recent years. Kulkarni *et al.* have contributed a chapter reviewing the relationship between MS and angiogenesis, inflammation, and identification of certain targets for the development of drugs against MS. The last review in this volume is centered on the role of angiogenesis in portal hypertension (PH), and strategic directions to treat PH and associated complications through the anti-angiogenic agents.

At the end, we would like to express our gratitude to all the contributors of the above cited review articles for their excellent contributions in this promising, and exciting field of biomedical and pharmaceutical research. The efforts of the efficient team of Bentham Science Publishers for the timely production of the 4th volume. We are particularly grateful to Ms. Mariam Mehdi (Assistant Manager Publications), and the excellent management of Mr. Mahmood Alam (Director Publications).

Prof. Dr. Atta-ur-Rahman, *FRS*
Honorary Life Fellow,
Kings College,
University of Cambridge,
Cambridge
UK

&

Prof. Dr. M. Iqbal Choudhary
H.E.J. Research Institute of Chemistry,
International Center for Chemical and Biological Sciences,
University of Karachi,
Pakistan

List of Contributors

Ali Alaseem
Rumbaugh-Goodwin Institute for Cancer Research, Nova Southeastern University, Fort Lauderdale, USA
College of Pharmacy, Nova Southeastern University, Fort Lauderdale, USA
College of Pharmacy, King Saud University, Riyadh, Saudi Arabia

Appu Rathinavelu
Rumbaugh-Goodwin Institute for Cancer Research, Nova Southeastern University, Fort Lauderdale, USA
College of Pharmacy, Nova Southeastern University, Fort Lauderdale, USA

Ankit P. Laddha
Shobhaben Pratapbhai Patel School of Pharmacy & Technology Management, SVKM's NMIMS, V.L. Mehta Road, Vile Parle (W), Mumbai-400056, India

Dmitry Victorovich Garbuzenko
South Ural State Medical University, Chelyabinsk, Russia

Evgeniy Leonidovich Kazachkov
South Ural State Medical University, Chelyabinsk, Russia

Georgios M. Iatrakis
Technological Educational Institute of Athens, Agiou Spyridonos, Athens, Greece

Ivan Cameron
Department of Cell Systems and Anatomy, University of Texas Health Science Center at San Antonio 7703, Floyd Curl Drive San Antonio, USA

Jesica Dimattia
Retina Department, Ophthalmology Service, Hospital Provincial del Centenario, Rosario, Argentina

Khalid Alhazzani
Rumbaugh-Goodwin Institute for Cancer Research, Nova Southeastern University, Fort Lauderdale, USA
College of Pharmacy, Nova Southeastern University, Fort Lauderdale, USA
College of Pharmacy, King Saud University, Riyadh, Saudi Arabia

Mohammad Algahtani
Rumbaugh-Goodwin Institute for Cancer Research, Nova Southeastern University, Fort Lauderdale, USA
College of Pharmacy, Nova Southeastern University, Fort Lauderdale, USA
College of Pharmacy, King Saud University, Riyadh, Saudi Arabia

Mitzy E. Torres Soriano
Retina Department, Ophthalmology Service, Hospital Provincial del Centenario, Rosario, Argentina
Clínica de Ojos "Dr. Carlos Ferroni", Rosario, Argentina

Maximiliano Gordon
Retina Department, Ophthalmology Service, Hospital Provincial del Centenario, Rosario, Argentina
Centro de la Visión Gordon-Manavella, Rosario, Argentina

Manisha J. Oza
Shobhaben Pratapbhai Patel School of Pharmacy & Technology Management, SVKM's NMIMS, V.L. Mehta Road, Vile Parle (W), Mumbai-400056, India
SVKM's Dr. Bhanuben Nanavati College of Pharmacy, V.L. Mehta Road, Vile Parle (W), Mumbai-400056, India

Mayuresh S. Garud　　Shobhaben Pratapbhai Patel School of Pharmacy & Technology Management, SVKM's NMIMS, V.L. Mehta Road, Vile Parle (W), Mumbai-400056, India

Nikolay Olegovich Arefyev　　South Ural State Medical University, Chelyabinsk, Russia

Rachel M Knott　　School of Pharmacy & Life Sciences, Robert Gordon University, Aberdeen, AB10 7GJ, UK

Sivanesan Dhandayuthapani　　Rumbaugh-Goodwin Institute for Cancer Research, Nova Southeastern University, Fort Lauderdale, USA

Sachin V. Suryavanshi　　Shobhaben Pratapbhai Patel School of Pharmacy & Technology Management, SVKM's NMIMS, V.L. Mehta Road, Vile Parle (W), Mumbai-400056, India

Sandip T. Auti　　Shobhaben Pratapbhai Patel School of Pharmacy & Technology Management, SVKM's NMIMS, V.L. Mehta Road, Vile Parle (W), Mumbai-400056, India

Thiagarajan Venkatesan　　Rumbaugh-Goodwin Institute for Cancer Research, Nova Southeastern University, Fort Lauderdale, USA

Yogesh A. Kulkarni　　Shobhaben Pratapbhai Patel School of Pharmacy & Technology Management, SVKM's NMIMS, V.L. Mehta Road, Vile Parle (W), Mumbai-400056, India

CHAPTER 1

Retinal Angiogenesis: Towards a Cure

Rachel M. Knott[*]

School of Pharmacy & Life Sciences, Robert Gordon University, Aberdeen, AB10 7GJ, UK

Abstract: Retinal angiogenesis is evident in a number of different pathological and degenerative conditions including proliferative diabetic retinopathy, retinopathy of prematurity and age-related macular degeneration. There have been numerous attempts to control retinal angiogenesis but the fragility of the tissue and the presence of the blood retinal barrier limiting the transport of pharmacological agents has proved problematic in the therapeutic regulation of this process. This chapter presents the structure of the retina in relation to the structure of the eye. In addition, the molecular initiators of angiogenesis are discussed and in particular how the hyperglycaemic environment leads to oxidative stress in proliferative diabetic retinopathy. The lack of perfusion due to damage from the diabetic milieu, the impaired retinal development in the case of retinopathy of prematurity and the aging of the retinal pigment epithelial cells are characteristics that are associated with angiogenesis. The consequent reduction in oxygen level that follows impaired perfusion creates an hypoxic environment that stabilises hypoxia inducible factor type 1 alpha and precipitates the activation of hypoxia inducible factor type 1. The activation of this transcription factor leads to the increased expression of a number of genes including vascular endothelial growth factor and this is central to the angiogenic process. The development of specific pharmacological inhibitors of aldose reductase, protein kinase Cβ, advanced glycated-end products, hypoxia inducible factor type 1 alpha and vascular endothelial growth factor are reviewed. Inhibition using small interfering RNAs to inhibit specific pathways and the use of cell replacement is discussed in terms of their therapeutic potential.

Keywords: Age-related macular degeneration, Angiogenesis, Diabetes, Diabetic retinopathy, Reactive oxygen species, Retina, Retinopathy of prematurity.

INTRODUCTION

In recent years there have been significant advances made regarding our understanding of the molecular mechanisms that drive new vessel formation. Particular interest in areas of angiogenic stimuli related to specific and significant clinical conditions have directed attention to the signals and potential solutions for

---

[*] **Corresponding author Rachel M. Knott:** School of Pharmacy & Life Sciences, Robert Gordon University, Garthdee, Aberdeen AB10 7GJ, UK; Tel: +44 (0) 1224 262524; E-mail: r.knott@rgu.ac.uk

Atta-ur-Rahman & Mohammad Iqbal Choudhary (Eds.)

the treatment of angiogenesis associated with disease. This chapter will focus upon retinal angiogenesis and an overview of the advances that have been made and the challenges that persist will be presented. Some relevant background information about the structure and function of the retina will be presented. In addition the role of angiogenesis in the context of diabetic retinopathy, macula degeneration and retinopathy of prematurity with respect to their known mechanisms of onset will be reviewed. The clinical impact of disease and treatment modalities will be discussed and the challenges and potential for future therapeutic interventions will be presented.

The Retina

The retina is a complex membranous structure that lines the optic cup (Fig. **1**). Light entering the eye is focussed on the retina where signals are received by the abundant rods and cones that lie at the base of the retina. The retina itself radiates out from the optic nerve and develops from the neural ectoderm during embryological development. This is important when we consider retinal angiogenesis because the retina is essentially an integral part of the central nervous system and thus the neurovascular networks are important in the consideration of the angiogenic process.

An additional feature of the eye that will be referred to later on in this chapter is the macula region. The fovea is located within the macular which is an avascular zone of the retina that contains a very high density of cones and is therefore essential for fine vision.

The retina lies between the vitreous and the pigmented epithelium, the latter being proximal to the choroidal circulation. The retina reduces in thickness towards the limbus region that lies towards the anterior of the eye as the sclera tapers towards the iris (Fig. **1**). The inner retina is a highly vascular tissue with a very high metabolic demand. The adequacy of the blood supply for retinal function, in both normal and pathological states depends on the magnitude of blood flow and how it is altered by autoregulation. The retina has two sources of blood supply: the central retinal artery and the choroidal blood vessels. Approximately 65 – 85% of the retina's needs arise from the faster choroidal blood flow and more extensive choroidal capillary network and this also allows for the diffusion of nutrients to the avascular outer retina [1].

Ultimately all tissue has an absolute requirement for nutrients and oxygen and these are supplied by the blood. Neurovascular mechanisms within the retina enable cells to be able to respond to inadequate supplies by the optimisation of blood flow due to the uncoupling of neuro- and vascular components [2]. Cell-cell communication and an intact blood retinal barrier are essential for the efficient and effective interaction between cells in the retina and any loss of this coupling may result in retinal damage and the appearance of ischemic microangiopathies [2].

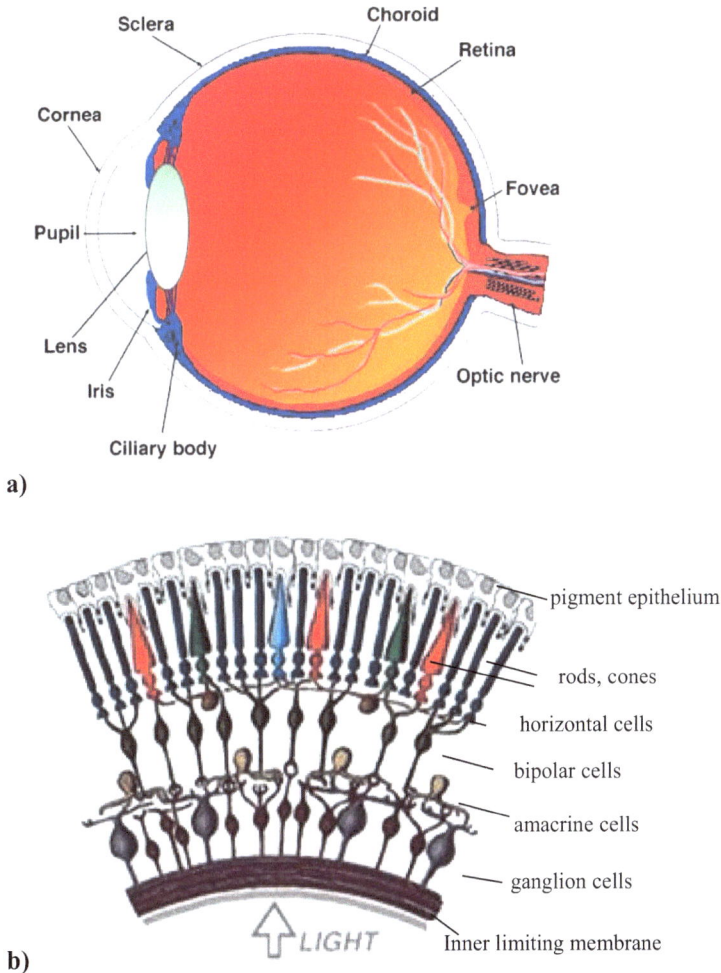

a)

b)

Fig. (1). Cross-section through the eye **a)** image shows position and relative location of retina **b)** detailed structure of retina illustrating cellular components.

Retinal Disease

Angiogenesis is driven by compensatory mechanisms that exist to respond to inadequate blood flow, and consequently the lack of retinal perfusion in regions of the retina where damage or dysfunction has taken place. The tissue response to these conditions may therefore contribute to the pathology of the disease process. Retinal disease and in particular retinal angiogenesis characterises a number of different conditions. Proliferative diabetic retinopathy (PDR) and retinopathy of prematurity (ROP) are both associated with retinal angiogenesis, and wet age-related macular degeneration (AMD) where choroidal angiogenesis is evident. In the case of ROP, a contributing factor is the requirement for a high concentration of oxygen during the birth of a premature infant with an associated decrease in vascular endothelial growth factor (VEGF) [3]. In the examples provided, the conditions that precede angiogenesis are distinct, but it is the consequence of the lack of perfusion and the loss of neurovascular integrity that drives angiogenesis.

Diabetic Retinopathy

Diabetic retinopathy (DR) is associated with progressive damage to the retinal vasculature, associated loss of neurovascular coupling and visual impairment/loss. DR represents a significant proportion of all retinal disease and the incidence has increased in accordance with the rise in both Type 1 and Type 2 diabetes mellitus with a third of the global estimate of 250,000,00 people with diabetes mellitus having DR [4]. Clinical trials dating back to the 1990s demonstrated incontrovertibly that there is a link between the control of glucose and the incidence and progression of diabetic retinopathy [5, 6]. Follow up analysis 20 years post trial demonstrates that even after convergence of glucose control measurements between the control and the intensive glucose controlled group; the latter is still reaping benefits with a significantly lower incidence of further progression of diabetic retinopathy [7].

Damage to the human retina in the early stages is recognised by pericyte loss and retinal neuronal degeneration [8]. Pericytes are specialised contractile cells that contribute to the regulation of blood flow within the retina [9]. Loss of this cell type results in reduced vascular contractile properties, associated loss of vessel wall integrity, and associated micro aneurysms [10]. Endothelial cells are damaged by increased levels of reactive oxidative stress resulting from high and/or fluctuating concentrations of glucose [11], and the enhanced activation and release of soluble factors from the endothelium and from activated leucocytes also contributes to enhanced adhesion of leucocytes [12]. Any disruption to blood flow in the form of a physical obstruction or loss of vessel integrity has the effect of reducing vessel diameter and therefore blood flow is also compromised ultimately leading to capillary dropout [13]. Pre-proliferative retinopathy is evident when there has been increasing and cumulative damage to the retina that results in the loss of perfusion to specific areas of the retina as evident in a fluorescein angiogram where the lack of fluorescent detection highlights non-perfused areas (Fig. **2**). Retinal angiogenesis is evident as vessels grow into the ischaemic areas of the retina (Fig. **2**) and can be seen as a consequence of the breakdown of the neurovascular network by the conditions created in the diabetic milieu [14].

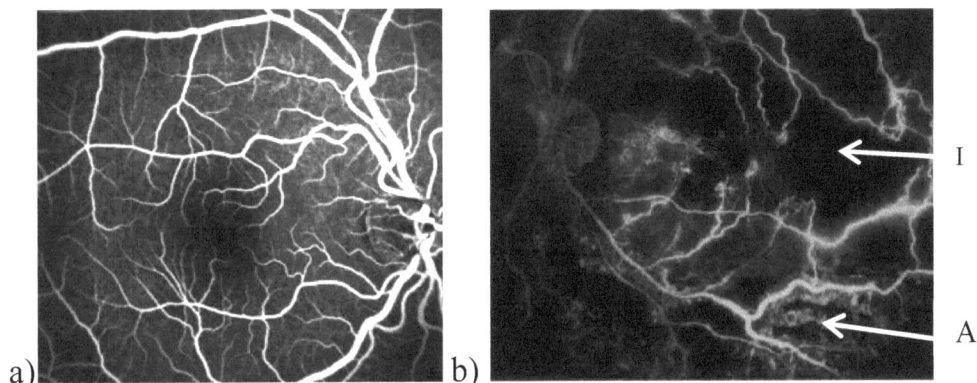

Fig. (2). Fluorescein angiogram: showing **a**) normal patterns of retinal vessels and **b**) dark areas where fluorescein dye is not evident resulting in ischemic areas (I), and the appearance of new vessels (A) is evident. The blurred vessels are indicative of vessel leakage and the tiny white dots are micro-aneurysms.

Several intracellular pathways that are activated as a result of hyperglycaemia have been shown to damage the endothelium resulting in the dysfunction of this important tissue and will be examined in more detail in the context of therapeutic options.

Retinopathy of Prematurity

Retinopathy of prematurity (ROP) is also characterised by retinal angiogenesis and is similarly driven by a lack of retinal perfusion. The incidence of ROP is increasing with the improvement of neonatal care and the increased survival rates of premature birth [3]. In this condition the retina of the premature infant does not complete the growth of blood vessels to the periphery of the retina prior to birth [15]. Vessel development extends from the optic nerve reaching the periphery of the retina by 38 – 40 weeks of gestation. If full gestation has not taken place the avascular regions of the retina become ischemic (Fig. **3**) and this initiates the formation of new blood vessels to compensate for the lack of perfusion to this area. As with PDR, it is the lack of perfusion that initiates the development of new vessels although the factors leading to non-perfusion are distinct. The trigger for the initiation of angiogenesis is the lack of oxygen supply to the tissue and this is mediated by specific intracellular processes that also must be considered in any attempt to affect a cure.

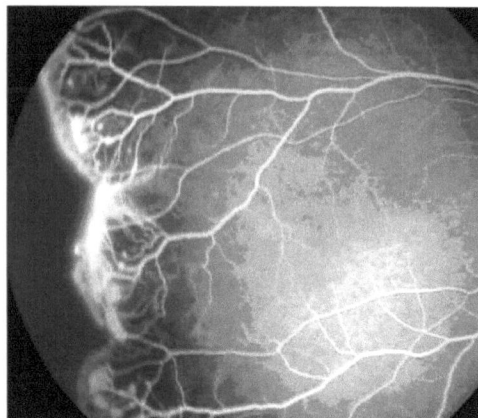

Fig. (3). Retinopathy of prematurity showing lack of perfusion to peripheral retina and new vessels starting to grow into the peripheral ischemic regions.

Age Related Macular Degeneration

Age related macular degeneration (AMD) affects the macular region of the eye and can result in major visual impairment resulting in this being a significant cause of sight loss in the population with over 50% of patients over 85 years of age with signs of AMD [16]. Retinal pigment epithelial (RPE) cells underlying the retina are very susceptible to ageing as they do not replicate throughout the lifetime [17]. Cumulative damage from ageing of the cells, and from other factors including smoking status, gender, cholesterol levels, body mass index, further exacerbates impaired RPE function [18]. In addition, underlying genetic factors are also known to play a role. The improvement in health care and associated longevity has resulted in an increased incidence of AMD as the age of the RPE is so central to the onset and progression of these conditions.

AMD may develop further into either 'wet', or 'dry' MD otherwise known as 'non-neovascular AMD', or 'neovascular AMD'. Non-neovascular AMD is characterised by the presence of a yellow deposition called drusen that lies between Bruchs membrane and the RPE layer (Fig. 4). Drusen may appear as a natural part of the aging process but it is also observed in a large and confluent form in association with AMD [19]. Drusen are composed of lipids and its deposition is increased with an associated loss of RPE function, photoreceptor death, increasing atrophy of the retina and associated visual loss. Neovascular or "wet" macular degeneration is characterised by new vessels developing in the choroid. In this condition angiogenesis does not originate in the retina but rather in the underlying choroid although the association of retinal inflammation and genetic factors are also known to contribute to choroidal neovascularisation The impact to the retina is still significant given the close dependency that these tissues have on each other and similar therapeutic approaches have been shown to be of benefit to the treatment of both retinal and choroidal angiogenesis [20].

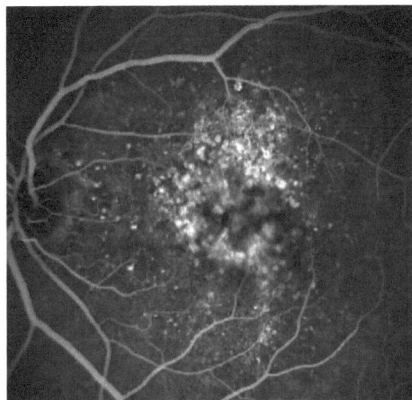

Fig. (4). Age related macular degeneration (wet) showing drusen deposition in the macular region and hyper-fluorescence indicating vessel leakage from damaged retinal vessels or from new vessels within the choroid.

Mechanism of Angiogenesis

In order to understand the therapeutic interventions that have been developed it is necessary to understand how and why angiogenesis is initiated and sustained.

Angiogenesis is initiated at a cellular level in response to hypoxia which is essentially an insufficient supply of oxygen to the tissue [21]. Central to this process is the activation of hypoxia inducible factor type 1(HIF1), a transcription factor responsible for the increased expression of a number of different proteins that have a role in the angiogenic process, coagulation, DNA damage/repair signalling, metabolism, apoptosis, cell proliferation, and a range of transporters, channels and receptors [22, 23]. HIF1 directly or indirectly activates or represses the expression of a number of different genes including those that relate directly to the cell cycle, angiogenesis and glucose metabolism and new roles for HIF1 continue to emerge [23]. HIF1 has been referred to as a central regulator of angiogenesis and it clearly has a very important role to play.

HIF1 is a heterodimer composed of the two sub-units HIF1α and HIF1β [22]. HIF1β is constitutively expressed while HIF1α is destabilised and does not remain for long within the cell if oxygen levels are satisfactory. In situations of oxygen insufficiency, HIF1α is stabilised and allows for dimerization with HIF1β to form the HIF1 transcription factor. Activation and mobilisation of HIF1 then follows as

it moves into the nucleus where it is possible for it to bind to the promotor regions of a range of genes (Fig. **5**).

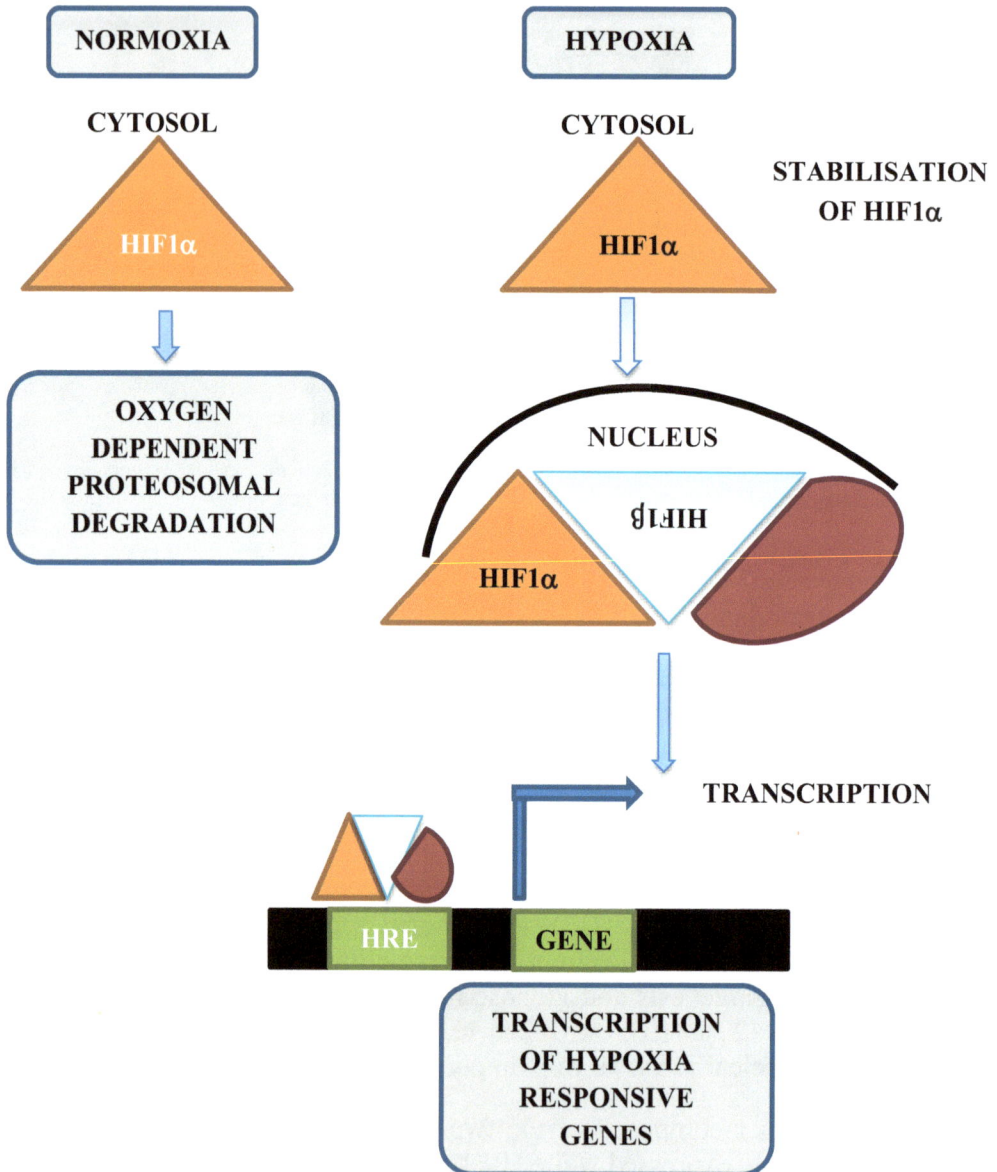

Fig. (5). Stabilisation of HIF1α due to oxygen insufficiency. Oxygen dependent proteosomal degradation of HIF1α protein occurs. When oxygen supply is limited it is stabilised and moves to the nucleus where it complexes with the ubiquitously expressed HIF1β and CBP/p300 where it binds to the hypoxia response element as an activation complex and facilitates the transcription of a number of different genes. **HRE**: hypoxia response element; **p300**: EP300 or E1A binding protein p300; **CBP**: CREB-binding protein.

The lack of perfusion within the retina and the consequent hypoxia initiates the angiogenic process *via* HIF1 activation and new vessels grow into the non-perfused area. The expression of vascular endothelial growth factor (VEGF) is increased following HIF1 activation and this is central to the ability of endothelial cells to migrate and proliferate as required at the initiation of angiogenesis [24]. The new vessels lack the robustness of the original vessels as they are generally thin, fragile and have unregulated growth with a lack of directionality.

Towards a Cure

The only way to effectively cure retinal angiogenesis is to prevent the activation of the molecular initiators of the angiogenic process. This can be achieved by the prevention of the onset of the events that lead to altered neurovascular communication and the consequent loss of perfusion. The prevention of these circumstances can be achieved by the management of the disease itself rather than any pharmacological intervention. For example, in the case of diabetic retinopathy a combination of good management of glucose control, regular screening and health promotion may prevent the onset of complications that lead to retinal angiogenesis [5], while for retinopathy of prematurity, post-partum screening and management is of importance for identifying those at risk [25]. General health advice and restriction of environmental factors *e.g.* smoking, may ameliorate the onset of AMD to some extent [26]. The reality is that there these are complex events and there are large numbers of individuals for whom retinal angiogenesis is a reality and the consequences can cause significant reduced quality of life. Thus, the pursuit of specific treatments for retinal angiogenesis remains a clinical priority.

Laser and Cryotherapy

Treatment of retinal angiogenesis for PDR, diabetic macula edema and ROP may take the form of argon laser photocoagulation therapy now increasingly replaced by micro-pulse lasers (MPL). MPL has the advantage over the argon laser as it limits the damage to the surrounding tissue [26, 27]. The pulsated delivery of the laser reduces the heat generation associated with the treatment and thus tissue damaged is minimised. Cryotherapy has also been used for the treatment of ROP with the similar aim of preventing retinal angiogenesis by destroying new vessels [28]. For the treatment of ROP, MPL or cryotherapy may be sufficient to save the central vision as the trigger for ROP angiogenesis is in the periphery. However, for PDR the stimulus may remain if hypoxia remains. There is a limit to the area of the retina that can be destroyed by laser and supplementation of treatment with pharmacological interventions also have an important role to play.

Pharmacology

The development of treatment for diabetic retinopathy has taken the course of seeking to identify the mechanism(s) that precipitate retinal damage from the diabetic milieu. Brownlee presented a 'unifying hypothesis' that brought together different work from previous decades [29] in which the production of mitochondrial reactive oxygen species (mtROS) was the common factor in hyperglycaemia mediated activation of the polyol pathway, increased production of protein kinase Cβ (PKCβ), increased flux through the hexosamine pathway and the production of advanced glycated end products (Fig. **6**).

The aim of a pharmacological approach is to inhibit any one, or several of the pathways activated by the hyperglycaemic conditions (Fig. **6**). However it is clear that hyperglycaemia is not the only contributor to retinal angiogenesis and inhibition of these identified pathways has received varying degrees of success.

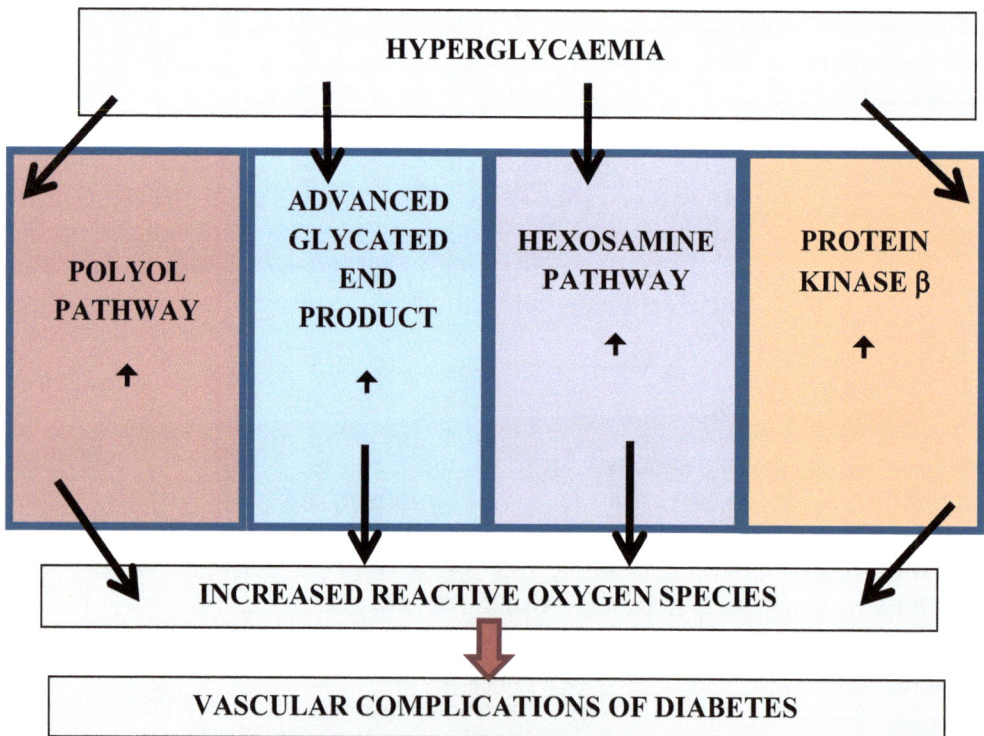

Fig. (6). Intracellular pathways activated by hyperglycaemia.

Inhibition of the polyol pathway can be achieved with the use of aldose reductase (AR) inhibitors [30]. AR is an NADPH-dependent enzyme and is a member of the aldo-keto superfamily [30]. Increased concentrations of glucose leads to increased flux through the sorbitol pathway and this ultimately leads to a build-up in cellular fructose. In addition it is also responsible for the increased levels of aldehydes within the cell *via* the generation of ROS. The rationale for the use of an AR inhibitor is clear as this essentially prevents the elevation of aldehydes and sorbitol within the cell and the consequent alteration of redox potential. It also reduces intracellular fructose thus limiting activation of the hexosamine pathway [31]. A number of inhibitors have been produced that have variously produced beneficial effects [32, 33] but overall there has been limited success in the full clinical implementation of the use of these inhibitors.

A common link with all identified biochemical changes is the elevation of VEGF which is a central driver in angiogenesis. AR inhibitors are believed to work by a reduction in VEGF induced angiogenesis [34]. However, VEGF(165) induces a phenotypic switch from increased vessel density associated with low VEGF concentration, to increased vessel diameter and increased eNOS activity at high VEGF concentration and the inconsistency of the results may be due to the dichotomy of concentration-dependent response with VEGF [35].

The lack of success of these compounds may also be due to the oxidation of the AR inhibitors and attention has now turned to development of inhibitors that are able to also act as anti-oxidants and be maintained in their reduced form until able to act at an intracellular level [36] with one particular compound phenolic 3,5-dihydroxylcompound also showing capacity as an inhibitor of lipid peroxidation [37]. There has been renewed enthusiasm to explore more fully these compounds for the treatment of the vascular complications of diabetes and other similar conditions.

Protein kinase C is a class of intracellular enzymes that are responsible for a wide range of metabolic activity within the cell [38]. Isoforms of this group are classified on the basis of the mode of activation. One isoform, PKCβ has been of particular interest in the context of vascular activation as it is activated by increased de novo synthesis of diacyl glycerol (DAG). DAG levels are increased due to un-metabolised triose that builds up in hyperglycaemic conditions [39]. The rationale for the development of inhibitors is that PKCβ is known to activate VEGF and therefore the aim is to limit activation of VEGF and remove this as an angiogenic stimulus.

However, as with the AR inhibitor studies there have been various degrees of success. In clinical trials inhibition of PKCβ has been reported with a net reduction in VEGF although translation to effectiveness in clinical studies has been less clear cut [40]. Minimal relief of symptoms is evident with the use of robuxistaurin but it is insufficient for the complete and sustained release of VEGF from the endothelium although hyperglycaemia induced pericyte derived VEGF is reduced [41]. These authors report an overall minimal benefit in terms of visual loss with a recommendation for the use of Ruboxistaurin prophylactically to prevent initiation of the process.

More specific inhibition of VEGF has also been used clinically in the context of diabetic macular edema (DME) and in combination with photo-coagulation therapy with PDR when DME is associated [42].There have been some safety concerns with the use of anti-VEGF therapy and the issue of inhibiting VEGF elsewhere in body but in general the positive benefits are well received [43]. These anti-VEGF inhibitors can also be used to inhibit choroidal angiogenesis in neovascular or wet AMD [44]. Aflibercept offers more hope as a VEGF antagonist as it inhibits both VEGF A and –B and also plasma placental derived growth factor (PlDGF) and has a longer half-life than either ranizumab or bevacizumab. Aflibercept has been used for the successful management of AMD and PDR [45]. Therefore while inhibition of the individual components appears to have yielded minimal success, VEGF activation, a downstream consequence of the activation of these pathways is significantly more promising.

Pharmacological treatment of retinal angiogenesis associated with ROP requires different considerations. It is possible to consider growth factor inhibitors *e.g.* VEGF inhibitors and platelet derived growth factors [46]. While the inhibitors of VEGF can potentially inhibit the proliferative stage of the disease, PDGF inhibitors can act earlier on in the angiogenic process following basement membrane thickening and prior to cell migration and also at later stages following new basement membrane deposition for new vessels and subsequent enrichment of pericytes and stabilisation of the angiogenic vessel [47].

If we go to the step preceding the activation of VEGF *i.e.* that of HIF1α and the activation of the HIF1 transcription factor we have this as a target for preventing both retinal and choroidal neovascularisation. Animal studies have demonstrated that HIF1 has been shown to be important in both retinal and choroidal neovascularisation [48]. Sustained delivery of a HIF-1 antagonist beta-lapachone for ocular neovascularization has been shown to be effective as a therapeutic target for retinal angiogenesis in ROP [49].

Pharmacological inhibition of AGE can be achieved using a number of compounds including aminoguanidine, pyridoximine, benfotiamine and angiotensin converting enzyme inhibitors [Reviewed 50]. Although not generally considered as directly anti-angiogenic *per se*, if they serve to maintain a robust vasculature then there is the potential to reduce the level of vascular dysfunction that leads to PDR. The anti-oxidant activity of compounds like Benfotiamine have been shown to reduce the activity of the polyol pathway [51], and this has been shown to block activation of AGE, PKCβ and the hexosamine pathway with corresponding beneficial effects seen in the retina of a diabetic animal model [52].

Interestingly, a down regulation of nuclear factor Kappa B (NFkB) has also been shown to occur when Benfotiamine is used and demonstrates the importance of the immune response to the vascular response in DR [52]. Other notable work linking the immune response with DR and PDR has demonstrated a key neurovascular immune element that contributes to the vascular changes that ultimately lead to the neurovascular uncoupling and the exacerbation of DR [53]. Chemokine response in the early stages of retinopathy has been shown to be important in the breakdown of the blood retinal barrier and the subsequent loss of 'normal' cell-cell contact [54].

VEGF induced reduction of tight junction proteins has been found to be reduced by another member of the PKC family, PKCzeta (ζ). Using isolated human retinal microvascular endothelial cells small interfering RNAs (si)PKCζ reduced the level of the specific tight junction proteins zonula occludin (ZO) – 1 and ZO-2 [55]. This same study used an animal model of diabetes to demonstrate *in vivo* efficacy of siPKCζ following intravitreal injection with a reported reduction of vascular leakage following fluorescein angiogram. While PKCζ inhibitors do not target the proliferating vessel it would potentially maintain vascular integrity and consequently delay/prevent onset of angiogenesis by maintaining retinal perfusion. An alternate approach which serves to rescue the ability of the cells to respond to VEGF is with the use of tyrosine kinase inhibitors that serve to block the VEGF receptor [56]. Evidence is also emerging for the role of specific miRNAs in retinal angiogenesis with an interdependence of VEGF and angiotensin 2 (ANG-2) with miR-351 [57]. A potential role of miR-351 in reducing the availability of these proteins and thus the hypoxia induced stimulus can be explored as a therapeutic option for both PDR and ROP.

Cell Replacement Therapy

Retinal pigmented epithelial cells (RPE) have been generated from embryonic and human stem cells [58] and given the lack of ability of these cells to regenerate *in vivo* it represents a potential source of treatment for diseases associated with retinal degeneration like AMD. The cells would need to be replaced prior to any irreversible damage occurring to the photoreceptors. Trials have shown promising effects [59] and as our understanding of the nuances of stem cell therapy and the complexities of retinal angiogenesis increases it has the potential to be a significance resource for positive therapeutic gain in the future.

CONCLUDING REMARKS

Attempts that have been made to target retinal angiogenesis have inevitably responded to only one part of what is a very complex pathway. Earlier studies that appeared to be promising *e.g.* aldose reductase inhibitors did not fulfil earlier promise. However, our greater understanding of the molecular events surrounding the neurovascular network, the angiogenic response and the role of the immune response has helped towards the development of more effective treatments. It has also facilitated the modification of previously used therapies with improved efficacy. This is both a challenging and exciting area which has the potential to have a significant impact for many who suffer from retinal angiogenesis and the sight loss and reduced quality of life that follows.

CONFLICT OF INTEREST

The author confirms that author has no conflict of interest to declare for this publication.

ACKNOWLEDGEMENTS

School of Pharmacy & Life Sciences, Robert Gordon University, Aberdeen UK

REFERENCES

[1]   Pournaras CJ, Riva CE. Retinal blood flow evaluation. Ophthalmologica 2013; 229(2): 61-74.
        [http://dx.doi.org/10.1159/000338186] [PMID: 23257770]

[2]   Pournaras CJ, Rungger-Brändle E, Riva CE, Hardarson SH, Stefansson E. Regulation of retinal blood
        flow in health and disease. Prog Retin Eye Res 2008; 27(3): 284-330.
        [http://dx.doi.org/10.1016/j.preteyeres.2008.02.002] [PMID: 18448380]

[3]   Hartnett ME. VEGF antagonist therapy for ROP. Clin Perinatol 2014; 41(4): 925-43.
        [http://dx.doi.org/10.1016/j.clp.2014.08.011] [PMID: 25459781]

[4]   Lee R, Wong TY, Sabanayagam C. Epidemiology of diabetic retinopathy, diabetic macular edema and
        related vision loss. Eye Vis (Lond) 2015; 2(2): 17.
        [http://dx.doi.org/10.1186/s40662-015-0026-2] [PMID: 26605370]

[5]   The effect of intensive treatment of diabetes on the development and progression of long-term
        complications in insulin-dependent diabetes mellitus. N Engl J Med 1993; 329(14): 977-86.
        [http://dx.doi.org/10.1056/NEJM199309303291401] [PMID: 8366922]

[6]   Tight blood pressure control and risk of macrovascular and microvascular complications in type 2
        diabetes: UKPDS 38. BMJ 1998; 317(7160): 703-13.
        [http://dx.doi.org/10.1136/bmj.317.7160.703] [PMID: 9732337]

[7]   Cefalu WT, Ratner RE. The diabetes control and complications trial/epidemiology of diabetes
        interventions and complications study at 30 years: the gift that keeps on giving! Diabetes Care 2014;
        37(1): 5-7.
        [http://dx.doi.org/10.2337/dc13-2369] [PMID: 24356590]

[8]   Fuchs U, Tinius W, vom Scheidt J, Reichenbach A. Morphometric analysis of retinal blood vessels in
        retinopathia diabetica. Graefes Arch Clin Exp Ophthalmol 1985; 223(2): 83-7.
        [http://dx.doi.org/10.1007/BF02150950] [PMID: 4007510]

[9]   Kelley C, DAmore P, Hechtman HB, Shepro D. Microvascular pericyte contractility *in vitro*: comparison with other cells of the vascular wall. J Cell Biol 1987; 104(3): 483-90.
        [http://dx.doi.org/10.1083/jcb.104.3.483] [PMID: 3818789]

[10]   Frank RN. On the pathogenesis of diabetic retinopathy. Ophthalmology 1984; 91(6): 626-34.
        [http://dx.doi.org/10.1016/S0161-6420(84)34258-0] [PMID: 6205341]

[11]   Giurdanella G, Anfuso CD, Olivieri M, *et al.* Aflibercept, bevacizumab and ranibizumab prevent glucose-induced damage in human retinal pericytes *in vitro*, through a PLA2/COX-2/VEGF-A pathway. Biochem Pharmacol 2015; 96(3): 278-87.
        [http://dx.doi.org/10.1016/j.bcp.2015.05.017] [PMID: 26056075]

[12]   Miyamoto K, Hiroshiba N, Tsujikawa A, Ogura Y. *In vivo* demonstration of increased leukocyte entrapment in retinal microcirculation of diabetic rats. Investigative Ophthalmology & Visual Science 1998; 39: 2190-4.

[13]   Bill A, Sperber GO. Control of Retinal and Choroidal Blood Flow Eye. 1990; 4: 319-25.

[14]   Ruhrberg C, Bautch Vl. Neurovascular development and links to disease. Cell Mol Life Sci 2013; 70: 1675-84.

[15]   Lundgren P, Kistner A, Andersson EM, *et al.* Low birth weight is a risk factor for severe retinopathy of prematurity depending on gestational age. PLoS One 2014; 9(10): e109460.
        [http://dx.doi.org/10.1371/journal.pone.0109460] [PMID: 25330287]

[16]   Jonasson F, Fisher DE, Eiriksdottir G, *et al.* Five-year incidence, progression, and risk factors for age-related macular degeneration: the age, gene/environment susceptibility study. Ophthalmology 2014; 121(9): 1766-72.
        [http://dx.doi.org/10.1016/j.ophtha.2014.03.013] [PMID: 24768241]

[17]   Bonilha VL. Age and disease-related structural changes in the retinal pigment epithelium. Clin Ophthalmol 2008; 2(2): 413-24.
        [http://dx.doi.org/10.2147/OPTH.S2151] [PMID: 19668732]

[18]   Kennedy CJ, Rakoczy PE, Constable IJ. Lipofuscinof the retinal pigment epithelium: a review. 1995; 9(6): 763-71.

[19]   Schlanitz FG, Sacu S, Baumann B, *et al.* Identification of Drusen Characteristics in Age-Related Macular Degeneration by Polarization-Sensitive Optical Coherence Tomography. Am J Ophthalmol 2015; 160(2): 335-344.e1.
        [http://dx.doi.org/10.1016/j.ajo.2015.05.008] [PMID: 25982973]

[20]   Shaw PX, Stiles T, Douglas C, *et al.* Oxidative stress, innate immunity, and age-related macular degeneration. AIMS Mol Sci 2016; 3(2): 196-221.
        [http://dx.doi.org/10.3934/molsci.2016.2.196] [PMID: 27239555]

[21]   Sutter CH, Laughner E. Hypoxia-inducible factor 1alpha protein expression is controlled by oxygen-regulated ubiquitination that is disrupted by deletions and missense mutations. Proc Natl Acad Sci 2000; 97(9): 4748-53.
        [http://dx.doi.org/http://dx.doi.org/ 10.1073/pnas.080072497]

[22]   Greijer AE, van der Groep P, Kemming D, *et al.* Up-regulation of gene expression by hypoxia is mediated predominantly by hypoxia-inducible factor 1 (HIF-1). J Pathol 2005; 206(3): 291-304.
        [http://dx.doi.org/10.1002/path.1778] [PMID: 15906272]

[23]   Kurihara T, Westenskow PD, Friedlander M. Hypoxia-inducible factor (HIF)/vascular endothelial growth factor (VEGF) signaling in the retina. Adv Exp Med Biol 2014; 801: 275-81.
        [http://dx.doi.org/10.1007/978-1-4614-3209-8_35] [PMID: 24664708]

[24]   Jo DH, An H, Chang DJ, *et al.* Hypoxia-mediated retinal neovascularization and vascular leakage in diabetic retina is suppressed by HIF-1α destabilization by SH-1242 and SH-1280, novel hsp90 inhibitors. J Mol Med 2014; 92(10): 1083-92.

[http://dx.doi.org/10.1007/s00109-014-1168-8] [PMID: 24875598]

[25] Austeng D, Källen KB, Ewald UW, Jakobsson PG, Holmström GE. Incidence of retinopathy of prematurity in infants born before 27 weeks gestation in Sweden. Arch Ophthalmol 2009; 127(10): 1315-9.
[http://dx.doi.org/10.1001/archophthalmol.2009.244] [PMID: 19822848]

[26] Yonekawa Y, Miller JW, Kim IK. Age-Related Macular Degeneration: Advances in Management and Diagnosis. J Clin Med 2015; 4(2): 343-59.
[http://dx.doi.org/10.3390/jcm4020343] [PMID: 26239130]

[27] Kiire C, Sivaprasad S, Chong V. Subthreshold Micropulse Laser Therapy for Retinal Disorders. Retina today 2011; 67-70.

[28] Iwase S, Kaneko H, Fujioka C, *et al.* A long-term follow-up of patients with retinopathy of prematurity treated with photocoagulation and cryotherapy. Nagoya J Med Sci 2014; 76(1-2): 121-8.
[PMID: 25129998]

[29] Brownlee M. The pathobiology of diabetic complications: a unifying mechanism. Diabetes 2005; 54(6): 1615-25.
[http://dx.doi.org/10.2337/diabetes.54.6.1615] [PMID: 15919781]

[30] Vedantham S, Ananthakrishnan R, Schmidt AM, Ramasamy R. Aldose reductase, oxidative stress and diabetic cardiovascular complications. Cardiovascular Hematol Agents Med Chem 2012; 10(3): 234-40.
[http://dx.doi.org/10.2174/187152512802651097] [PMID: 22632267]

[31] Marshall S, Garvey WT, Traxinger RR. New insights into the metabolic regulation of insulin action and insulin resistance: role of glucose and amino acids. FASEB J 1991; 5(15): 3031-6.
[PMID: 1743436]

[32] Hotta N, Kawamori R, Fukuda M, Shigeta Y. Long-term clinical effects of epalrestat, an aldose reductase inhibitor, on progression of diabetic neuropathy and other microvascular complications: multivariate epidemiological analysis based on patient background factors and severity of diabetic neuropathy. Diabet Med 2012; 29(12): 1529-33.
[http://dx.doi.org/10.1111/j.1464-5491.2012.03684.x] [PMID: 22507139]

[33] Sun W, Oates PJ, Coutcher JB, Gerhardinger C, Lorenzi M. A selective aldose reductase inhibitor of a new structural class prevents or reverses early retinal abnormalities in experimental diabetic retinopathy. Diabetes 2006; 55(10): 2757-62.
[http://dx.doi.org/10.2337/db06-0138] [PMID: 17003340]

[34] Yadav UC, Srivastava SK, Ramana KV. Prevention of VEGF-induced growth and tube formation in human retinal endothelial cells by aldose reductase inhibition. J Diabetes Complications 2012; 26(5): 369-77.
[http://dx.doi.org/10.1016/j.jdiacomp.2012.04.017] [PMID: 22658411]

[35] Parsons-Wingerter P, Chandrasekharan UM, McKay TL, *et al.* A VEGF165-induced phenotypic switch from increased vessel density to increased vessel diameter and increased endothelial NOS activity. Microvasc Res 2006; 72(3): 91-100.

[36] Zou Y, Qin X, Hao X, *et al.* Phenolic 4-hydroxy and 3,5-dihydroxy derivatives of 3-phenoxyquinoxalin-2(1H)-one as potent aldose reductase inhibitors with antioxidant activity. Bioorg Med Chem Lett 2015; 25(18): 3924-7.
[http://dx.doi.org/10.1016/j.bmcl.2015.07.048] [PMID: 26227780]

[37] Srivastava SK, Yadav UC, Reddy AB, *et al.* Aldose reductase inhibition suppresses oxidative stress-induced inflammatory disorders. Chem Biol Interact 2011; 191(1-3): 330-8.
[http://dx.doi.org/10.1016/j.cbi.2011.02.023] [PMID: 21354119]

[38] Wu-Zhang AX, Newton AC. Protein kinase C pharmacology: refining the toolbox. Biochem J 2013; 452(2): 195-209.
[http://dx.doi.org/10.1042/BJ20130220] [PMID: 23662807]

[39]   Geraldes P, King GL. Activation of protein kinase C isoforms and its impact on diabetic complications. Circ Res 2010; 106(8): 1319-31.
[http://dx.doi.org/10.1161/CIRCRESAHA.110.217117] [PMID: 20431074]

[40]   The effect of ruboxistaurin on visual loss in patients with moderately severe to very severe nonproliferative diabetic retinopathy: initial results of the Protein Kinase C beta Inhibitor Diabetic Retinopathy Study (PKC-DRS) multicenter randomized clinical trial. Diabetes 2005; 54(7): 2188-97.
[http://dx.doi.org/10.2337/diabetes.54.7.2188] [PMID: 15983221]

[41]   Deissler HL, Lang GE. The Protein Kinase C Inhibitor: Ruboxistaurin. Dev Ophthalmol 2016; 55: 295-301.
[http://dx.doi.org/10.1159/000431204] [PMID: 26501476]

[42]   Vaziri K, Schwartz SG, Relhan N, Kishor KS, Flynn HW Jr. New Therapeutic Approaches in Diabetic Retinopathy. Rev Diabet Stud 2015; 12(1-2): 196-210.
[http://dx.doi.org/10.1900/RDS.2015.12.196] [PMID: 26676668]

[43]   Amadio M, Govoni S, Pascale A. Targeting VEGF in eye neovascularization: Whats new?: A comprehensive review on current therapies and oligonucleotide-based interventions under development. Pharmacol Res 2016; 103: 253-69.
[http://dx.doi.org/10.1016/j.phrs.2015.11.027] [PMID: 26678602]

[44]   Semeraro F, Morescalchi F, Duse S, Gambicorti E, Cancarini A, Costagliola C. Pharmacokinetic and Pharmacodynamic Properties of Anti-VEGF Drugs After Intravitreal Injection. Curr Drug Metab 2015; 16(7): 572-84.
[http://dx.doi.org/10.2174/1389200216666151001120831] [PMID: 26424177]

[45]   Balaratnasingam C, Dhrami-Gavazi E, McCann JT, Ghadiali Q, Freund KB. Aflibercept: a review of its use in the treatment of choroidal neovascularization due to age-related macular degeneration. Clin Ophthalmol 2015; 9: 2355-71.
[PMID: 26719668]

[46]   Dong A, Seidel C, Snell D, *et al.* Antagonism of PDGF-BB suppresses subretinal neovascularization and enhances the effects of blocking VEGF-A. Angiogenesis 2014; 17(3): 553-62.
[PMID: 24154861]

[47]   Sadiq MA, Hanout M, Sarwar S, *et al.* Platelet derived growth factor inhibitors: A potential therapeutic approach for ocular neovascularization. Saudi J Ophthalmol 2015; 29(4): 287-91.
[http://dx.doi.org/10.1016/j.sjopt.2015.05.005] [PMID: 26586980]

[48]   Arduini A, Escobar J, Vento M, *et al.* Metabolic adaptation and neuroprotection differ in the retina and choroid in a piglet model of acute postnatal hypoxia. Pediatr Res 2014; 76(2): 127-34.
[http://dx.doi.org/10.1038/pr.2014.70] [PMID: 24819373]

[49]   Park SW, Kim JH, Kim KE, *et al.* Beta-lapachone inhibits pathological retinal neovascularizationin oxygen-induced retinopathy *via* regulation of HIF-1α. Cell Mol Med 2014; 18(5): 875-84.
[http://dx.doi.org/10.1111/jcmm.12235]

[50]   Nenna A, Nappi F, Singh SSA, Sutherland FW, Domenico FD, Chello M, *et al.* Res Pharmacologic Approaches Against Advanced Glycation End Products (AGEs) in Diabetic Cardiovascular Disease. Research in cardiovascular medicine 2015; 4(2): e26949.
[http://dx.doi.org/http://dx.doi.org: 10.5812/cardiovascmed.4(2)2015.26949]

[51]   Berrone E, Beltramo E, Solimine C, Ape AU, Porta M. Regulation of intracellular glucose and polyol pathway by thiamine and benfotiamine in vascular cells cultured in high glucose. J Biol Chem 2006; 281(14): 9307-13.
[http://dx.doi.org/10.1074/jbc.M600418200] [PMID: 16452468]

[52]   Hammes HP, Du X, Edelstein D, *et al.* Benfotiamine blocks three major pathways of hyperglycemic damage and prevents experimental diabetic retinopathy. Nat Med 2003; 9(3): 294-9.
[http://dx.doi.org/10.1038/nm834] [PMID: 12592403]

[53] Yu Y, Chen H, Su SB. Neuroinflammatory responses in diabetic retinopathy. J Neuroinflammation 2015; 12: 141.
[http://dx.doi.org/10.1186/s12974-015-0368-7] [PMID: 26245868]

[54] Rangasamy S, McGuire PG, Franco Nitta C, Monickaraj F, Oruganti SR, Das A. Chemokine mediated monocyte trafficking into the retina: role of inflammation in alteration of the blood-retinal barrier in diabetic retinopathy. PLoS One 2014; 9(10): e108508.
[http://dx.doi.org/10.1371/journal.pone.0108508] [PMID: 25329075]

[55] Song HB, Jun H-O, Kim JH, Yu Y-S, Kim KW, Kim JH. Suppression of protein kinase C-ζ attenuates vascular leakage *via* prevention of tight junction protein decrease in diabetic retinopathy. Biochem Biophys Res Commun 2014; 444(1): 63-8.
[http://dx.doi.org/10.1016/j.bbrc.2014.01.002] [PMID: 24434146]

[56] Hos D, Bock F, Dietrich T, *et al.* Inflammatory corneal (lymph)angiogenesis is blocked by VEGFR-tyrosine kinase inhibitor ZK 261991, resulting in improved graft survival after corneal transplantation. Invest Ophthalmol Vis Sci 2008; 49(5): 1836-42.
[http://dx.doi.org/10.1167/iovs.07-1314] [PMID: 18436817]

[57] Zhao R, Qian L, Jiang L. miRNA-dependent cross-talk between VEGF and Ang-2 in hypoxia-induced microvascular dysfunction. Biochem Biophys Res Commun 2014; 452(3): 428-35.
[http://dx.doi.org/http://dx.doi.org/10.1016/j.bbrc.2014.08.096]

[58] Buchholz DE, Hikita ST, Rowland TJ, *et al.* Derivation of functional retinal pigmented epithelium from induced pluripotent stem cells. Stem Cells 2009; 27(10): 2427-34.
[http://dx.doi.org/10.1002/stem.189] [PMID: 19658190]

[59] Song MJ, Bharti K. Looking into the future: Using induced pluripotent stem cells to build two and three dimensional ocular tissue for cell therapy and disease modeling. J Brain Res 2015; 2-14.
[http://dx.doi.org/http://dx.doi.org/10.1016/j.brainres.2015.12.011]

CHAPTER 2

Cancerous Tumor Growth, Driven by Hypoxia Induced Angiogenesis is Slowed by Brief Daily EMF Therapy

Ivan Cameron[*]

Department of Cell Systems and Anatomy, University of Texas Health Science Center at San Antonio 7703, Floyd Curl Drive San Antonio, TX 78229-3900, USA

Abstract: As cancerous tumors grow their continued increase in cancer cell number becomes dependent on an increased blood supply from the surrounding host non-tumor tissue. Tumor cancer cells furthest from the host blood supply become hypoxic and without an increased blood supply these cancer cells become necrotic and die. The cancer cells that become hypoxic are triggered to synthesize hypoxia inducible factor (HIF) and vascular endothelial growth factor (VEGF) that is released from the hypoxic cell to stimulate a major increase in sprouting of endothelial cells. Thus neoangiogenesis in the tumor is apparently hypoxia driven in tumors.

Our research group found that a brief daily therapeutic electromagnetic field exposure (TEMF) slowed breast cancer tumor growth in syngenetic mice. The optimal TEMF exposure dose for retardation of tumors growth and angiogenesis without harmful side effects was a 120 Hz semi-sine wave given at 15 mT for 10 minutes a day. This TEMF therapy gave the maximum antiangiogenic effect with no noticeable side effects. Although this TEMF slowed tumor growth it did not cause the tumors to shrink in size.

An experiment was done to find out if combining two different therapies, one targeting angiogenesis (TEMF) and the other targeting killing of rapidly dividing cells (gamma irradiation-IR), might have an additive tumor inhibitive effect. In short TEMF, combined with IR proved to have a significant additive tumor inhibiting effect and TEMF was judged to be a safe effective adjunct to IR therapy.

Keywords: Angiogenesis, Antiangiogenic therapy, Blood vessels, Blood vessel marker CD 31, Breast cancer, Electromagnetic field therapy, Endothelial cells, Gamma irradiation, Hypoxia, Hypoxia inducible factor, Metastasis, Morphometric analysis, Tumorous cancer, Tumor growth, Tumor structure.

[*] **Corresponding author Ivan Cameron:** Department of Cell Systems and Anatomy, University of Texas Health Science Center at San Antonio 7703, Floyd Curl Drive San Antonio, TX 78229-3900, USA; Tel/Fax: (210) 387-9434; E-mail: cameron@uthscsa.edu

Atta-ur-Rahman & Mohammad Iqbal Choudhary (Eds.)

INTRODUCTION

A team of six people came together to answer key questions on the use of therapeutic electromagnetic fields (TEMF) to inhibit growth of rapidly growing cancerous tumors. The team members were: M.S. Markov, C.D. Williams, I.L. Cameron, W.E. Hardman, L-Z Sun and N. Short.

This chapter gives an account of the experiments employed to answer the following key questions. The first question was, can a brief daily TEMF inhibit the growth of a rapidly growing cancerous tumor without harmful side effects to the tumor bearing host? If so, what is the best TEMF exposure condition needed for optimal inhibition of tumor growth and increase in host survival time? We then turned to the question of how does the TEMF work to bring about inhibition of cancerous tumor growth? The answer to this question pointed to the inhibition of the tumor vascularization (anti-angiogenesis) process which led us to investigate the mechanism of action of TEMF on angiogenesis. The research lead to the finding that tumor cell hypoxia stimulates the angiogenesis.

It has been reported in 13 publications [17] that brief daily exposure of a pulsating EMF significantly retarded tumor growth rate in a variety of cancer types (Table **1**) also see [11] and [12].

Table 1. A sample of literature reports on effects of electromagnetic field types on growth of cancerous tumors in animal hosts[a].

Type of Tumor	Frequency Hz and (pps)	Intensity m Tesla	Exposure min (m), (hr), or sec/day (d)	Significant Growth Retardation Yes or No	References
Melanoma	25	2-5 mT	3 hr/d	Yes	[7]
Hepatoma	100	0.7 mT	1 hr 3x/d	Yes	[8]
Colon	50	2.5 & 5.5 mT	70 m/d	Yes	[9]
Mammary	12 & 460	9 mT	10 m on alternate days	Yes	[2]
MX-1	50	15-20 mT	3 hr/d	Yes	
Carcinogen induced	0.8	100 mT	8 m/d	Yes	
Mammary	120	10-20 mT	10 m/d	Yes	
Mammary	120	10 & 20 mT	3 to 80 m/d	Yes	this report
Mammary	120	15 mT	10 m/d	Yes	[1]
Mammary	1	100 mT	60 to 180 m/d	No	[4]
	1		360 m/d	Yes	

(Table 1) cont.....

Type of Tumor	Frequency Hz and (pps)	Intensity m Tesla	Exposure min (m), (hr), or sec/day (d)	Significant Growth Retardation Yes or No	References
Sarcoma	0.16 – 1.3	0.6 - 2.0T	15 m/d	Yes	[5]
Melanoma	50	5.5 mT	70 m/d	Yes	[6]
Sarcoma	50	250 mT	80 sec/d	Yes	[13]

ªThis sample is not comprehensive but is judged to be a reasonably representative.
A semi sine wave was used in the 120 Hz studies; other studies used a sine wave signal.

However none of these studies demonstrated tumor regression. The most frequently used cancer therapy is to surgically remove the cancer cells or to kill rapidly dividing cancer cells.

Irradiation therapy and most chemotherapies kill rapidly dividing cancer cells but also kill rapidly dividing normal cell populations in the tumor bearing host with harmful side effects to the tumor bearing host.

Given that a pulsed electromagnetic field (PEMF) works to slow tumor growth by suppression of hypoxia induced angiogenesis, without harmful side effects to the host it was decided to combine PEMF therapy with gamma irradiation therapy to find out if the combination of these two therapies, focused on two different targets (angiogenesis and killing of rapidly dividing cells), might have an additive therapeutic benefit.

This idea was tested experimentally [17, 18]. The following section of this chapter summarizes experiments that our team did to determine an optimal EMF exposure condition to inhibit tumor growth and vascularity without harmful side effects on the host.

One of the animal models tested was a murine 16/c mammary adenocarcinoma. Tumor fragments were subcutaneously implanted between the scapula of 7-week old female C3H/HeJ mice [2, 14, 17, 18]. Once the tumor grew to 100 mm^3, the tumorous host mice were given daily EMF treatments. Fig. (**1**) illustrates the EMF machine and wave form used for the EMF therapy. The treatment was applied for 3 to 80 minutes either once or twice a day and ranged in intensity from 10-20 m Tesla (mT).

Tumors were measured for volume calculations every 3 to 4 days. The TEMF exposure conditions tested are listed in Table **2**.

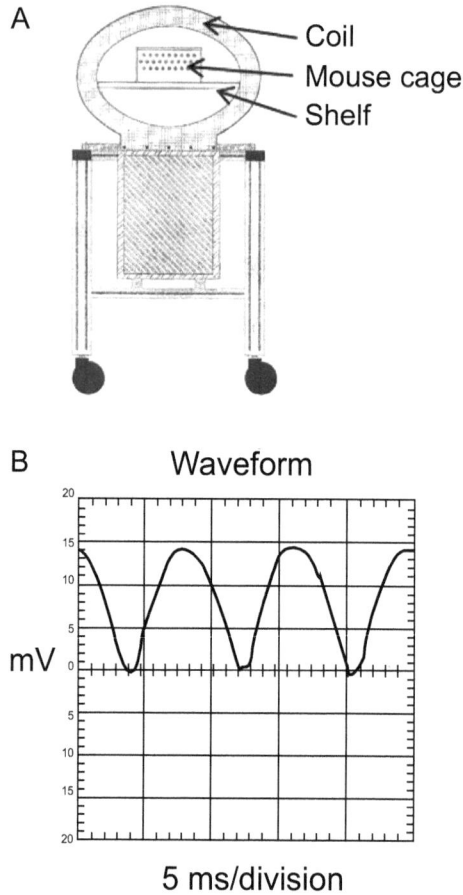

Fig. (1). The EMF exposure machine used has an ellipsoidal coil with diameter of 35 to 48 cm. The magnetic field measured in the mouse cage gave homogeneous flux density signal of 10, 15 or 20 mT and no measurable temperature change. The bottom illustrates the semi sine wave form that was given at 120 pulses per second [18].

Tumor size was measured on day 8 after tumor transplant just before the first TEMF exposure and again on days 10, 14, 17 and 20 (Table **3**).

Statistical analysis of the control and all of the TEMF groups revealed that the control group (with only sham TEMF exposure) had significantly larger tumor volume than each of the TEMF groups. Regression analysis of tumor volume increased by day 17, data revealed a significant linear regression of tumor growth rate in mice receiving 0, 10, 15 or 20 mT for 10 minutes per day indicated a clear TEMF dose response decrease on tumor growth rate. At termination of the experiment the tumors were removed, weighed and bisected then: rapidly frozen, cryosectioned at 12 μm thickness and used for immunohistochemical staining with anti-mouse CD-31 that specifically stains the surface of endothelial cells. The CD-31 stained tumor endothelial cells blood vessels are illustrated in Fig. (**2**).

Table 2. EMF exposure conditions used in this study.

Group number	EMF exposure condition
1.	Control (0 mT) sham exposure
2.	10 mT 3 minutes per day
3.	10 mT 10 minutes per day
4.	10 mT 40 minutes per day
5.	10 mT 40 minutes twice per day
6.	15 mT 10 minutes per day
7.	20 mT 10 minutes per day
8.	20 mT 10 minutes twice per day

There were 20 mice in group 1, all other groups had 10 mice.

Table 3. Tumor volumes (mm³, mean ±SD) for each group, at 8, 10, 14 and 17 days after implantation of tumors.

Group[a]	Day 8	Day 10	Day 14	Day 17
1	138.5 ± 37.2	370.3 ± 184.0	1602.0 ± 845.2	4089.1 ± 1341.6[b]
2	130.9 ± 39.2	282.3 ± 140.9	1320.8 ± 529.0	3149.8 ± 727.0
3	137.1 ± 37.0	308.0 ± 125.8	1207.2 ± 445.5	3081.9 ± 553.0
4	111.2 ± 36.6	294.9 ± 132.2	1095.2 ± 382.6	2901.9 ± 696.2
5	129.8 ± 39.2	275.4 ± 114.1	1306.7 ± 440.3	3194.5 ± 524.5
6	132.6 ± 43.3	264.9 ± 96.2	1181.5 ± 630.9	2742.2 ± 784.6
7	123.4 ± 44.0	261.1 ± 166.3	1057.5 ± 528.6	2473.0 ± 756.5
8	142.2 ± 44.3	225.9 ± 81.8	922.0 ± 303.7	2402.8 ± 562.6
P value[c]	0.71	0.24	0.05	0.0001

[a] see Table **2** for EMF exposure conditions
[b] Means of the tumor volume for each group were not significantly different until day 14. ANOVA followed by SNK showed that on Day 14 the tumor volume of group 1 was significantly greater than that of groups 7 and 8 and that on Day 17, the tumor volume of Group 1 was significantly greater than that of all other groups. Group 1 had 20 mice, all other groups had 10 mice.
[c] P value from the ANOVA. The decreasing p value with time indicates that the differences between groups were increasing with time.

Such immunohistochemical stained tumor slide sections were used for microscopic intercept point counting of areas of interest for tumor volume density analysis [14, 18].

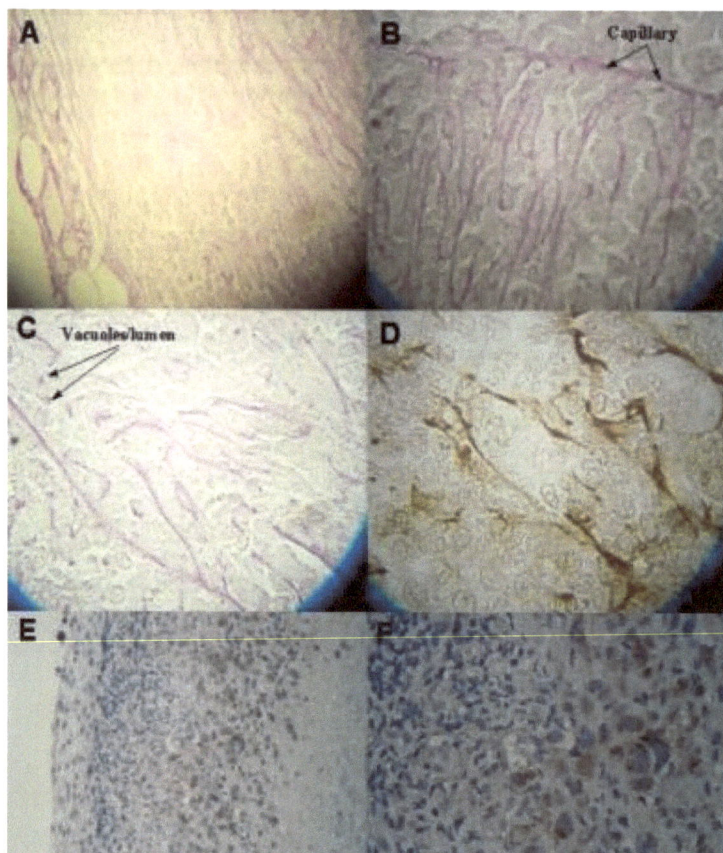

Fig. (2). Photomicrographs of histological sections of the mouse 16/c tumor. Photographs A-C are PSA stained images. A, shows the well vascularized capsule left, cortex middle and subcortex with capillaries with numerous endothelial pseudopod sprouts in the upper right corner. B shows a higher magnification of a subcortex field showing a capillary sprouting pseudopods. C illustrates pseudopods that branch and sometimes have a lumen. D illustrates that endothelial cells pseudopods stain positive as benign endothelial cell. E the viable cell area located just inside the tumor capsule (left) and area of tumor necrosis right, just to the right of the viable cell area in the subcortical endothelial rich area with tumor cell that stain a positive brown with the immunohistochemical hypoxia inducible factor (HIF) and F an enlarged image of this subcortical area revealing individual HIF positive cells [14].

Histopathological analysis was performed to access host side effects on the small intestine, brain, spleen, and kidney of all mice using 5 μm thick hematoxylin and eosin stained sections. The only evidence of histopathology was extramedular hematopoiese in mice in all of the groups. This was attributed to non-specific stimulation of the host immune system by presence of the tumor not to the TEMF therapy.

The host survival percentage at 20 days after tumor inoculation in the non-TEMF treated group was 60% while survival in the TEMF treated groups had a significant dose dependent increase to 93% (p value=0.017).

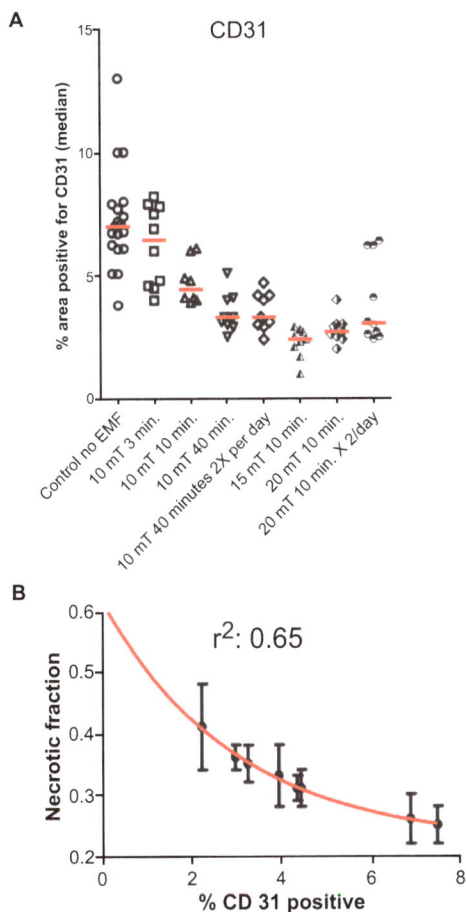

Fig. (3). A. The percent of CD-31 positive (tumor vascular volume density fraction) for each tumor in the 8 groups reveal the following statistical analysis results: control group was significantly higher than all but the 3 minutes TEMF group. The 15 minutes TEMF had the lowest volume density of all other groups. B, illustrates a significant one phase decay relationship between the necrotic volume fraction and the vascular (CD-31) density fraction after TEMF therapy [1].

The results of TEMF treatments on the vascular (CD-31 positive), necrotic and viable tumor volume density fractions in mice following 12 days of treatment are summarized next. Mice that died before day 12 were not included in the analysis. Statistical analysis (ANOVA followed by the SNK post (test) showed the mean CD-31 positive vascular area of the control mice to be significantly greater than in the TEMF treated groups. The group given 15 mT for 10 minutes had the lowest vascular positive volume density fraction (Fig. **3-A**) and had the highest necrotic volume density fraction (Fig. **3-B**). Fig. (**3-B**) also illustrates a significant one phase exponential decay curve relationship between the necrotic area and the CD-31 vascular area in tumors after 12 days of TEMF.

Morphometric findings indicate that the viable tumor volume density fraction is significantly related of the percent of CD-31 positive (vascular) volume density and that vascular area is not significantly related to tumor growth rate. These findings demonstrate that blood supply (vascular area) is related to tumor viable tumor area but is not shown to be related to tumor growth rate [14].

In summary TEMF therapy was given to groups of breast cancer bearing host mice. Treatment was daily exposure to a 120 Hz semi sine wave pulse given at 10 to 20 m Tesla (mT) for 3-80 minutes. Tumor volume was measured every 3 to 4 days. The TEMF therapy significantly slowed tumor growth in all of the TEMF treatment groups. Tumors were excised at termination by euthanasia and the extent of necrosis, viable and vascular (CD-31) areas of cryosectioned tumor were measured and subjected to statistical analysis. A major finding was that TEMF reduced the blood vessel volume fraction.

The maximum antiangiogenic effect was TEMF at 15 mT for 10 minutes per day. Given that the 15 mT for 10 minutes per day treatment gave the maximum antiangiogenic TEMF effect it was selected for use in our subsequent TEMF tumor antiangiogenic studies as reported below. But first it seems helpful to review angiogenesis in growth of untreated tumors.

Recruitment of New Blood Vessels (Angiogenesis) by Growing Tumors

Tumor vascularization was studied in female athymic nude mice (strain C3H) that had been inoculated in the inguinal mammary fat pad with two million human breast cancer cells (MDA-MB-231) [1, 14, 17]. Tumors <35 mm^3, observed through the skin, were white while tumors >35 mm^3 were pink. Histology of white and pink tumors showed that the pink color was associated with development of a well vascularized connective tissue capsule not present in the white tumors. Histological sections of tumors greater than 35 mm^3 were stained by the periodic acid-Schiff (PAS) technique for glycoprotein or with CD-31 antibody (a marker of endothelial cells) or with hypoxia inducible factor 1 alpha antibodies (HIF). The volume fraction density of blood vessels and endothelial pseudopods was measured by the ocular grid intercept point counting method using PAS stained eight micron thick slides. The PAS technique for glycoproteins gave an unexpected abundance of PAS endothelial cells and their pseudopods which also staining positive for CD-31 (Fig. **2-A, B, C**).

The non-random distribution of PAS pseudopods in the tumor caused us to focus on this non-random pattern of endothelial cell pseudopods during angiogenesis of the rapidly growing tumor. Endothelial cell pseudopods and blood vessels were sparse in the tumor cortical region located adjacent to the well vascularized tumor connective tissue capsule while areas greater than 100 μm (the subcortical area) showed more blood vessels, capillaries and an abundance of endothelial pseudopods sprouting from capillaries (Fig. **2-B**). Quantitative morphometric analysis of the volume density of endothelial pseudopods located within 100 μm of the capsule cortical area were significantly (p<0.001) lower 1.24 ±, 0.30% *vs.* in the subcortical regions further (>100mm) from the capsule 5.57± .09% or a 4.5 fold difference. See Fig. (**2-A**) for illustrated example. In regions greater than 150 to 200 μm the tumor cells undergo death resulting in a necrotic area. How can these observations be explained? The subcortical region was rich in pseudopods, some with a lumen (Fig. **2-C**). This is the same subcortical region found to be rich in hypoxia inducible factor (HIF) cells as revealed by immunohistochemical location (Fig. **2-E.F**). Thus the extent of endothelial cells appears to indicate tissue hypoxia [1, 14].

Apparently, tumor cells in the subcortical area become hypoxic because they are too distant (>100 μm) for the vascular rich connective tissue capsule. These hypoxic tumor cells then produce HIF presumably related to synthesis and secretion of vascular endothelial growth factor (VEGF) which results in the formation of endothelial cell sprouting of pseudopod that forms new blood vessels (neo-angiogenesis). One can conclude from this account that tumor angiogenesis is a hypoxia-driven process. It is also hypothesized that inhabitation of growth and vascularization of tumor growth is the mechanism by which TEMF works to slow tumor growth and to increase survival of the host. The findings of no regression in tumor size also indicate that TEMF, used as the sole therapy, is not a likely cancer cure. TEMF may however have value as an adjunct to more commonly use cancer therapies (gamma irradiation-IR and chemothcrapy). Given that IR and most commonly used chemotherapies work by killing rapidly dividing cancer cell populations in the host tissues with harmful side effects. The question posed was would therapy that targets two different tumor growth inhibitor mechanisms (anti-angiogenesis and killing of dividing cell) have an additive beneficial cancer therapy effect. This question is addressed in the next section.

Effects of Combining TEMF and Gamma Irradiation (IR) on Human Breast Cancer Xenograph Growth, Angiogenesis and Metastasis

Nude mice bearing human MDA MB231 breast cancer cells transfected with a green fluorescence protein gene were injected into the mammary fat pad of young female mice. Six weeks after injection these mice were divided into the following groups: 10 minutes a day exposure to a semi-sinewave signal of 15 mT at 120 pulses per second (TEMF), 200 cG of gamma irradiation (IR) every other day for a total of 800 cG, given both TEMF and IR and sham exposed controls. Some mice in each group were euthanized one day after 8 days of therapy while others were euthanized 20 days later.

The body weight increase continued in the control and TEMF groups of mice while the two IR groups demonstrated a significant mean body weight loss during the 8 days of IR therapy but started to regain weight after the 8 day of IR therapy. The tumor growth rates in mm^3/day from day 7 through day 15 post IR treatment are: control 12.8± 1.1 SEM, TEMF 4.3± 0.09, IR 1.9± 0.5, TEMF x IR 0.8± 0.3. Statistical analysis by the ANOVA and SNK found the control group tumor growth rate to be significantly higher than the other treated groups and the TEMF + IR group to be significantly less than the other three groups. This indicates that the combination of TEMF + IR therapies has a significant additive tumor growth inhibiting effect.

The ocular grid intercept point counting morphometric method was used to determine the percent areas (volume density) of blood vessels and endothelial pseudopods in 8 μm thick mid tumor histological sections stained with periodic acid-Schiff (PAS). The blood vessel area data from one day after the end of IR treatment are: control 2.63± 0.35% area, TEMF 1.09± 0.30%, IR 0.98± 0.28%, TEMF + IR 1.09± 0.31%. Statistical analysis revealed TEMF and IR to be significantly less than the control but the TEMF + IR was not quite significantly less than the control.

The endothelial pseudopod area volume density fraction data from the PAS stained slides of tumors of all four groups that were sacrificed one day after the last dose of IR are: control 7.50 ± 1.90%, TEMF 10.18 ± 1.91%, IR 13.98 ± 2.01%, TEMF + IR 11.82 ± 1.89%. These data show all three treatment groups to have a higher mean percent more endothelial pseudopod area than the controls but the mean values were not quite significantly different. However statistical analysis of the mean blood vessel area *vs.* the pseudopod area indicated that as blood vessel area decreases the endothelial pseudopod area increases.

In past reports [12, 16 - 18] tumor cell metastasis has been linked to the extent of tumor vascularity. Based our finding that each of our TEMF treated groups significantly reduced the percent of tumor vascularity it was decided to test if the decrease in tumor metastasis might be reduced in our three therapy groups *vs.* the control group. The experiment involved the metastasis of the green fluorescence protein (GFP) containing tumor cancer cells from their site of inoculation in the inguinal mammary fat pad to the lungs of mice in each of the four experimental groups. The entire lung in each of 12 to 14 mice in each group was removed and smashed between microscope slides. These slides were observed using illuminated blue light to detect the pressure of green fluorescence microcolonies of cancer cells. The lungs of sham treated control mice had a higher number of GFP positive microcolonies than did all three of the therapy treated groups (control 2.0 per lung, IR 0.61, TEMF 0.42, IR + TEMF 0.25). Clearly all three of the therapy groups had significantly reduced lung metastasis varying from 70 to 87% and this reduction can be linked to their significantly decreased tumor vascularization.

The possible side effects of TEMF and IR therapy are an important concern for the application of treatments to patients. As summarized in Table **4** the IR treatment caused a significant decrease in WBC, RBC, and Platelet and spleen weight one day after the last IR treatment. There were no other significant differences. Thus TEMF therapy was without harmful side effects as illustrated in Table **4**.

Another measure of possible harmful side effect was to score the cell proliferation (mitotic) activity by measuring the metaphase figures per mid axial histological section in the duodenal intestinal crypts one day after IR therapy. Gamma irradiation (IR) significantly decreased the crypt metaphase figures but TEMF did not. It was also observed that IR but not TEMF caused a tan skin color eight days after the course of IR but normal skin color returned by 22 days. As mentioned earlier in this report IR therapy resulted in loss of body weight which then returned to the control level by 22 days after the last IR treatment.

Table 4. Host side effects of IR and TEMF treatments.

Therapy Group	WBC x $10^3/\mu L$	RBC x $10^6/\mu L$	Platelets x $10^3/\mu L$	Spleen wt.g
Control	2.91 ± 0.83	9.08 ± 0.07	584 ± 76	0.107 ± 0.0009
IR	0.11 ± 0.01	7.50 ± 0.16	389 ± 17	0.031 ± 0.004
TEMF	2.89 ± 0.60	9.05 ± 0.12	505 ± 61	0.110 ± 0.006
TEMF/IR	0.23 ± 0.06	7.68 ± 0.13	443 ± 34	0.033 ± 0.004

Results of mice sacrifice one day after last irradiation (IR) or therapeutic electromagnetic field (TEMF). Gamma irradiation caused significant decreases in WBC, RBC, platelet counts and spleen weight. No other significant differences.

A major conclusion of our tumor growth and angiogenesis studies is that angiogenesis in the tumor is a hypoxia driven process that is inhibited by TEMF. The question is, does TEMF inhibit angiogenesis under normoxic condition? This question was tested by application of TEMF on development of zebra fish embryos. Observation of zebra fish embryo tissue section for presence of HIF found no evidence of hypoxia. Daily exposure of the embryos during their development to the pro-mouth stage at 147 hours showed no evidence of growth retardation. Neither early cell division at an early stage of development or angiogenesis at the prime stage were retarded compared to the non-TEMF control embryos. It was concluded that TEMF is not antiangiogenic under normoxic growth conditions [17].

A review of recent reports on use of a TEMF signal for treatment of human cancer patients found three reports indicating that TEMF therapy of patients with advanced liver cancer increased their life expectation. No noticeable side effect of the TEMF used was observed [3, 15, 16]. Thus the TEMF used was judged safe for use in humans. A review of this topic indicated the need for funding for additional human cancer TEMF therapy research [19].

SUMMARY AND CONCLUSION

This chapter deals with the following questions. Can a brief daily exposure to a pulsed electromagnetic field slow, stop or decrease the size of a growing cancerous tumor? If so how does this EMF field work to accomplish such inhibition? Experimental research proved that EMF therapy did slow growth but did not shrink tumor size with no harmful side effects to the tumor bearing host. What then is the optimal EMF exposure? The answer was a pulsed therapeutic electromagnetic field (TEMF) of 120 pulses per second semi-sinewave signal of 15 mT given for 10 minutes once a day.

How does this therapeutic field work to slow tumor growth? Tumor growth involves an increase in cancer cell numbers that requires nutrients and oxygen from the vascular system of the host. Cancer cells furthest from the host blood supply become hypoxic and begin production of hypoxia inducible factor leading to secretion of vascular endothelial growth factor resulting in formation of endothelial cell pseudopods that then form lumens and new blood vessels. It is concluded from the experimental results that TEMF works to inhibit hypoxia driven tumor angiogenesis without harmful side effects. It also reduced tumor cell metastasis and increased host survival time. Further research found that the TEMF did not inhibit angiogenesis in normoxic fish embryos implying that the hypoxia driven pathway is the target of TEMF's tumor growth inhibition.

An experiment was done to determine if combining TEMF that works to inhibit tumor angiogenesis with gamma irradiation (IR) that works to kill rapidly dividing cells would have a significant additive effect on tumor growth. In short, TEMF plus IR did have a significant additive inhibiting effect on the tumor growth rate. TEMF therefore proved a safe adjunct to therapy that targets killing of rapidly dividing cells.

CONSENT FOR PUBLICATION

Not applicable.

CONFLICT OF INTEREST

The author confirms that he has no conflict of interest to declare for this publication.

ACKNOWLEDGEMENTS

This work supported by NIH grant CA 7553 and EMF Therapeutics, Inc.

Figs. (**1**, **2**, **3**) and Tables **2**, **3**, **4** were originally published under license to Bio Med Central Ltd under terms of the Creative Commons Attribution Licenses (http://creativecommons.org/license/by/12.0) which permits unrestricted use, distribution, and reproduction in any medium, provided work is properly cited.

ABBREVIATIONS

ANOV = Analysis of variances

CD-31 = Also known as platelet endothelial cell adhesion molecule (PECAM-1) is used as an angiogenesis maker

GFP = Green fluorescence protein

HIF = Hypoxia inducible factor

IR = Gamma irradiation

PAS = Periodic acid-Schiff

PEMF = Pulsed electromagnetic field

RBC = Red blood cells

SE = Standard error

SNK = Student Newman Kesel

TEMF = Therapeutic electromagnetic field

VEGF = Vascular endothelial growth factor

WBC = White blood cells

REFERENCES

[1]   Cameron IL, Sun LZ, Short N, Hardman WE, Williams CD. Therapeutic electromagnetic field (TEMF) and gamma irradiation on human breast cancer xenograft growth, angiogenesis and metastasis. Cancer Cell Int 2005; 5: 23-8.
[http://dx.doi.org/1186/1475-2867-5-23]

[2]   Williams CD, Markov MS, Hardman WE, Cameron IL. Therapeutic electromagnetic field effects on angiogenesis and tumor growth. Anticancer Res 2001; 21(6A): 3887-91.
[PMID: 11911264]

[3]   Markov MS. Expanding use of pulsed electromagnetic field therapies. Electromagn Biol Med 2007; 26(3): 257-74.
[http://dx.doi.org/10.1080/15368370701580806] [PMID: 17886012]

[4]   Hu JH, St-Pierre LS, Buckner CA, Lafrenie RM, Persinger MA. Growth of injected melanoma cells is suppressed by whole body exposure to specific spatial-temporal configurations of weak intensity magnetic fields. Int J Radiat Biol 2010; 86(2): 79-88.
[http://dx.doi.org/10.3109/09553000903419932] [PMID: 20148694]

[5]   Wen J, Jiang S, Chen B. The effect of 100 Hz magnetic field combined with X-ray on hepatoma-implanted mice. Bioelectromagnetics 2011; 32(4): 322-4.
[http://dx.doi.org/10.1002/bem.20646] [PMID: 21452362]

[6]   Tofani S, Cintorino M, Barone D, *et al.* Increased mouse survival, tumor growth inhibition and decreased immunoreactive p53 after exposure to magnetic fields. Bioelectromagnetics 2002; 23(3): 230-8.
[http://dx.doi.org/10.1002/bem.10010] [PMID: 11891753]

[7]   Bellossi A, Desplaces A. Effect of a 9 mT pulsed magnetic field on C3H/Bi female mice with mammary carcinoma. A comparison between the 12 Hz and the 460 Hz frequencies. *in vivo* 1991; 5(1): 39-40.
[PMID: 1932623]

[8]   Berg H, Günther B, Hilger I, Radeva M, Traitcheva N, Wollweber L. Bioelectromagnetic field effects on cancer cells and mice tumors. Electromagn Biol Med 2010; 29(4): 132-43.
[http://dx.doi.org/10.3109/15368371003776725] [PMID: 21062126]

[9]   Seze R, Tuffet S, Moreau JM, Veyret B. Effects of 100 mT time varying magnetic fields on the growth of tumors in mice. Bioelectromagnetics 2000; 21(2): 107-11.
[http://dx.doi.org/10.1002/(SICI)1521-186X(200002)21:2<107::AID-BEM5>3.0.CO;2-6]   [PMID: 10653621]

[10]   Tatarovo I, Panda A, Petkov D, *et al.* Effect of magnetic fields on tumor growth and viability. Comp Med 2011; 61(4): 339-45.
[PMID: 22330249]

[11]   Zhang X, Zhang H, Zheng C, Li C, Zhang X, Xiong W. Extremely low frequency (ELF) pulsed-gradient magnetic fields inhibit malignant tumour growth at different biological levels. Cell Biol Int 2002; 26(7): 599-603.
[http://dx.doi.org/10.1006/cbir.2002.0883] [PMID: 12127939]

[12]   Tofani S, Barone D, Berardelli M, *et al.* Static and ELF magnetic fields enhance the *in vivo* anti-tumor efficacy of cis-platin against lewis lung carcinoma, but not of cyclophosphamide against B16 melanotic melanoma. Pharmacol Res 2003; 48(1): 83-90.
[PMID: 12770519]

[13]   Yamaguchi S, Ogiue-Ikeda M, Sekino M, Ueno S. Effects of pulsed magnetic stimulation on tumor development and immune functions in mice. Bioelectromagnetics 2006; 27(1): 64-72.
[http://dx.doi.org/10.1002/bem.20177] [PMID: 16304693]

[14]   Cameron IL, Short N, Sun L, Hardman WE. Endothelial cell pseudopods and angiogenesis of breast cancer tumors. Cancer Cell Int 2005; 5: 10-7.
[http://dx.doi.org/1186/1475-2867-5-17]

[15]   Hannan CJ Jr, Liang Y, Allison JD, Pantazis CG, Searle JR. Chemotherapy of human carcinoma xenografts during pulsed magnetic field exposure. Anticancer Res 1994; 14(4A): 1521-4.
[PMID: 7979179]

[16]   Salvatore J, Markov M. Electromagnetic fields as an adjuvant therapy to antineoplastic chemotherapy. In: Rosch P, Markov MS, Eds. Bioelectromagnetic Medicine. NY: CRC Pr I Llc/Taylor & Francis 2004; pp. 613-24.

[17]   Cameron I, Markov MS, Hardman WE. Daily exposure to a pulsed electromagnetic field for inhibition of cancer growth. In: Markov MS, Ed. Electromagnetic Fields in Biology and Medicine. NY: CRC Pr I Llc/Taylor & Francis 2015; pp. 311-8.

[18]   Cameron IL, Markov MS, Hardman WE. Optimization of a therapeutic electromagnetic field (EMF) to retard breast cancer tumor growth and vascularity. Cancer Cell Int 2014; 14(1): 125-32.
[http://dx.doi.org/10.1186/s12935-014-0125-5] [PMID: 25530714]

[19]   Blackman CF. Treating cancer with amplitude-modulated electromagnetic fields: a potential paradigm shift, again? Br J Cancer 2012; 106(2): 241-2.
[http://dx.doi.org/10.1038/bjc.2011.576] [PMID: 22251967]

CHAPTER 3

Angiogenesis in Cancer Treatment: 60 Years' Swing Between Promising Trials and Disappointing Tribulations

Khalid Alhazzani[1,2,4], **Ali Alaseem**[1,2,3], **Mohammad Algahtani**[1,2,4], **Sivanesan Dhandayuthapani**[1], **Thiagarajan Venkatesan**[1] and **Appu Rathinavelu**[*, 1,2]

[1] *Rumbaugh-Goodwin Institute for Cancer Research, Nova Southeastern University, Fort Lauderdale, Florida, USA*

[2] *College of Pharmacy, Nova Southeastern University, Fort Lauderdale, Florida, USA*

[3] *College of Medicine, Al Imam Mohammad Ibn Saud Islamic University, Riyadh, Saudi Arabia*

[4] *College of Pharmacy, King Saud University, Riyadh, Saudi Arabia*

Abstract: Pathological angiogenesis plays essential role in tumor progression, invasiveness, and metastasis. This process is highly stimulated by VEGF/VEGFR signaling pathway(s). Additional players such as Ang/Tie-2, FGF/FGFR, and Notch signals are also involved in this complex process by stabilization and maturation of blood vessels. As a result of the identification of molecular pathways and various targets driving angiogenesis, several agents have been developed for cancer treatment. Among various pathways, targeting VEGF/VEGFR2 has been proven to be the most effective to inhibit tumor angiogenesis and subsequent tumor growth in preclinical and clinical settings. This chapter highlights on the ramification of some of the crucial events that leads to the maturation of angiogenesis, explore the perplex process of angiogenesis and discuss the amenable strategies for intervention. We will discuss about the myriad number of current therapeutic agents based the target selectivity, preclinical findings, clinical application, and toxicity profile.

Keywords: Ang/Tie-2, Notch Signals, Pathological Angiogenesis, Toxicity profile, Tumor Growth, Tumor Progression.

---

[*] **Corresponding author Appu Rathinavelu:** 3321 College Avenue, CCR 6th Floor, Fort Lauderdale, FL-33328, USA; Tel: +19542620400; Fax: +19542620401; E-mail: appu@nova.edu

Atta-ur-Rahman & Mohammad Iqbal Choudhary (Eds.)

TUMOR ANGIOGENESIS: OVERVIEW OF SIGNALING PATHWAYS IN TUMOR PROGRESSION

Introduction

In 1902, Theodor Boveri described that malignant tumors arise from a single cell with abnormal chromosomes or gene defects and such abnormality causes uncontrolled cell growth. The observation made by Boveri was one of the milestones that shaped the contemporary cancer research [1]. However, accumulated knowledge of cancer biology reveals that it is a tangled disease with complex pathological phenomenon [2]. In fact, there are more than 100 distinct cancer subtypes found within the same organ with different pathological basis and characteristics [3]. Therefore, it is widely accepted that cancer is so diverse where finding two identical specimens will be nearly impossible. This heterogeneity of cancer is attributed to the unique genetic variations that accumulate during the course of the disease also, which allows cancer cells to breach all defense mechanisms. Despite cancer heterogeneity, nearly all cancers, no matter where the tumor is originated from or which genes are mutated, share essential capabilities and characteristics. Hanahan and Weinberg have described these common capabilities as "The Hallmarks of Cancer" [3]. One of these hallmarks is the ability of cancer to induce sustained angiogenesis. This chapter will summarize the perplex process of angiogenesis and also discuss about the benefits and pitfalls of anti-angiogenic therapies.

Angiogenesis and Cancer Growth

The term angiogenesis was coined by John Hunter in 1787 [4]. Angiogenesis can be defined as a multi-step process that triggers the growth and development of new blood vessels from pre-existing vasculature. The contemporary field of tumor angiogenesis was established by several of pioneers who have shaped the field with their influential hypotheses and experimental observations. The first association between tumor growth and increased observations of angiogenesis was made in 1863 by Rudolf Virchow [5]. He observed infiltration of leukocytes into the malignant tissues linking inflammation to tumor growth. Another significant observation was made by Warren Lewis in 1927, when he was analyzing the vascularization patterns of various tumor types, he came to the conclusion that tumor microenvironment could influence different types and patterns of angiogenesis [6]. Several other scientists have corroborated the finding that tumor growth was accompanied with rapid induction of blood vessel formation. In 1939, Gordon Ide and colleagues provided the first *in vivo* image of tumor angiogenesis, supporting Lewis' observation. Subsequently, Gordon Ide *et al* took a step forward by postulating that these blood vessels are stimulated by factors released from the tumor mass. Even though the previous observations were significant yet, they did not outline the exact role of angiogenesis in tumor growth, and therefore, the concept of secreted factors remained just speculations in the context of tumor angiogenesis.

Angiogenesis as a Target for Cancer Treatment

Judah Folkman was the first scientist to postulate that inhibition of angiogenesis would be an effective approach for cancer treatment. In 1971, Folkman proposed a field shifting idea of inhibiting angiogenesis as a venue for treatment of human cancer when cytotoxic chemotherapy at that time was widely used and accepted as the main form of cancer treatment [7]. Folkman built his initial hypothesis based on the observation that tumor growth would be dependent on angiogenesis. This new concept was initially perceived with considerable skepticism. However, A few months' latter, when Folkman and colleagues reported the isolation of tumor angiogenesis factor (TAF) from many animal and human tumors, his team was able to prove that TAF could stimulate angiogenesis in rat and chick embryo models [8]. Folkman's contribution did not stop at TAF discovery; he further proved that tumor angiogenesis is critical for tumor progression and hence, in the absence of angiogenesis; tumor size would not expand beyond 1 or 2 mm^3. In support of this hypothesis Folkman was able to demonstrate that only tumor mass with 1 or 2 mm^3 in the vicinity of blood vessels could obtain the essential nutrients and oxygen through simple diffusion. For the tumors to grow beyond 2 mm^3 limit, the cancer cells have to send signals to establish new blood vessels in order to support their exponential growth [9]. Also, Folkman was burgeoning the field of angiogenesis by developing bioassays that provided sensitive methods for studying *in vitro* angiogenesis such as long-term culturing of capillary endothelial cells, and chick-embryo chorioallantoic membrane assays and rabbit cornea assays [10]. Therefore, Folkman's proposals and discoveries became a strong trigger point that encouraged scientists to extensively invest their time and efforts in exploring angiogenesis biology as evidenced by the surge in publications from this time onwards.

As the field of angiogenesis was steadily advancing with the efforts from Folkman, the discovery of vascular endothelial growth factor (VEGF), was one of the major breakthroughs that the researchers were awaiting further shaped the field towards discovering new strategies for cancer treatment. In fact, VEGF was discovered independently by two research groups in the eighties. In 1983, Donald Senger and colleagues reported the isolation of a protein from conditioned media of a guinea pig's tumor cell line [11]. Subsequently, Senger and colleagues demonstrated that the isolated protein induced vascular leakage and therefore, they proposed to name it vascular permeability factor (VPF). It is worth mentioning that, because VPF was partially purified by Senger's team, without sequencing the protein or the corresponding gene, the identity of VPF remained debatable for some time. Five years later, Napoleon Ferrara and his team isolated a protein from a conditioned media of bovine pituitary follicular cells, and his team observed that their isolated protein possesses a mitogenic activity only towards endothelial cells. Based on this observation, they proposed to name it as vascular endothelial growth factor (VEGF). Since VEGF was purified to homogeneity by Ferrara's team, subsequently the N-terminal sequencing was performed to reveal the protein identity of VEGF [12]. Interestingly, the sequence studies indeed have revealed that VPF and VEGF were the same molecules [13, 14]. Another important discovery that was made around the same time period was the identification of vascular endothelial growth factor receptor-2 (VEGFR-2) that mediates VEGF signaling [15]. These discoveries were the cornerstone for the maturation of angiogenesis field towards cancer treatment which paved the way for the successful development of the first angiogenesis inhibitor.

Angiogenesis Process

Vasculogenesis and angiogenesis are the two major successive processes implicated in the development of the vascular system. Vasculogenesis, which is defined as the *de novo* synthesis of primitive vascular plexus that takes place during early embryonic stages through differentiation of mesoderm to angioblasts (endothelial progenitor cells) and assembly of angioblasts to form primitive blood vessels. Following vasculogenesis, angiogenesis takes place during both embryonic and adulthood to expand and remodel the primitive blood vessels [16]. Since cancers occur, most often during adulthood, much attention was focused understanding the process that triggers tumor angiogenesis.

The process of angiogenesis is immensely complicated, as evidenced by multiple steps that endothelial cells have to undergo to form new branching vessels, and by the redundancy of signaling pathways that are responsible for initiation and coordination of angiogenesis (Fig. **1**). In cancer, tumor microenvironment (TME) sends several signaling molecules to nearby blood vessels in order to initiate angiogenesis (see pages 7−19). The process typically begins with vasodilation in response to signals sent from TME. Also, tumor signals activate endothelial cells, which in turn secrete proteases to degrade the basement membrane of the existing vessels. The degradation of the basement membrane allows the detachment and migration of endothelial cells towards tumor cells [17]. Following this step, endothelial cells are differentiated into three distinctive phenotypes (*tip, stalk, tube cells*) during the process of angiogenesis. The endothelial *tip cells*, located at the top of the new blood vessels, are non-proliferative and highly motile cells whose function is to guide the direction of the migration of the endothelial cells (*stalk and tube cells*) towards the tumor site. During angiogenesis, the endothelial cells compete dynamically against each other for the *tip* cell site, and those with lower VEGFR-1 and higher VEGFR-2 levels have a better opportunity to win the competition and occupied the leading position [18]. On the other hand, endothelial *stack cells* are highly proliferative cells that follow the *tips cells*. Endothelial *tube cells* are non-proliferative lumen containing cells whose function is to construct the final shape of blood vessels. Lastly, pericytes, which are specialized supportive cells, cover the new capillaries that ultimately join together to form new blood vessels carrying oxygen and nutrients necessary for tumor propagation [19].

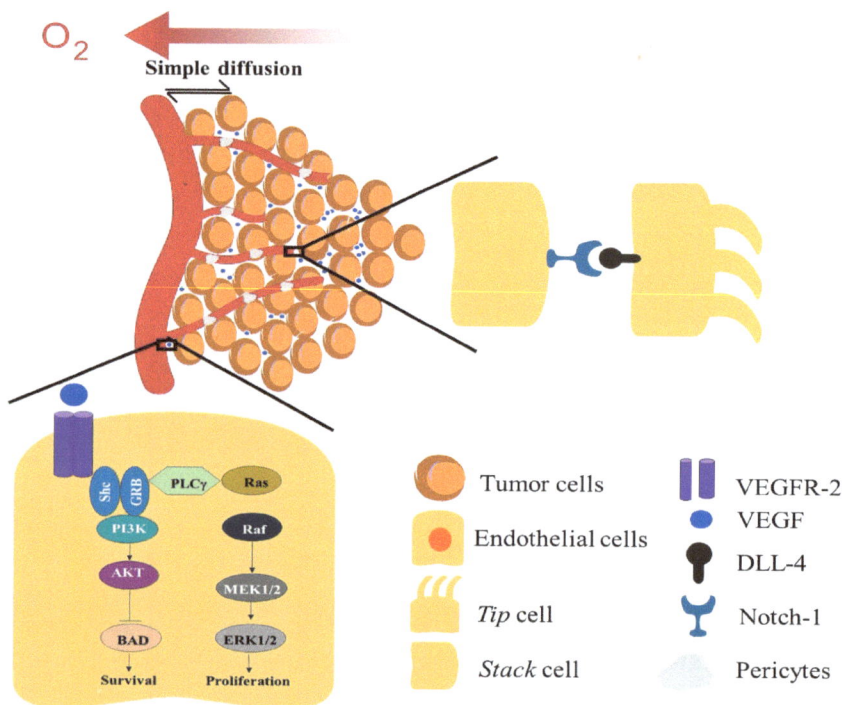

Fig. (1). Illustration of endothelial cells passing through various steps to make new blood vessel. This process is supported by multi signaling pathways predominantly through VEGF binding to its receptor VEGFR-2. The VEGF binding supports VEGFR-2 dimerization, autophosphorylation and initiation of the downstream signaling cascades such as PI3K/AKT, FAK, and MAPK/ERK1. The angiogenesis process starts when TME sends signals to adjacent vessels. During the process of angiogenesis, the endothelial cells dynamically differentiate into three different types tip, stalk, and tube cells. These cell types along with pericytes, by working together, can form new blood vessels. In this process, activated VEGFR-2 induces DLL-4 expression in the tip cells, which in turn triggers Notch-1 receptors on the stalk endothelial cells to support the migration process.

Vascular architecture around tumor is distinctive from any other normal vascular walls. Unlike normal vessels, tumor vessels are structurally and functionally abnormal. Tumor vasculature is chaotic, disorganized, immature with leaky and irregular branching, whereas normal vasculature is highly orchestrated and organized [17].

Angiogenesis Switch Hypothesis

The hypothesis states that the normal blood vessels remain dormant due to a balance between pro- and anti-angiogenic factors. The shift from this balance by increasing pro-angiogenic signals will initiate the process of tumor angiogenesis. The below stated hypothesis explains the difference between angiogenesis that is occurring in physiological and pathological conditions. For instance, angiogenesis is essential for normal physiological conditions such as pregnancy, embryonic development, menstrual cycle, and wound healing. During these physiological conditions, angiogenesis is initiated by secretion of more pro-angiogenic factors, which tilt the balance towards angiogenic phenotype switch. These changes are temporary and time-limited; however, once the equilibrium between pro- and anti-angiogenic factors is reached that will restore the dormancy of blood vessels.

In cancer, however, angiogenesis is continuously activated by the pro-angiogenic signals secreted from TME [20]. Several experimental models have demonstrated that dormant *in situ* cancer cells can grow exponentially if the cancer cells can attract new blood vessel formation by releasing the pro-angiogenic signals. Among these experimental models, a convening observation was noticed by Harry Greene, when a small fraction of the tumor was implanted into a guinea pig's eye [21]. The tiny fraction of tumor remained dormant with limited size for more than one year. However, when this tiny dormant tumor was removed and transplanted into rabbit muscles, the tumor was growing exponentially by attracting blood vessels. This observation of tumor dormancy due to lack of vascularization by Greene was substantiated by Brem's team [22]. Also, the levels of pro-angiogenic factors were undetectable in healthy subjects whereas their levels were significantly high in serum, urine, and cerebrospinal fluid in patients with cancer [23]. These observations highlighted the importance of identifying pro-angiogenic molecules responsible for tumor growth and expansion.

Pro-Angiogenic Pathways

Before 1971, angiogenesis was a mysterious process with little information known. Folkman's conjecture was the foundation that started a new field of cancer treatment. Since 1971, researchers have focused their attention on profoundly understanding the signaling pathways that are involved in angiogenesis. Their goal is to delineate angiogenesis pathways in order to develop pharmacological inhibitors. As a result, numerous extracellular, cell surface, and intracellular molecules have been discovered as modulators of angiogenesis. In cancer, the excess production of pro-angiogenic molecules is triggered by metabolic stresses such as hypoxia, or acidosis and also by genetic aberrations such as oncogenes activation and inactivation of tumor suppressor genes [24]. One or more of these cohesive mechanisms support the existence and growth of cancers, which eventually undergo metastasis also with the support of the tumor angiogenesis.

VEGF/ VEGFR Pathway

VEGF, which was previously known as vascular permeability factor, is the major and the best-characterized factor among all pro-angiogenic factors. In fact, VEGF family includes five structurally related molecules: VEGF-A, VEGF-B, VEGF-C, VEGF-D, and placenta-derived growth factor (PIGF). VEGF-A, simply known as VEGF, is the primary contributor to tumor angiogenesis. In fact, VEGF gene has several spliced variants that differ in total amino acid content (VEGF$_{121}$, VEGF$_{145}$, VEGF$_{165}$, VEGF$_{189}$, VEGF$_{205}$) [25].

Based on the splice variant information available in the literature, two families of VEGF isoforms have been identified, which are (i) the pro-angiogenic family and (ii) the anti-angiogenic family. The members of the pro-angiogenic family, which is named as VEGFxxx, are formed by splicing at the proximal sites found in the terminal exon. On the other hand, the members of the anti-angiogenic family that is named as VEGFxxxb, are formed by splicing of the distal sites found in the terminal exon, where xxx refers to the total amino acids in the isoforms [26]. The most remarkable isoforms of VEGFxxx found in humans are VEGF$_{121}$, VEGF$_{165}$, and VEGF$_{189}$. These isoforms have different effects on the formation of blood vessel due to the difference in their affinities for VEGF receptors and heparan sulfate proteoglycans (HSPGs). In contrast, the murine isoforms (VEGF$_{120}$, VEGF$_{164}$, VEGF$_{188}$) are one amino acid shorter than the human isoforms, with equal component and biological functions [25]. Both VEGF$_{165}$ and VEGF$_{189}$ contain a highly basic heparin-binding domain (HBD) and they are tightly bound to the extracellular heparin-containing proteoglycans, which produce a branching network with narrow vessels. However, VEGF$_{121}$ is a non-heparin-binding acidic protein and freely diffusible upon secretion, therefore it can stimulate the formation of poorly branching and leaky blood vessels [27, 28]. Angiogenesis is regulated by the spatial distribution of VEGF which is controlled by both matrix binding and proteolytic release. For instance, VEGF$_{165}$ and VEGF$_{189}$ have a sharp gradient and tight pericellular sequestration, since they bind strongly to the extracellular matrix (ECM) [29 - 32]. The expression of VEGF isoform also varies between different tissues as well as in various pathological condition, which may help to generate vascular networks matching each tissue specific needs [33]. The growth of tumor cells overexpressing VEGF$_{164}$, the predominant isoform typically found in normal adult tissues, appears to be fast compared to the non-expressing cells [31]. On the other hand, substantial defects in cardiac and pulmonary development were observed in mice that were expressing only $VEGF_{120}$ and lacking $VEGF_{164}$ and $VEGF_{188}$. The above mentioned developmental defects were because of insufficient angiogenesis due to the lack of $VEGF_{164}$ and $VEGF_{188}$ [33].

Interestingly, the VEGFxxxb isoforms (*e.g.* $VEGF_{121}b$, $VEGF_{165}b$, and $VEGF_{189}b$) have been shown to be present in normal tissues as well as in tumor cells [34, 35]. Except in placenta, VEGFxxxb isoforms represent half or more than half of the total level of VEGF-A that can be found in the normal tissues [36, 37]. These isoforms are considered to be anti-angiogenic, and they are downregulated in some tumors, such as renal and prostate cancer [38, 39]. Among the various isoforms, the $VEGF_{165}b$ is the most widely studied, and has been shown to inhibit formation of new blood vessels, cell migration and proliferation under both *in vitro* and *in vivo* conditions by inhibiting hypoxia and VEGF expression [40, 41]. In addition, tumor cells which express $VEGF_{165}b$ have been shown to grow slower than the tumor cells that express $VEGF_{165}$ [40].

Unlike VEGF-A, both VEGF-B and PIGF are dispensable for vascular development. VEGF-B is essential for fatty acid uptake in endothelial cells whereas PIGF mediates inflammation associated with angiogenesis [42]. On the other hand, lymphangiogenesis, a process of sprouting lymphatic vessels, is mediated by VEGF-C and VEGF-D. These growth factors, which are secreted as dimeric glycoproteins, transduce intracellular signals by binding to one or more members of the VEGF receptors (VEGFR-1, VEGFR-2, VEGFR-3) and Neuropilin co-receptors (NRP-1, NRP-2).

The basic structure of all VEGFRs is composed of extracellular, transmembrane, and intracellular regions. The extracellular region is the N-terminal part that is composed of seven immunoglobulin (IgG) repeats which provide an extracellular ligand binding site whereas the intracellular region contains C-terminal with two tyrosine kinases [42]. The transmembrane is a single helix, which connects the extracellular region to the cytoplasmic domain. Despite the structural similarity, all VEGFRs have different binding affinity for VEGF ligands. For instance, VEGF-A, VEGF-B, and PIGF can bind to VEGFR-1. In contrast, ligands for VEGFR-2 are mainly VEGF-A and to less extent VEGF-C and VEGF-D. The VEGFR-3 binds mainly to VEGF-C and VEGF-D that are classically involved in lymphangiogenesis. Vascular endothelium expresses VEGFR-1 and VEGFR-2 while lymphatic endothelium expresses mainly VEGFR-3. The expression of VEGFR-3 is associated with metastasis of tumor cells to the lymph nodes [43].

Genetic studies have revealed the crucial role for VEGF/VEGFRs in vascular development during early embryonic stages. One of the roles of VEGFR-1 during embryonic development is believed to be negative regulation of angiogenesis by ligand-trapping. In this connection, homozygous gene knockout mice embryos (VEGFR-1$^{-/-}$) were found to die prematurely due to increasing VEGF availability for VEGFR-2 leading to uncontrolled cell proliferation and disorganized vasculature. Similarly, mice with VEGFR-2 $^{-/-}$ genetic makeup were also found to die during embryonic development due to severe malformation of the vascular system [42]. Mice deficient in NRP-1 also died due to abnormal cardiovascular and central nervous system (CNS) development whereas NRP-2 deficient mice were alive with the apparently normal cardiovascular system [42].

VEGF signaling is the most potent inducer of angiogenesis through promoting endothelial proliferation, migration, survival, and differentiation. In addition, VEGF signaling increase vascular dilation and permeability, which facilitates extravasation and migration of endothelial cells to initiate angiogenesis [44]. Among the sub-types of VEGF receptors, VEGF signaling *via* VEGFR-2 is the critical step in mediating angiogenesis. When VEGF binds to VEGFR-2 that promotes dimerization, autophosphorylation, and activation of multiple downstream signaling cascades, which eventually leads to increase in vascular permeability, endothelial cell proliferation, survival and migration. The VEGFR-2 phosphorylation results in activation of several downstream signaling pathways through recruitment of signaling proteins containing SH2 domain such as PI3K, PLC-γ, SHP-2, and GRB-2 [43]. For example, PLC-γ is recruited by activated VEGFR-2 to transduce the signals by phosphorylating a range of kinase and non-kinase signaling molecules. Activation of PLC γ triggers MAPK/ERK1 pathway which in turn activates a variety of transcription factors that induce endothelial cell proliferation processes. On the other hand, VEGFR-2 mediates endothelial cell survival through recruiting SHB protein. This interaction between SHB and VEGFR-2 activates PI3K/AKT survival pathway. Once activated, the PI3K catalyzes the conversion of PIP2 to PIP3 by adding a phosphate group. The latter recruits AKT to the cell membrane where AKT binds through its plextrin homology domain with PIP3 resulting in AKT phosphorylation and activation [42]. Activated PI3K/AKT phosphorylates and inactivates the pro-apoptotic protein BAD (Bcl-2 associated death promoter) and also inhibits the release of caspase 9 [43]. In addition, activation of VEGFR-2 mediates endothelial cell migration through regulating focal adhesion turnover and actin reorganization. The focal adhesion turnover triggered by VEGFR-2 is mediated through focal adhesion kinase (FAK) phosphorylation and activation. Also, FAK activation is implicated in vascular leakage that is commonly observed in tumor vasculatures. VEGFR-2 also induces the expression of MMPs in endothelial cells, which facilitates degradation of extracellular matrix allowing detachment and migration of endothelial cells [45]. Furthermore, VEGF signaling increases vascular permeability through inducing eNOS production and activation [43].

VEGF overexpression has been attributed to several genetic variations and epigenetic alterations in cancer cells [46]. One of the major epigenetic inducers of VEGF expression is hypoxia, which is considered as the principal regulator of VEGF expression. As a solid tumor grows exponentially, the environment surrounding tumor mass suffers from oxygen deprivation. This hypoxic environment stabilizes and activates hypoxia-inducible factor (HIF-1α), which functions as a transcriptional factor to promote the expression of VEGF, and many other pro-angiogenic factors such as angiopoietin (Ang-1, Ang-2) and their receptor (Tie-2). In contrast, the level of HIF-1α in the presence of oxygen (normoxia) is kept low due to the fact that oxygen activates prolyl-hydroxylase (PHD) enzymes which hydroxylate HIF-1α leading to proteasomal degradation mediated by Von Hippel-Lindau (VHL) ubiquitin ligase protein [47]. Besides hypoxia, VEGF expression is induced by paracrine or autocrine release of several growth factors including epidermal growth factor (EGF), fibroblast growth factor (FGF), insulin-like growth factor (IGF-1), transforming growth factor (TGF), and platelet-derived growth factor (PDGF) *etc.* that are known to promote tumor growth *via* activation of angiogenesis [19]. Therefore, over-expression of VEGF is correlated well with of microvessels density, poor prognosis and overall survival (OS) in patients with colorectal [48], ovarian [49], prostate [50], and breast cancers [51]. Hence, inhibition of angiogenesis triggered by VEGF/VEGFR-2 is accepted as a valuable approach in cancer treatment.

Ang/Tie-2 Pathway

Another crucial signaling pathway implicated in vascular remodeling, maturation, and tumor angiogenesis is angiopoietin (Ang) / tunica intima endothelial receptor-2 (Tie-2). The human Ang family includes three secreted ligands (Ang-1, Ang-2, and Ang-4) and two related receptor tyrosine kinases (Tie-1 and Tie-2) [52]. These receptors are expressed predominantly on the surface of endothelium layer that is lining the interior surface of blood vessels. Tie-1 is considered as an orphan receptor due to the fact that no endogenous ligand has been identified yet that is specific for this receptor. In contrast to Tie-1, Ang-1 and Ang-2 bind with similar affinity to Tie-2 [53].

Each ligand has differential effects on Tie-2 signaling. For instance, Ang-1 acts as a Tie-2 agonist by inducing receptor phosphorylation and activation of downstream signaling. Ang-1 signaling *via* Tie-2 tends to stabilize blood vessels and facilitate endothelial cells sprouting and network maturation. Moreover, Ang-1 is constitutively expressed by pericytes, smooth muscle cells, and some of the tumor cells; thereby Ang-1 exerts pro-survival, anti-inflammatory, and anti-permeability effects on endothelial cells [52]. In contrast, Ang-2 is primarily produced by endothelial cells at vascular remodeling sites [53]. Ang-2 was originally thought to be a naturally occurring Tie-2 antagonist competing with Ang-1 for Tie-2 binding. In addition, Ang-2 mediates destabilization of blood vessels *via* degradation of vascular membrane facilitating endothelial cell migration [54]. Recent data suggest that Ang-2 has a dual mechanism and exerts context-dependent effects. In other words, Ang-2 can activate and deactivate Tie-2 signaling. It has been shown through *in vitro* experiments that Ang-2 can activate Tie-2 signaling in the absence of Ang-1. Additionally, exogenous administration of Ang-2 can also activate Tie-2 signaling [55]. These findings support the hypothesis that Ang-1 is a potent agonist whereas Ang-2 is a partial agonist for Tie-2. Hence, targeting Ang/ Tie-2 pathway has been more challenging than targeting VEGF/ VEGFR pathway due to the complexity of Ang ligand interactions for the same receptor.

PDGF/PDGFR Pathway

The family of PDGF is comprised of four structurally related ligands: PDGF-A, PDGF-B, PDGF-C, PDGF-D and two corresponding receptors namely PDGFR-α, and PDGRF-β. The PDGF ligands are expressed by many cell types as dimeric proteins with five identified compositions (PDGF-AA, PDGF-BB, PDGF-AB, PDGF-CC, PDGF-DD). On the other hand, PDGFRs are mostly expressed on the cell surface of fibroblasts, pericytes, endothelial, and smooth muscle cells [56]. The basic structure of PDGFRs consists of five extracellular IgG loops connected through a single transmembrane domain to the intracellular tyrosine kinase domain [57].

PDGF signaling has major mitogenic activity towards fibroblast and smooth muscle cells. This family is essential for recruitment of pericytes and smooth muscle to the newly formed blood vessels during tumor angiogenesis. Such recruitment ensures maturation and stability of the recently created vasculature. In particular, PDGF-B signaling through its cognate receptor PDGFR-β is essential for the development of the vascular system [56]. Certain genetic alterations of PDGF-B and its receptor PDGFR-β in mice have been reported to result in the loss of pericytes coverage that was leading to vascular hyperplasia, leakage, and hemorrhage [58]. However, the effect of PDGF on initiation of angiogenesis seemed to be weaker compared to that of VEGF and FGF, as evidenced by the absence of major vascular abnormality in mice with genetic mutation of PDGF or PDGFRs [58]. Under *in vitro* conditions, PDGF-B was reported to elicit endothelial cell proliferation and migration that was mediated by PDGFR-β whereas PDGF-A had no such effects on endothelial cells [59].

Different homo- or hetero-dimeric PDGF ligands have different affinities for their receptors PDGFR-α and PDGFR-β. The *In vivo* experiments revealed that PDGF-AA and PDGF-CC have high affinity for PDGFR-α whereas PDGF-BB and PDGF-DD bind to PDGFR-β [57]. Binding of PDGF ligands to PDGFRs induces receptor homo- or hetero- dimerization (PDGFR-αα, PDGFR-ββ, or PDGFR-αβ) which leads to auto-phosphorylation of the receptor tyrosine kinase residues and subsequent activation of the several signaling pathways by recruitment of SH-2 domain-containing proteins such as PLC, PI3K, Grb2, GAP and STAT [56]. However, it is not clear whether all of the PDGF isoforms are effective in promoting angiogenesis under *in vivo* conditions [60]. Current literature indicates that PDGFR heterodimer formation may occurs under *in vivo* conditions as seen by crossing of mice carrying PDGFR-α and PDGFR-β signaling mutants. Though, some level of crosstalk between VEGF and PDGF have been reported for the *in vitro* conditions, their physiological significance under *in vivo* conditions, specifically during tumor angiogenesis, is not clear at present [61].

FGF/FGFR Pathway

The FGF/FGFR family is by far the largest group of pro-angiogenic factors, which contains 18 members of FGF ligands and 7 tyrosine kinase receptors. FGF ligands are secretable glycoproteins named FGF1−10 and FGF16−23. The ligand-receptor bindings are stabilized by heparan sulfate proteoglycans (HSPGs) located on the cell surface which protect FGF ligands from proteolytic degradation [62].

The basic structure of FGFRs is composed of an extracellular N-terminal domain, a single transmembrane domain, and an intracellular tyrosine kinase domain. Uniquely, FGFR-5 lacks an intracellular kinase activity [62]. The extracellular domain of FGFRs consists of three IgG like loops compared to seven loops that are found on VEGFRs [63]. The FGFRs are expressed in a wide range of normal tissues also owing to a unique regulation of cellular hemostasis, which differs from VEGFRs that are highly expressed on endothelial cells. Among the subtypes, both FGFR-1 and FGFR-2 are widely expressed on the surface of endothelial cells whereas FGFR-3 and FGFR-4 have not been reported to be expressed in endothelial cells. Besides angiogenesis, FGFR signaling is essential for glucose, lipid, and bile acid metabolism [43] and also for maintaining vitamin D and phosphate levels [63].

FGF/FGFR signaling affects angiogenesis both directly and indirectly. The direct effect arises from the ability of FGF/FGFR interaction to promote endothelial remolding whereas the indirect effect comes through synergizing VEGF and PDGF signaling pathways [63]. The Ligand FGF-2 is essential to sustain VEGFR-2 expression in endothelium, therefore, it becomes unresponsiveness to

VEGF in the absence of FGF-2 [64]. In addition, FGF-2 mediates angiogenesis by inducing endothelial cell migration and proliferation. Studies have shown that FGF-2 supports vascular maturation by inducing proliferation of fibroblasts and smooth muscle cells [65]. Upon FGF-2 binding to its receptor, FGFR Substrate 2 (FRS2) is recruited to the complex, which acts as an adaptor protein to activate downstream signals such as MAPK and PI3K signaling pathways. Interestingly, FGFR can activate MAPK and PI3K pathways in a FRS2 independent manner, through recruitment of PLC-γ . Once recruited, the PLC-γ transduces the signals down to PKC, which in turn activates MAPK pathway by phosphorylating RAF. Other signaling pathways related to FGF/FGFR are activated in a context-dependent manner and support angiogenesis [63].

Notch Signaling

The Notch signaling pathway consists of five ligands (Jagged-1, Jagged-2, DLL-1 [Delta Like Canonical Notch Ligand 1], DLL-3, DLL-4) and four Notch receptors (Notch 1–4). Unlike the tyrosine kinase receptors, Notch receptors are single-pass transmembrane proteins [66] composed of an extracellular ligand binding site (NECD), a transmembrane (TM), and an intracellular domain (NICD). The role of Notch signaling in vascular development was highlighted by genetic studies in mice which indicates the importance of Notch signaling for artery-vein specification, and for endothelial *tip* and *stalk* cell regulation. Therefore, genetic inactivation of DLL-4, DLL-1, Jagged-1, or Notch-1 were embryonically lethal due to severe vascular abnormality caused by the above mentioned mutations [42, 44]. In addition, Notch signaling is crucial for cell-cell communication, regeneration of stem cell survival leading to differentiation of postnatal tissues [42].

Upon ligand binding, Notch singling is activated through proteolytic cleavage of Notch receptors by γ-secretase and tumor necrosis factor-alpha converting enzyme (TACE), which results in the release of NICD. The latter is translocated to the nucleus and acts as a transcription activator along with RBP-JK/CBF-1 to induce the gene expression of HES 1, HES 5, HES 7 and HESR/Hey 1,2, L [19]. The crosstalk between Notch and VEGFR pathways are necessary to guide endothelial cells during angiogenesis. Among Notch ligands, DLL-4 is highly expressed in vascular endothelium [67] and therefore, during angiogenesis, activation of VEGFR-2 induces DLL-4 expression in the *tip* cells. Subsequent to DLL-4 expression, the endothelial *tip* cells activate Notch-1 receptors on the *stalk* endothelial cells guiding them to follow the *tip* cells during the migration process [68].

MMPs

Blood vessels are covered with basement membrane (BM) and extracellular matrix (ECM), which provide support and stability for blood vessels. These supportive structures are rich in collagens, laminin, and fibronectin [69]. Matrix metalloproteinases (MMPs) are a family of 24 enzymes that are capable of degrading various component of ECM. The MMPs are sub-divided into five major groups [70] based on structure, location, and/or subtract specificity as follows: collagenases (MMP-1, MMP-8, MMP-13), gelatinases (MMP-2, MMP-9), matrilysins (MMP-7, MMP-26), stromelysin-3 (MMP-11), and membrane-bound MMPs (MMP-14, MMP-15, MMP-16, MMP-24).

MMPs activity is essential for ECM breakdown, which takes place during angiogenesis. MMPs are well known to facilitate remolding of vascular networks *via* degrading BM and remolding ECM allowing endothelial cells and pericytes to migrate towards tumor mass. Also, MMPs plays crucial roles in cellular adhesion and signaling through release of membrane-bound growth factors. For example, growth factors such as FGFs, IGF, TGF-β, and VEGFs are held inactive when bound to HSPGs expressed on the ECM. Hence, MMPs proteolytic activity is required for release of active growth factors [71]. Among MMPs, MMP-9 has a critical role in triggering "angiogenic switch" during carcinogenesis [72]. Interestingly, MMPs expression and activity were found to correlate with invasive characteristics also [70]. Therefore, effective targeting of MMPs would result in suppression of tumor angiogenesis and invasive phenotypes.

MDM2

MDM2 is one of the recently discovered protoncogenic proteins, which has drawn significant level of importance in the contest of tumor growth and metastasis mainly because it is a negative regulator of p53 [73]. MDM2 overexpression has been found in many tumors with high metastatic and angiogenic ability. MDM2 can produce several p53-independent mechanisms and, consequently, is emerging as a significant therapeutic target more than ever before. In addition, some of the differentially expressed genes in MDM2 overexpressing cancers can be utilized as a biomarker in conjunction with their master regulators. Hence, identifying the exact mechanisms by which MDM2 is impacting cancer progression at the molecular level would offer greater benefits towards treating cancers that are overexpressing MDM2 [74]. As mentioned earlier, the process of angiogenesis is intricate with involvement of multiple signaling pathways. These complex signals act either directly by inducing endothelial cell remodeling or indirectly by inducing expression of pro-angiogenic molecules. Therefore, identifying and perturbing these pathways represent an opportunity for targeting angiogenesis and subsequently developing cancer treatments. In the last decade, MDM2 has been hypothesized to be implicated in the induction of tumor angiogenesis in a p53 independent manner. The hypothesis was initially faced with considerable skepticism, which usually happens with novel ideas that are 'outside the box', due to the widespread belief at the time that MDM2 has only p53-dependent functions. Therefore, any notion of MDM2 out of its relationship with p53 was immediately rejected. To prove our hypothesis, we had co-expression of MDM2 and VEGF in different cancer cell lines including HL-60, a leukemia cell line harboring p53 mutations [75 - 77]. Furthermore, we demonstrated that treatment with MDM2 gene-specific antisense inhibitor could reduce VEGF expression, which resulted in inhibition of tube-formation in human umbilical vein endothelial cells (HUVECs). At the molecular level, we demonstrated that MDM2 could mediate VEGF expression though induction of HIF-1α levels [78]. Besides the impact of MDM2 on VEGF expression, we have also demonstrated a positive correlation between MDM2 and MMP-9 levels. Our research findings which confirmed the fact that MDM2 has more oncogenic activity beyond the grips of p53 has been substantiated by different research groups around the world in last ten years [79 - 81].

Endogenous Anti-Angiogenic Molecules

Several endogenous signaling molecules were found to impact angiogenesis negatively. The equilibrium between these molecules and pro-angiogenic molecules are necessary to prevent superfluous angiogenesis. The discovery of platelet factor-4 and Interferon α was the proof of concept that endogenous angiogenesis inhibitors existed [82]. Several cleaved forms of collagens such as endostatin, arresten, tumstatin, and canstatin were shown to inhibit endothelial cell proliferation and migration through binding to integrin receptors expressed on the surface of endothelial cells [71]. Similarly, angiostatin, a 38 kDa endogenous molecule generated by proteolytic fragmentation of plasminogen, was reported as a potent inhibitor of endothelial cell proliferation and migration. Consequently, *in vivo* administration of angiostatin resulted in a significant reduction in tumor growth and metastases. Angiostatin was also able to induce apoptosis in endothelial cells [83]. Other endogenous angiogenesis inhibitors such as circulating VEGFR-1, Ang-2, mutltimerin 2 (MMRN-2), and thrombospondin-1 (THBS-1) were reported to sequester and disrupt the growth factor signals leading to angiogenesis suppression [54]. Pharmacological application of THBS-1 as anti-angiogenic agent is restricted due to its huge molecular weight. Given the important role of THBS-1 in preventing angiogenesis, the THBS-1 mimetic proteins such as ABT-510 were developed for the therapeutic use, which was subcutaneously administered in phase II clinical trial for treating non-small cell lung carcinoma (NSCLC) in combination with Carboplatin and Taxol. The clinical trial was prematurely terminated upon interim analysis showing failure of ABT-510 to reach the primary endpoint of increasing progression free survival (PFS) of the patients [84]. Thus, the clinical use of endogenous anti-angiogenic molecules showed disappointing results, thereby the interest shifted towards antagonizing pro-angiogenic signals using exogenous agents and molecules.

Mode of Action for Angiogenesis Inhibitors

Nowadays, targeting angiogenesis as a therapeutic option for patients with cancer is widely accepted. Till today, many angiogenesis inhibitors are clinically proven efficacious against diverse type of cancers. Since angiogenesis is implicated in virtually all types of cancers, angiogenesis inhibitors can be given in an undiscriminating manner to cancer patients, unlike other targeted molecules that are given to only a subset of patients on the basis of biomarker presence [85]. However, the mode of action of angiogenesis inhibitors is still debatable. In fact, there are two hypotheses depicting the role of angiogenesis inhibitors in cancer treatment which are discussed in the following sections.

Starve Tumor to Death Hypothesis

Starving tumor to death is the classic hypothesis that was based on the concept of antagonizing angiogenesis by using endogenous or exogenous inhibitors. The strength of this hypothesis was relying on the fact that angiogenesis inhibitors would starve the tumor cells by cutting-off the strategic supplies (oxygen and nutrients) from reaching the tumor sites [86]. This hypothesis was supported by several experimental observations of a decrease in vascular networks in the tumor following the administration of angiogenesis inhibitors. In conjunction with this observation, we have observed a significant decrease in vascular biomarker levels in mice treated with our anti-angiogenic agent F16. Similarly, a clinical study with a small cohort of NSCLC patients (n=10) showed that Bevacizumab, an anti-VEGF therapeutic antibody, reduced blood tumor perfusion using positron emission tomography (PET). In addition, Bevacizumab significantly reduced the influx rate of radiolabeled Docetaxel to tumor sites as a result of reducing blood perfusion [87]. Thus, several pre-clinical and clinical studies of angiogenesis inhibitors have demonstrated a decrease in blood vessel density and tumor growth supporting the "starve to death" hypothesis [88 - 90]. However, this hypothesis is refuted by the results of some of the clinical trials that showed an additive effect when cytotoxic agents were combined with angiogenesis inhibitors. Consequently, the major question asked by scientists is, if angiogenesis inhibitors decrease blood perfusion to tumor sites, how is it possible for the combination of angiogenesis inhibitors with cytotoxic agents to improve the efficacy of treatment outcome? To address some of these conflicting findings, scientists proposed an alternative hypothesis called "normalization" hypothesis.

Normalization Hypothesis

In 2001, Rakesh Jain introduced the concept of vascular normalization [91]. This concept may seem to be counter-intuitive to the "starve to death" hypothesis. However, the normalization hypothesis states that angiogenesis inhibitors would transiently normalize the tumor blood vessels leading to the alleviation of hypoxia through increasing oxygen and nutrient delivery to tumor sites. Angiogenesis inhibitors would also decrease intra-tumoral tissue pressure by preventing vascular leakage. Though this hypothesis is contradictory to the typical effects of anti-angiogenic agents, it is supported by the observations of increased oxygenation to the tumor sites after administration of angiogenesis inhibitors [92, 93]. Clinically, the use of Cediranib, a multi-tyrosine kinase inhibitor, was reported to increase blood perfusion in a subset of patients with glioblastoma who survived longer (26.3 *Vs.* 17 months) compared to patients received the same regimen and showed low blood perfusion [94]. In addition, the normalization hypothesis could be indirectly supported by the results from some of the clinical trials that showed an additive effect when cytotoxic agents were combined with angiogenesis inhibitors. Winkler and colleagues following Jain's footstep has introduced a concept of "normalization window" based on experimental observations of combining angiogenesis inhibitor with radiation for treating orthotopic glioblastoma model [95]. The above-described concept basically states that angiogenesis inhibitors will transiently normalize tumor vasculature increasing tumor oxygenation and opening a therapeutic window. Administration of chemotherapy or radiation during this window will achieve the best outcome [95]. However, the concept of normalization fails to answer the following questions. If angiogenesis inhibitors increase oxygen perfusion by normalizing blood vessels, would that not increase tumor growth? Why do angiogenesis inhibitors alone decrease tumor growth? While attempting to find an answer for this question, it is important to recognize the fact that, when endothelial proliferation and migration is inhibited, the organization of the cells in the vasculature is left undisturbed, and that could be the reason for improved vascular permeability until the vascular density is reduced.

In view of this prevailing knowledge, it is believed that angiogenesis inhibitors may exert dual effects. Anybody could argue that 'starve - normalize' dual effects of angiogenesis inhibitors may seem logical given the fact that VEGF was first discovered as a vascular permeability factor increasing vascular leakage and later as an endothelial mitogen for increasing vascular networks. Therefore, it is anticipated that angiogenesis inhibitors would antagonize normal functions of VEGF resulting in: i) reduction of vascular leakage, which would increase blood and oxygen perfusion to the tissues; ii) inhibition of VEGF mitogenic activity, which would reduce the number of newly formed blood vessels. Even though angiogenesis inhibitors would increase oxygen perfusion that could support tumor growth, the limited number of blood vessels would not be sufficient to support continued growth and eventually would force tumor cells to cease growth and die (Fig. **2**). Therefore, supporting the dual hypothesis would be reasonable since the evidence for both starve/normalization were strong and combining these observations in one hypothesis brings better logic.

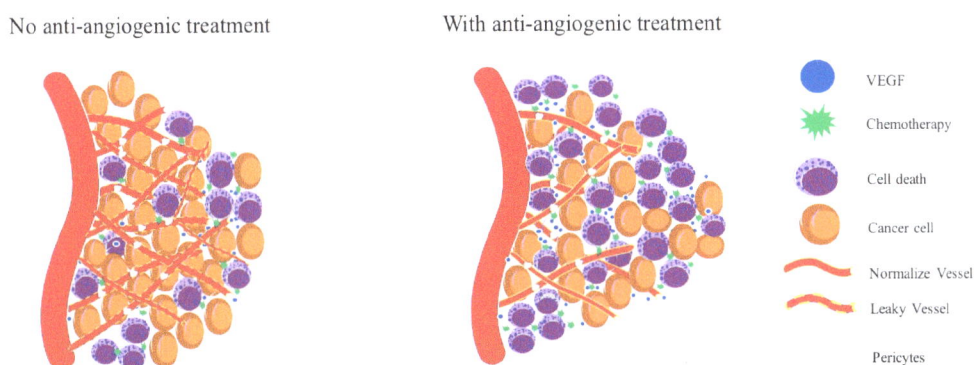

Fig. (2). Tumor vasculature is not arranged or functioned typically unlike normal vessels. This atypical phenotype is displayed by not fully matured, disordered vascular architecture. As a result, angiogenesis inhibitors would counteract normal functions of VEGF leading to increase blood and oxygen supplementation as a result of a reduction in vascular permeability and inhibition of VEGF mitogenic activity. However, ultimately the angiogenesis process will be compromised due to the overall reduction of newly endothelial cells formation.

Failure of Angiogenesis Inhibitors

Treatment failure is common and considered as a significant challenge in cancer treatment. Drug resistance, severe toxicities, and lack of efficacy are other reasons for the failure of chemotherapeutic agents. Anti-angiogenic agents have no exceptions for facing primary or acquired resistance, and therefore the clinical outcome is less than what is originally anticipated.

Drug Resistance

Several mechanisms are implicated in chemotherapy drug resistance such as increased drug efflux, enzymatic inactivation, DNA repair, and target mutations [96]. Although anti-angiogenic therapies have been widely acknowledged to produce antitumor activity, a few studies have shown that some of the anti-angiogenic agents could increase the invasiveness and metastatic ability in tumors such as, pancreatic neuroendocrine cancers, breast carcinoma, melanoma, and glioblastoma [97, 98]. Interestingly, one of the recent studies have indicated that the treatment of healthy mice with VEGF inhibitors displayed unfavorable aggressive phenotype behavior after implanting xenograft tumors to these animals [99]. However, mechanisms of resistance to angiogenesis inhibitors are different than that are seen with chemotherapy. The initial thought was that anti-angiogenic agents were less likely to develop drug resistance due to the fact that these agents target endothelial cells which are genetically stable rather than genetically unstable cancer cells [100]. However, the emergence of drug resistance to anti-angiogenic agents was evident in pre-clinical and clinical settings. One of the most common observations with anti-angiogenic agents is transitory tumor regression followed by inevitable tumor progression. In some cases, anti-angiogenic agents fail from the beginning to produce any clinical benefits [101]. Bergers and Hanahan have classified modes of resistance to angiogenesis inhibitors into adaptive (evasive) and intrinsic (pre-existing) resistance. Both modes of resistance are attributed mainly to up-regulation of other pro-angiogenesis pathways to compensate VEGF inhibition, and to the recruitment of pericytes and inflammatory cells to protect tumor vasculature from anti-VEGF agents [102]. Clinically, a subset of patients with colorectal cancer who were non-responding to Bevacizumab showed higher plasma levels of FGF2, MMP-9, and PDGF. Such up-regulation of alternative pro-angiogenic cytokines supporting angiogenesis can negatively compensate for VEGF inhibition by Bevacizumab and pave the basis for resistance [103].

Toxicity

The initial expectation is that modulation of angiogenesis would result in low toxicity compared to chemotherapy. However, currently available anti-angiogenic agents are associated with severe toxicity. These toxicities range from bleeding, gastrointestinal perforation, fatigue, hypertension, myelosuppression, life-threatening hepatotoxicity, and sudden death. Another set of treatment induced toxicities such as hypothyroidism, posterior leukoencephalopathy syndrome, and nephrotoxicity are also reported in a subset of patients. Therefore, the severe toxicities that are observed with several VEGFR-targeted small molecule inhibitors might limit the therapeutic benefits of these agents.

Lack of Efficacy

Angiogenesis inhibitors are primarily believed to be cytostatic agents even through several *in vitro* and *in vivo* studies have demonstrated a direct cytotoxic effect. Therefore, clinical studies with anti-angiogenic agents should be designed carefully and take into consideration the fact that these agents are cytostatic, thereby the primary endpoints to evaluate the effectiveness based on the reduction of tumor volume will not be far below the levels with angiogenesis inhibitors as much as with cytotoxic chemotherapy. In fact, there are no markers that are clinically validated to predict the drug response of angiogenesis inhibitors other than traditional endpoints [104]. Using circulating VEGF levels as a biomarker has yielded a conflicting result. In some clinical cases, circulating VEGF levels unexpectedly increased in response to anti-VEGF treatment [105]. We believe that using one biomarker to predict drug response is not reliable. Instead, an array of biomarkers associated with angiogenesis might have a paramount impact on the evaluation of drug response, selection, and dosing schedule.

Cancer metastasis to multiple organs is one of the primary causes of mortality. Indeed, multiple reports have demonstrated the substantial role of anti-angiogenic drugs in impeding primary tumor development with less consideration towards the control of cancer metastasis. In fact, modifications in the primary tumor and surrounding tumor microenvironment (TME) can increase the revascularization and subsequent metastasis development. In addition to the earlier unfavorable outcomes, commonly observed rebound vascularization of tumors suggest that, sustained inhibition of tumor angiogenesis is essential for better clinical outcomes in targeting primary and secondary tumor development. Consequently, the continuous administration of antiangiogenic therapies using sustained-release formation could be a more useful approach compare to overcoming the resistance caused by anti-angiogenic drugs [106].

In addition, angiogenesis by known definition is the process of branching of blood vessels from existing vasculature. Thus, angiogenesis inhibitors will prevent new blood vessel formation whereas existing vessels will continue to supply tumor mass with the necessary nutrients and oxygen for growth and survival. It should be taken into account once vessels are fully formed; they are less likely to regress. One discrepancy between pre-clinical studies and clinical trials is that angiogenesis inhibitors were tested on different stages. Most angiogenesis inhibitors were pre-clinically examined on early stages of tumor whereas in clinical trials angiogenesis inhibitors were mostly evaluated in patients with highly aggressive and/or late stage tumors. Therefore, giving angiogenesis inhibitors in late stages is more likely to be ineffective since the tumor mass is generally large with extensive network of blood supplies. Hence, use of angiogenesis inhibitors in early stages of cancer may be more beneficial than late stages. In conclusion, these obstacles necessitate the discovery of novel approaches that can simultaneously influence various pro-angiogenic mechanisms, identify the ideal time for anti-angiogenic treatments, and discover prognostic tools that can predict treatment responsiveness.

CURRENT STATUS OF ANTI-ANGIOGENIC DRUGS AVAILABLE FOR CANCER TREATMENT

Introduction

Over the last 40 years, active research in the field of angiogenesis and TME has yielded several angiogenesis inhibitors entering clinical trials. A landmark was established when the Food and Drug Administration (FDA) approved Bevacizumab as the first angiogenesis inhibitor. Since then, a significant quantity of angiogenesis inhibitors has demonstrated clinical benefits in patients with advanced cancer. This chapter will discuss the myriad number of current therapeutic agents used for anti-angiogenic therapy, based upon target selectivity, preclinical findings, clinical application, and toxicity profile.

Therapeutic Strategy

Remarkably, inhibition of angiogenesis illustrates a unique approach in fighting cancer since it targets the growing blood vessels rather than tumor cells. This approach of treatment can initially delay the tumor growth (cytostatic) rather than eradicating them with direct cytotoxic attack. Since the angiogenesis inhibitors are considered selective for endothelium around tumor mass that are proliferating compared to normal endothelium, the toxicities are minimal. The normal endothelial cells are highly quiescent and are characterized by a very low proliferation rate and long doubling time ranging from 47-23,000 days. In contrast, tumor endothelial cells proliferative ability has short doubling time ranging from 3-13 days [82]. Hence, combining angiogenesis inhibitor with other anti-cancer agents are typically intended to increase therapeutic efficacy and reduce the risk of developing drug resistance. Therefore, the maximum efficacy of angiogenesis inhibitors is achieved when they are combined with another therapy, especially cytotoxic chemotherapy.

Monotherapy

The rationale for using angiogenesis inhibitors as monotherapy is to delay cancer progression in patients who were previously treated with first line or second line of treatment for growth arrest. In this regard, Bevacizumab monotherapy demonstrated an increase in response rate in patients with recurrent glioblastoma [107] and therefore, Bevacizumab monotherapy was approved by the FDA as a second line of treatment for glioblastoma. On the other hand, use of angiogenesis inhibitors as monotherapy has two disadvantages. First, angiogenesis inhibitors are not cytotoxic, so that complete tumor remission is not typically achieved. Secondly, drug resistance is more likely to occur when angiogenesis inhibitors are used for monotherapy.

Combination Therapy

The strategy of combining angiogenesis inhibitor with anti-cancer agents is the most promising to achieve therapeutic outcomes with less frequency of drug resistance. Several signaling pathways are highly expressed or activated in cancers. Therefore, defining the key targets would be crucial for selecting the combination regimen to achieve the maximum therapeutic response. In this strategy, however, the incident of severe toxicity may emerge, and combining different agents would broaden the toxicity.

Recently, combining angiogenesis inhibitor with immunotherapy have emerged as a novel strategy to potentiate the treatment effectiveness [108]. Given the fact that cancer cells escape immune surveillance, by creating an abnormal hypoxic and acidic microenvironment that attenuates immune cells patrolling and protecting activity against anomaly in cellular behavior [109]. Thus, it has been shown that combining immunotherapy with anti-VEGF therapy had more therapeutic efficacy than using these agents alone in a mouse model [110]. Clinically, combining Sunitinib (anti-VEGF) with Nivolumab (anti-PD-1) showed an encouraging anti-tumor activity in patients with metastatic renal cell carcinoma [111].

Prevention Therapy

In 1976, the concept of chemoprevention was proposed and defined as the use of drugs to prevent cancer from development [112]. Since then, several natural or synthetic compounds have been reported to reduce the risk of carcinogenesis. For instance, a follow-up study that lasted for 20 years revealed that daily administration of Aspirin, a non-selective COX-1 and COX-2 inhibitor, can significantly reduce the incident and mortality of colorectal cancer [113]. Similarly, Celecoxib, a selective COX-2 inhibitor, was also shown to significantly reduce the incidence of colorectal adenomas in a randomized placebo-controlled clinical trial with a follow-up for 3 years [114].

In addition, daily administration of branched-chain amino acids (BCAAs) for 60 months was shown to reduce the risk of hepatocellular carcinoma recurrence in patients (n=51) with liver cirrhosis and obesity [115]. BCAAs treatment was found to be associated with a significant reduction in the serum levels of soluble VEGFR-2. Since angiogenesis is pre-requisite for tumor growth and expansion, use of angiogenesis inhibitors to prevent cancer development or treat cancer in patients with high risk seems promising. This strategy is supported by a relative safety of angiogenesis inhibitors when administered over extended periods. However, use of anti-angiogenic agents for prevention is unchartered territory, which requires full evaluation of the benefits with the careful consideration for safety during long-term use.

Targeting VEGF/VEGFR

No doubt that angiogenesis is essential for tumor growth and targeting angiogenesis will be an effective therapeutic approach. There is a consensus that VEGF signaling plays a central role in the induction of angiogenesis, therefore targeting VEGF and its signaling pathway are expected to antagonize angiogenesis and consequently stop cancer growth. In fact, two approaches approved by FDA are used to antagonize tumor angiogenesis as shown in Table **1**. These approaches are classified, based on the nature and the molecular structure of the therapeutics into: *monoclonal antibodies* or *small molecule tyrosine kinase inhibitors*. Since monoclonal antibodies are relatively large molecules, their targets are either expressed on the cell surface or secreted in the plasma. Thus, monoclonal antibodies act only extracellularly. In contrast to monoclonal antibodies, tyrosine kinase inhibitors are able to cross the cell membrane and act intracellularly due to the hydrophobic nature of these small molecules. Also, small molecule tyrosine kinase inhibitors can be administrated orally in a salt form. Therefore, small molecule tyrosine kinase inhibitors have better oral bioavailability compared to monoclonal antibodies.

Bevacizumab

Bevacizumab is a fully humanized monoclonal antibody which binds to all human VEGF-A isoforms [117]. In both pre-clinical and clinical studies, Bevacizumab had shown a significant reduction in tumor growth, irrespective of tumor types, which gave further proof for the effectiveness and benefit of anti-angiogenic therapy. Furthermore, *in vitro* studies evaluating the impact of Bevacizumab on the growth of several cancer cell lines showed no direct cytotoxicity suggesting that the anti-cancer activity of Bevacizumab is a consequence of inhibition VEGFR mediated angiogenesis mechanisms [118]. Bevacizumab treatment was significantly associated with low incidence of brain metastases in pre-clinical models. In consistence with pre-clinical observations, a retrospective analysis of three clinical trials of NSCLC suggested a preventive effect of Bevacizumab against brain metastases [119]. Bevacizumab was extensively evaluated in several clinical trials for advanced cancer types. In those clinical trials, Bevacizumab demonstrated a significant increase in objective response rate, PFS, and/or OS. In a randomized phase III clinical trial, patients with metastatic colorectal cancer receiving Bevacizumab in combination with Irinotecan, Fluorouracil, and Leucovorin showed a significant increase in OS which ultimately led to the approval of Bevacizumab by FDA as a first anti-angiogenic agent with significant clinical outcomes [120]. The successful clinical application of Bevacizumab for metastatic colorectal cancer was extended to the other cancer types. As a result, FDA subsequently approved Bevacizumab for treatment of metastatic NSCLC,

Table 1. Overview of FDA approved VEGF/VEGFR targeted agents , corresponding indications, and side effects [116].

	Generic Name	FDA Proven Indication(s)	FDA Warnings/Reported Side Effects
Monoclonal antibody	**Bevacizumab** (Avastin®)	1. Metastatic CRC 2. Non-squamous NSCLC 3. Metastatic breast cancer 4. Glioblastoma 5. Metastatic RCC 6. Metastatic cervical cancer	1. Gastrointestinal perforations 2. Wound healing complications 3. Hemorrhage 4. Hypertension 5. Proteinuria 6. RPLS
	Ramucirumab (Cyramza®)	1. Advanced gastric adenocarcinoma 2. Metastatic NSCLC 3. Metastatic CRC	1. Fatal hemorrhage 2. Hypertension 3. Cirrhosis 4. ATE 5. RPLS
Small tyrosine kinase inhibitor	**Sorafenib** (Nexavar®)	1. Unresectable hepatocellular carcinoma 2. Advanced RCC 3. Metastatic DTC	1. Cardiac ischemia 2. Dermatological toxicities 3. Gastrointestinal perforation 4. Bleeding 5. Hypertension
	Sunitinib (Sutent®)	1. GIST 2. Metastatic RCC 3. Advanced PNET	1. Hepatotoxicity 2. Thyroid dysfunction 3. Left ventricular dysfunction 4. QT interval prolongation & torsade de Pointes 5. Hemorrhage 6. Adrenal dysfunction
	Pazopanib (Votrient®)	1. Advanced RCC 2. Advanced soft tissue sarcoma	1. Hepatotoxicity 2. Cardiac dysfunction 3. QT interval prolongation & torsade de Pointes 4. Gastrointestinal perforation/fistula 5. RPLS 6. ATE
	Axitinib (Inlyta®)	Advanced RCC	1. Hypertensive crisis 2. Hepatic impairment 3. RPLS 4. Thyroid dysfunction 5. TAE 6. Hemorrhage
	Cabozantinib (Cometriq®)	Metastatic medullary thyroid cancer	1. Gastrointestinal perforation/ fistula 2. Jaw osteonecrosis 3. Wound complication 4. RPLS 5. Hypertension 6. Palmar-Plantar erythrodysesthesia syndrome
	Vandetanib (Caprelsa®)	Metastatic medullary thyroid cancer	1. Sudden death 2. Hypothyroidism 3. Steven-Johnson syndrome 4. Interstitial lung disease 5. QT interval prolongation and Torsade de Pointes 6. Heart failure and Ischemic cerebrovascular events
	Lenvatinib (Lenvima®)	Metastatic iodine refractory thyroid cancer	1. Cardiac dysfunction 2. Hepatotoxicity 3. Renal failure 4. QT interval prolongation 5. Embryo-fetal toxicity 6. Proteinuria 7. Hypertension 8. Hypocalcaemia 9. RPLS
	Regrofanib (Stivarga®)	1. Advanced GIST 2. Metastatic CRC	1. Dermatological toxicity 2. Cardiac ischemia and infraction 3. RPLS 4. Gastrointestinal perforation 5. Hypertension

metastatic renal cell carcinoma, metastatic HER2 negative breast cancer, metastatic cervical cancer, glioblastoma, and platinum-resistant recurrent epithelial ovarian cancer. Generally, Bevacizumab is considered safe with observations of less complicated side effects such as hypertension, hemorrhage, gastrointestinal perforation, proteinuria, venous and arterial thromboembolic events, wound healing and headache [121].

Ramucirumab

Ramucirumab is another monoclonal antibody, which targets VEGFR-2. It binds to the extracellular domain of VEGFR-2 blocking the ligand-induced receptor activation. Ramucirumab was well tolerated and demonstrated clinical benefits in patients with late stage/advanced cancer. In phase III clinical trial, Ramucirumab as monotherapy demonstrated a statistically significant increase in OS by 1.4 month in comparison to placebo for patients with metastatic gastric or gastroesophageal junction adenocarcinoma [122]. Similarly, the combination of Ramucirumab with Paclitaxel increased OS by 2.3 months compared to Paclitaxel plus placebo for treatment of metastatic gastric or gastroesophageal junction adenocarcinoma [123]. Despite the modest increase in OS, Ramucirumab monotherapy or in combination with Paclitaxel was approved by FDA for advanced gastric cancer as a second line of treatment. Furthermore, Ramucirumab in combination with Docetaxel was approved by FDA for metastatic NSCLC based on a statistically significant increase in OS (10.5 *Vs.* 9.1 months) compared to placebo plus Docetaxel combination [124]. FDA also approved Ramucirumab in combination with FOLFIRI as a second line of treatment for metastatic colorectal cancers. The approval was based on a statistically significant increase in OS (13.3 *Vs.* 11.7 months) in Ramucirumab plus FOLFIRI compared to FOLFIRI plus placebo combination [125]. Recently, Ramucirumab treatment with Docetaxel showed promising results in metastatic urothelial carcinoma with a significant in increase in PFS (5.4 *Vs.* 2.8 months) compared to Docetaxel monotherapy [126]. As a result, Ramucirumab plus Docetaxel treatment was advanced into global, randomized, double-blinded placebo-controlled phase III clinical trial (NCT02426125).

IMC-3C5

IMC-3C5 is a monoclonal antibody directed against VEGFR-3 [127]. The rationale behind the development of IMC-3C5 was to prevent VEGFR-3 mediated lymphangiogenesis, which in turn would prevent metastasis of solid tumors to lymph nodes. It was not possible to test IMC-3C5 activity using a mouse model since it recognized only human VEGFR-3 and did not cross-react with murine

VEGFR-3. However, a murine-specific VEGFR-3 antibody (mF4-31C1) was developed and tested to predict the physiological activity of IMC-3C5. Administration of mF4-31C1 demonstrated a complete and specific inhibition of lymphangiogenesis with no effect on blood angiogenesis in mice implanted with human breast carcinoma [128]. In another study, blocking VEGFR-3 using mF4-31C1 inhibited tumor metastases to regional lymph nodes, implying the crucial role of VEGFR-3 signaling in promoting tumor metastasis [129]. These studies provided solid evidence to support clinical development of IMC-3C5. In a phase I clinical trial, when IMC-3C5 was given to patients with advanced solid tumors or CRC, to evaluate the safety, maximum tolerated dose, pharmacokinetic parameters, and anti-tumor efficacy, it was well tolerated. However, nausea, vomiting, peripheral edema, fatigue and urinary tract infection were observed in patients. However, a small fraction of patients with CRC (19%) showed a marginal increase in PFS of only 6.3 weeks [127] and therefore, no clinical trials were planned to pursue further testing of IMC-3C5.

Icrucumab

Icrucumab is a monoclonal antibody that binds to the extracellular domain of VEGFR-1, precluding VEGF-A, VEGF-B, and PIGF binding, that leads to the inhibition of VEGFR-1 downstream signals. The *in vitro* studies showed that Icrucumab prevents ligand-induced VEGFR-1 phosphorylation [130]. Similarly, Icrucumab inhibited *in vivo* growth of the breast xenograft through a reduction of MAPK and AKT activation and induction of apoptosis. In a phase I clinical trial, Icrucumab was well tolerated with observations of peripheral edema, anemia, fatigue, nausea, and dyspnea. Surprisingly, hypertension, hemorrhage, and cardiovascular side effects were not observed in a cohort treated with Icrucumab, insinuating that blockade of VEGFR-2 not VEGFR-1 is associated with these side effects [131]. On the other hand, Icrucumab failed so far to achieve significant clinical benefits. In a phase II trial, combination of Icrucumab with Docetaxel showed no significant increase in PFS in patients with advanced urothelial carcinoma [126]. Similar disappointing results were observed in combination of Icrucumab with mFOLFOX-6 for treatment with metastatic CRC [1132]. A recently published phase II clinical results also revealed that Icrucumab in combination with Capecitabine showed no significant increase in PFS and OS in patients with metastatic breast cancer [133], which excluded the hope for future clinical applications.

Semaxanib

Semaxanib was the first small molecular VEGFR inhibitor tested clinically. Semaxanib showed high selectivity against VEGFR-2 associated tyrosine kinase

[134]. Pre-clinical studies have demonstrated a potent anti-angiogenic activity both in *in vitro* and *in vivo* experiments, which prompted clinical evaluation. In a phase I trial to evaluate safety, severe headache, nausea and vomiting were the dose-limiting toxicities. Pharmacokinetic studies revealed poor oral bioavailability with a very low half-life which necessitated more frequent parenteral administration of Semaxanib to achieve active plasma levels [135]. However, Semaxanib was also prematurely discontinued in phase III clinical trials for treatment of advanced CRC due to disappointing results. However, Semaxanib remains as an experimental drug and not licensed for any human use.

Orantinib

Orantinib is a small molecule tyrosine kinase inhibitor with a relatively broad targeting profile. It competitively inhibits VEGFR-2, PDGFR-β, FGFR-1, and c-KIT [136]. Orantinib showed a significant reduction of tumor growth in several xenograft models of melanoma, glioma, lung, and ovarian cancers [137]. During evaluation of safety in phase I clinical trials, Orantinib showed good tolerability for once daily dosing compared to twice daily dosing, which yielded dose-limiting toxicities including dyspnea, chest pain and pericardial effusions [138]. In a phase III trial, Orantinib plus transcatheter arterial chemoembolization (TACE), a minimally invasive procedure to restrict tumor blood supply, was tested in patients with un-resectable hepatocellular carcinoma. Independent interim analysis revealed that Orantinib plus TACE did not show any superiority in OS over TACE plus placebo, which led to the termination of the trial (NCT01465464). Further development of Orantinib was ceased due to disappointing clinical results.

Sunitinib

Sunitinib is a multi-target receptor tyrosine kinase inhibitor which targets VEGFR-1, VEGFR-2, VERGR-3, PDGFRs, c-KIT, CSF-1R, FLT-3, EGFR, FGFR-1, and Met [139]. Since Sunitinib has broad targeting profile, it exerts a direct anti-tumor activity alongside with its anti-angiogenic activity. In xenograft models, Sunitinib not only inhibited tumor growth but also induced tumor regression [140]. Sunitinib is metabolized by cytochrome P450 system into an active metabolite called N-Desethyl sunitinib, which has equivalent potency and activity as the parent Sunitinib. The N-Desethyl Sunitinib is further metabolized by CYP 3A4 into an inactive moiety [140]. Clinically, Sunitinib has demonstrated efficacy against wide range of solid malignancies. In phase III clinical trial, patients with metastatic RCC exhibited longer PFS (11 *Vs.* 5 months) in Sunitinib arm compare to INF-α arm [141]. In addition, patients treated with Sunitinib experienced better quality of life and longer OS compare to INF-α (26.4 *Vs.* 21.8

months) [142]. Thus, FDA initially approved Sunitinib for treatment of metastatic RCC. Later, Sunitinib was approved by FDA for treating patients with Imatinib resistant gastrointestinal stromal tumors based on a significant increase in PFS (27.3 *Vs.* 6.4 weeks) with Sunitinib compared to placebo treatment [143]. Similarly, Sunitinib was approved by FDA, due to a significant increase in PFS (11.4 months) compared to placebo arm (5.5 months), for treating patients with pancreatic neuroendocrine tumors [144]. On the other hand, Sunitinib failed to meet the primary and secondary endpoints in 4 clinical trials of metastatic breast cancer [145]. The most clinically relevant side effects of Sunitinib were fatigue, hypertension, hypothyroidism, bleeding, and hand-foot syndrome, a severe skin toxicity which negatively impacts the patients' quality of life [146]. Other significant toxicities induced by Sunitinib include hepatotoxicity, cardiotoxicity, and nephrotoxicity apart from the hematotoxicity [147].

Sorafenib

Sorafenib is a small molecule tyrosine kinase inhibitor, which is a potent inhibitor of the intracellular RAF serine kinase family (RAF-1 and RAF-B). Also, Sorafenib inhibits VEGFR-2, VEGFR-3, PDGFR-β, and FLT-3 [148]. Sorafenib has a direct anti-proliferative effect on several cancer cell lines as a result of inhibiting of RAF-mediated MEK/ERK phosphorylation. Sorafenib demonstrated anti-tumor and anti-angiogenic activity against breast, colon, and NSCLC xenograft models [148, 149]. Sorafenib monotherapy demonstrated significant clinical benefits that led to FDA approval for treatment of patients with advanced RCC, un-resectable hepatocellular carcinoma, and radioactive iodine-refractory advanced thyroid carcinoma. Sorafenib-induced side effects include hypophosphatemia, hypertension, alopecia, weight loss, hand-foot syndrome, and hemorrhage which could be accommodated by dose interruptions or reductions [150, 151].

Regorafenib

Regorafenib is a small molecule multi-kinase inhibitor. Its chemical structure is similar to Sorafenib but Regorafenib has potent inhibitory effects against VEGFR-1, VEGFR-2, VEGFR-3, PDGFR-β, FGFR-1, c-KIT, RET, Tie-2, and RAF-B. Regorafenib demonstrated a potent *in vivo* anti-angiogenic activity by reducing tumor blood perfusion and reducing extravasation of the contrast agent during dynamic contrast magnetic resonance imaging (DCEMRI). Moreover, Regorafenib exhibited a potent tumor growth inhibition and in some cases tumor regression in several xenograft models [152]. Clinically, Regorafenib was approved by FDA for treatment of HCC, relapsed CRC, and gastrointestinal stromal tumors. Similar to previous agents, Regorafenib treatment was associated with increased incidents of hand-foot syndrome, hypertension, and diarrhea [153].

Pazopanib

Pazopanib is also a multi-target small molecule tyrosine kinase inhibitor. It potently inhibits VEGFR-1, VEGFR-2, VEGFR-3, PDGFR, FGFR, c-KIT and c-Fms. Pazopanib strongly inhibits VEGF induced VEGFR-2 phosphorylation leading to the inhibition of HUVECs proliferation [154]. In addition, Pazopanib demonstrated a direct anti-proliferative activity, mediated through suppression of PI3K-AKT pathway, against several cancer types including multiple myeloma, breast carcinoma, lung carcinoma, chronic lymphocytic leukemia, and sarcoma cells [155 - 157]. Clinically, Pazopanib was approved by FDA for treatment of metastatic RCC and advanced soft tissue sarcoma based on a significant increase in PFS [158, 159]. However, a follow-up study showed no significant increase in OS (22.9 *Vs.* 20.5 months) in patients with metastatic RCC compared to placebo [160]. Treatment with Pazopanib is associated with severe hepatotoxicity that requires continuous monitoring of the liver function. Other adverse reactions associated with Pazopanib include arterial and venous thromboembolic events, hypertension, hemorrhage, gastrointestinal perforation, hair hypopigmentation, musculoskeletal pain, and left ventricular dysfunction [159]. The use of Pazopanib as monotherapy or in combination with anticancer agents was under clinical investigation in over 24 clinical trials for the treatments of metastatic advanced angiosarcoma, glioblastoma multiforme, advanced prostate, breast, ovarian, and pancreatic neuroendocrine cancers. Recently, in phase I clinical trial, Pazopanib in combination with Cyclophosphamide showed promising results in patients with recurrent platinum-resistant ovarian cancer [161].

Vandetanib

Vandetanib is a small molecule with dual VEGFR-2 and EGFR inhibition [162]. Vandetanib has low activity against MEK, FAK, c-KIT, PDGFR-β, and Tie-2 compared to VEGFR-2. In the *in vitro* conditions, Vandetanib has direct inhibitory effects on the growth of several cancer cell lines, through inhibition of EGFR. Similarly, in the *in vivo* experiments, Vandetanib exhibited anti-VEGF activity by reversing VEGF induce hypotensive status in rats [162]. Also, Vandetanib demonstrated a significant efficacy against the growth of several human xenograft models at a dose $\geq$ 50 mg/kg/day [162]. In clinical settings, Vandetanib demonstrated significant improvements in objective response and PFS compared to placebo in patients with inoperable aggressive medullary thyroid cancer [163]. Despite no increase in OS, Vandetanib was approved by FDA as a first targeted therapy for treatment of surgery ineligible patients with advanced medullary thyroid cancer. Currently, Vandetanib is being tested as monotherapy for treatment of patients with breast cancer (NCT01934335), and patients with head and neck cancer (NCT01414426). Treatment with Vandetanib, however, was associated with severe toxicities and side effects, which might require discontinuation of Vandetanib. These toxicities include prolong QTc, torsades de pointes, heart failure, hemorrhage, Stevens-Johnson syndrome, and sudden death [164].

Cabozantinib

Cabozantinib is a small molecule receptor tyrosine kinase inhibitor, which inhibits broad spectrum of tyrosine kinases including MET, RET, c-KIT, VEGFR-2, FLT-3, AXL, and Tie-2 [165]. Pre-clinical evaluation of Cabozantinib revealed potent anti-tumor, anti-angiogenic, and anti-metastatic activities against several xenograft models. Also, Cabozantinib treatment was shown to overcome the acquired drug resistance associated with chronic Sunitinib treatment in pre-clinical model of RCC, due to the ability of Cabozantinib to potently inhibit the up-regulation of MET and AXT receptors [166]. The promising pre-clinical results gave the rationale for the clinical evaluation of Cabozantinib. Cabozantinib was also evaluated in over 22 clinical trials for the treatment of a wide range of aggressive or metastatic tumors such as thyroid, ovarian, prostate, non-small cell lung, kidney, liver, breast, glioblastoma, melanoma, and osteosarcoma. Results from phase I clinical studies revealed that Cabozantinib was well-tolerated with promising clinical activity and response against multiple tumor types [153, 167, 168]. In a phase III clinical trial, patients with aggressive medullary thyroid cancer receiving Cabozantinib showed improvement in PFS compared to placebo (11.2 *Vs.* 4 months) which eventually led to the FDA approval [169]. Recently, Cabozantinib showed a significant increase in PFS (7.4 *Vs.* 3.8 months) and OS (21.4 *Vs.* 18.7 months) compared to Everolimus in patients with advanced RCC, who were previously treated with one or more VEGF-tyrosine kinase inhibitors [170]. Based on this study, Cabozantinib was approved by FDA as a second line of treatment for patients with RCC who were previously treated with other anti-angiogenic therapies. A recent clinical study demonstrated a superior clinical benefit of Cabozantinib over Sunitinib as first line of treatment for patients with metastatic RCC [171]. Despite the encouraging clinical benefits that were observed initially, Cabozantinib failed to meet the primary clinical endpoint (increase in OS) in heavily treated patients with metastatic, castration-resistant prostate cancer [172].

Cediranib

Cediranib, also known as AZD21721, is yet another small molecule tyrosine kinase inhibitor with a potent and selective inhibitory activity against VEGFR-2.

It also inhibits other tyrosine kinases including c-KIT, PDGFR-α, and PDGFR-β at 2, 10, and 16-fold higher concentration than VEGFR-2 respectively [173]. Thus, Cediranib at nanomolar concentrations showed a strong inhibition of VEGF induced HUVEC proliferation and tube formation whereas at micro-molar concentrations it directly inhibited *in vitro* tumor growth. Pre-clinical efficacy studies showed that Cediranib was an orally active agent with potent and broad-spectrum anti-tumor activity against different human xenograft models. Also, Cediranib showed a strong *in vivo* inhibition of VEGF-driven angiogenesis using Matrigel plugs containing VEGF in xenograft implanted nude mice. Pre-clinical toxicity assessments in rat and non-human primate showed that Cediranib was well-tolerated with increased observations of hypertension [174]. In clinical trials, hypertension was a common adverse reaction of Cediranib which was manageable by anti-hypertensive agent [174]. Also, left ventricular dysfunction was observed in patients receiving Cediranib [175]. Similar to previous agents, Cediranib treatment was associated with increased risk of bleeding and hemorrhage. Recently, Cediranib was evaluated in phase I and II clinical trials for advanced solid tumors (NCT02484404, NCT02498613). In particular, Cediranib treatment showed a promising clinical result in patients with ovarian cancer. In a phase II clinical trial, combination of Cediranib with Olaparib, an FDA approved agent as a PARP inhibitor for BRCA positive ovarian cancer, showed a significant increase in PFS compared to Olaparib monotherapy (17.7 *Vs.* 9 months) in patients with recurrent platinum-sensitive ovarian cancer [176]. Thus, the combination of Cediranib plus Olaparib is advanced to phase III clinical trial for platinum sensitive or platinum-resistant ovarian cancer (NCT02446600, NCT02502266). On the other hand, Cediranib in combination with chemotherapy failed to meet the primary endpoint for patients with metastatic CRC [177]. Similarly, the clinical development of Cediranib was suspended in patients with recurrent glioblastoma due to lack of efficacy [178].

Vatalanib

Vatalanib is a small molecule tyrosine kinase inhibitor of VEGFR-2 with sub-micro-molar concentrations. It also inhibits all other VEGFRs, PDGFR-β c-KIT, and c-Fms at relatively higher concentrations [179]. Besides tyrosine inhibition, Vatalanib was shown to inhibit aromatase activity in both *in vitro* and *in vivo,* which significantly inhibited the growth of breast cancer xenograft [180]. Vatalanib inhibited both *in vivo* VEGF and PDGF induced angiogenesis in mice [181]. Similarly, Vatalanib induced clinical response was associated with a reduction of tumor blood flow, measured by DCEMRI, due to inhibition of tumor vasculature in patients with metastatic RCC [182]. However, Vatalanib showed a modest result in CRC with only a subset of patients who were benefited from Vatalanib treatment [183]. The clinical development of Vatalanib, in patients with recurrent glioblastoma multiforme, was prematurely discontinued upon sponsor's request due to unexpected complications [184].

Targeting Ang/Tie-2

In addition to the pro-angiogenic stimuli through VEGF, activation of Tie-2 signals by Ang-1 was also reported to increase pericytes recruitment to the tumor vasculature, which decreases vascular leakage and ultimately increases vascular normalization. Such activation is believed to increase drug delivery to the tumor mass [185]. Therefore, one of the strategies for anti-angiogenic therapy is to restore Tie-2 signals by blocking its natural antagonist Ang-2. VEGF signaling acts mainly on early steps of angiogenesis by increasing vascular permeability, endothelial proliferation and migration. Whereas, Ang-1/Tie-2 acts on late stages of vascular remolding by increasing vascular maturation and stabilization [186].

As of now there is no FDA approved drugs that mainly target Ang/Tie-2. However, four novel Ang/Tie-2 targeted therapies are currently being tested in clinical settings. First, Nesvacumab (REGN-910) is a monoclonal antibody against Ang-2 [187]. Nesvacumab has just completed an open-label, multicenter phase I clinical trial in patients with advanced solid malignancies (NCT01271972). During the initial testing Nesvacumab was well tolerated with no dose-limiting toxicity [188]. Second, MEDI-3617 is another monoclonal antibody directed against Ang-2 [189]. MEDI-3617 is currently under phase I clinical trial to evaluate its safety and anti-tumor activity in patients with advanced solid tumors (NCT01248949, NCT02141542). Third candidate tested for Ang/Tie-2 target was CEP-11981, which is a small molecule with tyrosine kinase inhibitor ability. This compound has completed an open-label, phase I clinical trial that was designed to determine the maximum tolerated dose and dose-limiting toxicity (NCT00875264). Some of the CEP-11981 related adverse effects were neutropenia, chest pain, dyspnea, headache and dizziness [190]. Fourth experimental drug, code named CVX-241, is a fusion protein that targets both Ang-2 and VEGF [191]. In phase I clinical trial with solid tumors, CVX-241 was prematurely discontinued since no significant pharmacological effects were achieved (NCT01004822).

Targeting FGF/FGFR

In addition to VEGF, Ang-2 and Tie-2 mediated effects, FGF/FGFR signaling is also implicated in tumor proliferation, migration, survival, and angiogenesis. Pre-clinical and clinical studies showed that FGF signaling is activated as a means of resistance to anti-VEGF therapy [103]. All currently available FGF/FGFR inhibitors are either monoclonal antibodies that inhibit FGFs binding or small molecules that inhibit FGFRs tyrosine kinase activity. Since all tyrosine kinase receptors share structure homology, small molecule tyrosine kinase inhibitors may inhibit more than one kinase. The first generation of FGFRs inhibitors is non-selective tyrosine kinase inhibitors including Brivanib, Cediranib, Nintedanib, Lenvatinib, Sulfatinib, Dovitinib, Ponatinib, and Lucitanib [63]. These agents exhibited potent anti-angiogenic and anti-tumor activities in different pre-clinical cancer models. However, recent interest has been shifted towards development of a relatively selective FGF-targeted therapy. Several novel compounds with high potency and selectivity for FGF/FGFR signaling are currently being evaluated in clinical trials as shown in Table **2**. Unlike VEGFR inhibitors, FGFR selective inhibitors are not associated with elevation of blood pressure and proteinuria. In fact, FGFR selective inhibitors are associated with hyperphosphatemia and ectopic mineralization and calcification due to antagonizing the crucial role of FGFRs signals in calcium/phosphate homeostasis [192].

Table 2. Overview of the FGF/FGFR inhibitors undergoing clinical trials. The symbol (*) indicates discontinued trial due to safety concerns.

Agents	Target	Ongoing Clinical Trial	Reference
BAY1179470	mAB FGFR-3	Advanced solid tumors	NCT01881217
FPA144	mAB FGFR-2	Advanced solid tumors	NCT02318329
LY3076226	FGFR-3 antibody drug conjugate	Advanced solid tumors	NCT02529553
B-701	mAB FGFR-3	Metastatic urothelial cell carcinoma	NCT03123055 NCT02925533 *NCT02401542
MFGR1877S	mAB FGFR-3	Advanced solid tumors Multiple myeloma	NCT01363024 NCT01122875
U3-1784	mAB FGFR-4	Advanced solid tumors	NCT02690350
ASP5878	RTK	Solid tumors	NCT02038673
INCB054828	RTK	Myeloid lymphoid Cholangiocarcinoma Urothelial carcinoma Advanced malignancies	NCT03011372 NCT03011372 NCT02872714 NCT02393248
TAS-120	RTK	Advanced solid tumors	NCT02052778
BLU-554	FGFR4	Hepatocellular carcinoma	NCT02508467
H3B-6527	FGFR4	Advanced hepatocellular carcinoma	NCT02834780
Erdafitinib	panFGFR	Urothelial cancer Advanced hepatocellular carcinoma Multiple myeloma	NCT02365597 NCT92421185 NCT02952573
Rogaratinib	panFGFR	Advanced solid tumors	NCT01976741

AZD4547

AZD4547 is a potent selective FGFR-1, FGFR-2, FGFR-3 tyrosine kinase inhibitor. Though AZD4547 showed a relatively week inhibitor activity for VEGFR-2, FGFR-4, and IGF1R, in pre-clinical models it reduced the growth of lung xenograft derived from a patient with FGFR1 overexpression, in a dose-dependent manner. The AZD4547 also showed a significant reduction of tumor growth in myeloma and leukemia xenografts [193]. However, in safety studies, AZD4547 treatment was associated with serious adverse effects such as asthenia, bilateral central subfoveal edema, hyponatremia, mucositis, and general deterioration [194]. Currently, AZD4547 is under clinical investigation in 3 clinical trials; a phase I safety study in patients with muscle invasive bladder cancer (NCT02546661); a phase II trial for treatment of patients with advanced refectory lymphomas, or multiple myeloma (NCT02465060); and a phase III clinical trial for patients with recurrent squamous cell lung cancer (NCT02154490).

BGJ398

BGJ398 is a potent pan inhibitor of FGFR-1, FGFR-2, FGFR-3, and FGFR-4. In addition to the above listed targets, BGJ398 has shown inhibitory activities against VEGFR-2, c-KIT, and LYN at sub-micro-molar concentrations. In a bladder xenograft model, BGJ398 reduced tumor growth after oral administration [195]. In addition, BGJ398 showed a potent inhibition of FGFR2-amplified gastric and FGFR2-mutant endometrial cancer models [196]. In a recent phase I clinical trial, BGJ398 treatment was associated with hepatotoxicity, hyperphosphatemia, and corneal toxicity [192, 197]. Presently, BGJ398 is under clinical evaluation in 3 ongoing clinical trials. BGJ398 is being evaluated for treatment of patients with invasive urothelial bladder cancer (NCT02657486), recurrent head and neck cancer (NCT02706691), and advanced cholangiocarcinoma (NCT02150967).

LY2874455

LY2874455 is also a potent selective inhibitor of all FGFRs. It tested in different tumor xenograft models with aberrant FGFR expression. In these studies, LY2874455 showed rapid and dose-dependent reduction of tumor growth. Even though, it inhibited VEGFR-2 under *in vitro* conditions, LY2874455 treated rats showed no signs of VEGFR-2 inhibition such as increasing blood pressure. In a phase I clinical trial, LY2874455 was well tolerated with observations of hyperphosphatemia, diarrhea, and stomatitis. Currently, LY2874455 is being tested in combination with Merestinib for treatment of patients with relapsed or refractory AML (NCT03125239).

Targeting PDGF/PDGFR

Over-expression of PDGF/PDGFRs is reported in many human malignancies derived from mesenchymal tissues such as glioblastoma, sarcomas, and gastrointestinal stromal tumors [198]. Such overexpression was correlated with poor response to chemotherapy and shorter OS rates [199, 200]. Several agents were developed to antagonize PDGF/PDGFR signaling which showed promising results in pre-clinical and clinical studies. In fact, targeting PDGFR-β showed reduction of interstitial fluid pressure increasing the delivery of concomitantly administered drugs [201]. A selected example of PDGF/PDGFR inhibitors will be discussed below.

Imatinib

Imatinib, a 2-phenyl amino pyrimidine derivative, is used in targeted therapy, which works by blocking the action of PDGF protein that signals cancer cells to multiply. Imatinib was invented in the late 1990's by Nicholas Lyndon and used for treating both chronic myeloid leukemia (CML) and acute lymphoblastic leukemia (ALL) at the Dana-Farber Institute [202]. Imatinib specifically targets several protein tyrosine kinases, including Abl-related gene (Arg), the stem cell factor receptor (c-KIT), platelet-derived growth factor receptor (PDGF-R), and their oncogenic forms, most particularly BCR-ABL [203]. The first clinical trial of Imatinib took place in 1998 and the drug received FDA approval in May 2001 for oral therapy in the treatment of patients with CML during the blast crisis phase, accelerated phase or in chronic phase after failure of interferon-alpha (IFN-α) therapy. Imatinib was found to produce a similar effect in some of the other cancers where the above mentioned tyrosine kinases were overexpressed. Similar to many other tyrosine kinase inhibitors, Imatinib works by binding to the ATP binding site, locking it in a closed or self-inhibited conformation that leads to the inhibition of the enzyme activity in a semi-competitive manner [204]. Imatinib is well absorbed and tolerated after oral administration with a bioavailability exceeding 90% [205]. Common side effects for this drug include fluid retention, headache, diarrhea, loss of appetite, weakness, nausea and vomiting, abdominal distention, edema, rash, dizziness, and muscle cramps. Serious side effects reported in the literature include myelosuppression, heart failure, and liver function abnormalities [206]. The major drawback with Imatinib is development of resistance which is therapeutically challenging. However, understanding the underlying mechanisms of resistance has led to the development of new second- and third-generation tyrosine kinase inhibitors which has helped to overcome this challenge [203].

Tovetumab

Tovetumab, also known as MEDI-571, is a monoclonal antibody directed against PDGFR-α [198]. Tovetumab selectively binds to human PDGFR-α inhibiting ligand-induced receptor auto-phosphorylation and activation of downstream signaling. In pre-clinical settings, Tovetumab reduced the robust growth of glioma in mice models by interfering with PDGFR-α autocrine signaling. In addition, Tovetumab suppressed tumor growth in Calu-6 model of NSCLC with no significant effect on blood vessel content [198]. In phase I clinical trials, Tovetumab was well tolerated with no dose-limiting toxicity in patients with advanced solid tumors [207]. However, data from phase II clinical trial was disappointing because MEDI-575 showed limited clinical outcomes in patients with first recurrence of glioblastoma [208]. Currently, no clinical trial is ongoing and clinical development of Tovetumab was discontinued [209].

Olaratumab

Olaratumab is a monoclonal antibody directed against PDGFR-α. Olaratumab selectively hinders the ligand binding of PDGF-AA, PDGF-BB, and PDGF-CC to PDGFR-α. Such interaction inhibits ligand-induced receptor activation and subsequent activation of mitogenic signaling pathways including PI3K/AKT, MAP, and JAK/STAT. By targeting human PDGFR-α, Olaratumab was found to reduce the tumor growth of glioma and sarcoma in several pre-clinical models [210]. Administration of Olaratumab was associated with inhibition of angiogenesis and tumor cell proliferation. Under phase I trials, Olaratumab exhibited a safe profile in patients with advanced malignancies [211]. Data from phase II clinical trial of Olaratumab with Doxorubicin showed a significant increase in PFS from 4.4 to 8.2 months and OS from 14.7 to 26.5 months in patients with metastatic soft tissue sarcoma compared to doxorubicin monotherapy. These significant results led to accelerated approval of Olaratumab by FDA for treatment of soft tissue sarcoma [212]. Currently, Olaratumab in combination with Pembrolizumab, anti-PD-1 receptor, is being evaluated in patients with advanced soft tissue sarcoma (NCT03126591). Also, Olaratumab is being tested in combination with standard chemotherapy in pediatric patients with relapsed or refractory solid tumors (NCT02677116).

Crenolanib

Crenolanib is a small molecule tyrosine kinase inhibitor with high selectivity for PDGFR-α, PDGFR-β, and FLT-3 [213]. Uniquely, Crenolanib inhibited both the wild-type and constitutively active mutated isoforms of PDGFRs and FLT-3 [213, 214]. It has been shown that Crenotanib was more potent than Imatinib in inhibiting the mutated isoforms of PDGFR-α kinases (D842I, D1842-843IM,

D842Y, D842V, and deletion of I843) associated with gastrointestinal stromal tumor [213]. Similarly, Crenolanib showed a high affinity and a potent inhibition against the mutated isoform of FLT-3 (FLT3-ITD, FLT3-D835V, FLT3-D835Y) associated with acute myeloid leukemia [215]. Therefore, Crenolanib is considered mutant-specific with high efficacy against constitutively active or mutated forms of PDGFRs and FLT-3. In a phase I clinical trial, Crenolanib was tolerated and the dose-limiting toxicities included increased gamma-glutamyl transferase (GGT) or alanine aminotransferase (ALT), hematuria, and insomnia [216]. Currently, Crenolanib is under clinical investigation for treatment of AML, glioma, and gastrointestinal stromal tumors. In a single arm phase II clinical trial, Crenolanib use was tested as a maintenance therapy for patients with FLT-3 positive AML who have achieved complete remission after allogeneic stem cell transplantation (NCT02400255). Also, Crenolanib was evaluated for efficacy and tolerability in patients newly diagnosed with AML or patients with relapsed or refractory AML with FLT3 mutation (NCT02283177; NCT01657682) respectively. Combination therapy of Crenolanib with standard chemotherapy or with 5-Azacitidine was also tested in a phase II trial for patients with AML (NCT02400281). Additional studies with Crenolanib included monotherapy in patients with refractory glioblastoma (NCT02626364) and in patients with advanced or metastatic GIST containing PDGFRA gene mutation (NCT02847429).

DCC-2618

DCC-2618 is an orally available small molecule tyrosine kinase inhibitor which has high affinity for PDGFR-α and c-KIT [217]. It binds to the switch pocket binding sites of the wild type and the mutated isoforms of PDGFR-α and c-KIT. By binding to these receptors, DCC-2618 prevents the switch of the receptors from inactive to active conformations abrogating tumor cell signaling mediated by c-KIT/PDGFR-α. Thus, DCC-2618 inhibits the proliferation of c-KIT/PDGFR-α driven cancers such as gastrointestinal stromal tumors (GIST), mast cell leukemia (MCL) and systemic mastocytosis (SM), and AML [218, 219]. DCC-2618 is under phase I clinical trial to evaluate its safety, tolerability, pharmacokinetics and pharmacodynamics in patients with advanced solid tumors (NCT02571036). Preliminary results from this study showed that DCC-2618 treatment was associated with a rapid decrease of circulating tumor cells (CTCs) with c-KIT mutations in patients with GIST. Also, DCC-2618 was well tolerated with common observations of fatigue, anemia, dyspnea and decrease in appetite [220].

BLU-285

BLU-285 is a small molecule tyrosine kinase inhibitor with high potency and selectivity for mutant PDGFR-α (D842V) and c-KIT (Exon 17 mutants such as D816V, D816Y, and N822K) in the targeted cancers [221]. Daily dosing of patients with BLU-285 showed in *vivo* tumor growth inhibition in KIT D816Y driven GIST and mastocytoma xenograft models [222, 223]. In patient-derived xenograft (PDX) models of GIST also, BLU-258 reduced tumor growth in a dose-dependent manner, even in Imatinib-resistant model [224]. Currently, BLU-285 is being evaluated in phase I clinical trials that were designed to evaluated safety, tolerability, pharmacokinetic and antineoplastic activity in patients with GIST and myeloid malignancy (NCT02508532; NCT02561988). So far, the primary results have shown that BLU-285 was well tolerated in patients with GIST with no dose-limiting toxicity but the early efficacy results are still not available.

Targeting Notch Pathway

Notch signaling is implicated in several cancer-related functions such as tumor angiogenesis, cancer stem maintenance, cell fate specification, EMT, and differentiation of embryonic and postnatal tissues [225]. The Notch protein spans the cell membrane, with the binding extracellular domain that induces proteolytic cleavage and release of the intracellular domain, which enters the cell nucleus to modify gene expression and cell proliferation. Currently, Notch signaling is targeted by three approaches. First, targeting γ-secretase, an enzyme that catalyzes the cleaving of Notch receptor that leads to the release of NICD (Notch Intracellular Domains) and induction of the transcription of Notch targeted genes. Second, targeting Notch receptor with specific monoclonal antibodies. Third, neutralize Notch ligands using monoclonal antibodies.

Targeting Notch signaling to antagonize angiogenesis is a challenging task due to the ubiquitous role of Notch in tumorigenesis. Since Notch signaling is so complex with conflicting roles based on the cellular context, where it can act as an oncogene or tumor suppressor, the expected outcome also differs [226]. For example, specific targeting of DLL-4 with neutralizing antibodies resulted in increased angiogenesis around tumor mass [227]. Whereas, dual targeting of VEGFR-2 and DLL-4 with monoclonal antibodies seems to be more efficacious. Also, inhibition of notch signaling *via* inhibiting γ-secretase was reported to be efficacious in neuroblastoma. However, the therapeutic application of γ-secretase inhibitors is limited due to severe gastrointestinal toxicity [228].

Brontictuzumab

Brontictuzumab is a humanized monoclonal antibody which selectively binds to Notch-1 receptor. Aberrant Notch-1 signaling is prevalent in several cancer types including T-acute lymphoblastic leukemia (T-ALL), colorectal, pancreatic, non-small cell lung, and adenoid cystic carcinomas [229, 230]. Under *in vitro* condition, Brontictuzumab binds to Notch-1 receptors that are expressed on the cell surface, thereby antagonizing Notch-mediated signaling. Brontictuzumab demonstrated a significant growth inhibition in PDX models of adenoid cystic carcinomas with Notch-1 mutation [231]. Safety studies showed that Brontictuzumab treatment was associated with frequent diarrhea in 73% of the patients which was caused by the blocking of Notch signaling in the gut epithelial cells [232].

BMS-906024

BMS-906024 is a synthetic dual inhibitor of pan-Notch receptors (Notch-1, Notch-2, Notch-3, Notch-4) and γ-secretase. When BMS-906024 was tested preclinically, against wide range of human cancer xenografts including triple negative and HER2 positive breast carcinoma, colon carcinoma, pancreatic carcinoma, neuroblastoma, and T-cell Acute Lymphocytic leukemia (T-ALL) it revealed promising anti-neoplastic activities [233]. BMS-906024 was also tested in a phase I clinical trial designed to evaluate safety in patients with relapsed/refractory T-ALL. Similar to other γ-secretase inhibitors, diarrhea was common among the patients receiving BMS-906024. Also, BMS-906024 was associated with several drug-related adverse reactions such as anemia, hypophosphatemia, thrombocytopenia, pancytopenia, febrile bone marrow aplasia, and hepatotoxicity [234]. Despite the above listed side effects, BMS-906024 revealed a strong anti-leukemia activity leading to a complete hematologic remission of T-ALL patient following treatment with BMS-906024 [235]. Currently, BMS-906024 is undergoing three clinical trials to evaluate safety and tolerability in patients with advanced or metastatic solid tumors (NCT01653470; NCT01363817; NCT01292655).

MK0752

MK0752 is another γ-secretase inhibitor, which blocks the cleavage of NICD and subsequent nuclear translocation. Under *in vitro* conditions, MK-0752 inhibited Notch-1 and its downstream effectors such as MDM2, c-Myc, XIAP, and HES1 leading to cell cycle arrest and apoptosis in ovarian cancer cell lines [236]. Subsequently, MK0752 was clinically tested for treatment of T-ALL, which was prematurely terminated based on the preliminary results showing a limited anti-tumor activity with the observation of gastrointestinal toxicity (diarrhea, nausea, and vomiting). However, use of MK-0752 in intermittent dosing schedule (3 days on and 4 days off) was well tolerated with signs of clinical benefits in patients with solid tumors [237]. Besides cancer treatment, MK-0752 has potential for treating Alzheimer's disease since γ-secretase, along with β-secretase, catalyzes the cleavage of amyloid precursor protein into amyloid beta (Aβ) subunits [238].

Accumulation of Aβ variants such as Aβ-40 in the brain region is considered as one of the pathological hallmarks of Alzheimer's disease. In response to γ-secretase inhibition by MK-0752, the secretion of Aβ-40 was reduced in human neuroblastoma cell line. In guinea pigs, MK-0752 significantly reduced the plasma, brain, and cerebrospinal fluid (CSF) levels of Aβ-40 in dose-dependent manner [239]. Similarly, MK-0752 was able to reduce Aβ-40 levels in the CSF of humans. However, MK-0752 was clinically discontinued for the treatment of Alzheimer's disease owing to its poor tolerability [240].

Tarextumab

Tarextumab is a monoclonal antibody directed against both Notch-2 and Notch-3 receptors. Pre-clinical studies of Tarextumab showed anti-tumor activity against different PDX models including pancreatic, small cell lung, breast, and ovarian cancers [241]. Also, *in vivo* treatment using Tarextumab significantly reduced the levels of cancer stem cells (CSCs) and delayed tumor recurrence after chemotherapy discontinuation. Tarextumab also increased pericytes recruitment to endothelial cells leading to vascular maturation and increased blood perfusion [241]. Final data from phase I clinical trials revealed a safe profile for Tarextumab with no dose-limiting toxicity [242]. Recently, Tarextumab has received orphan drug designation by FDA for the treatment of pancreatic and small cell lung cancer based on two clinical trials where Tarextumab in combination with chemotherapy showed encouraging clinical benefits in those patients (NCT01647828; NCT01849741).

RO4929097

RO4929097 is another experimental drug with potent and selective γ-secretase inhibitory activity that was initially developed for the treatment of Alzheimer's disease. Later, RO4929097 was found to have anti-tumor activity through inhibition of Notch receptor activation and Aβ secretion. Further explorations with RO4929097 revealed its ability to reduce *in vivo* tumor growth along with inhibition of the expression of several angiogenesis-related genes [243, 244]. In a phase I clinical trial, RO4929097 treatment was associated with observations of several side effects such as nausea, vomiting, diarrhea, and hypophosphatemia in patients with refractory metastatic or locally advanced solid tumors [245]. Also, RO4929097 monotherapy failed to achieve significant clinical benefits in patients with metastatic colorectal, platinum-resistant ovarian, and pancreatic cancers [246 - 248]. Thus, RO4929097 is no longer clinically investigated and its development has been discontinued.

Miscellaneous Anti-Angiogenic Agents

In addition to the above discussed drugs, there are several agents that have demonstrated strong inhibition of tumor vasculature with significant impact of cancer growth. Pre-clinically, many of these agents have been shown to occlude tumor vasculature that was eventually leading to tumor cell death due to ischemia or apoptosis. However, the mode of action of these agents require further investigation. For example, Thalidomide was initially used in Europe to treat morning sickness and was withdrawn from the market in 1950s due to serious birth defects. Later, Thalidomide was found to possess anti-angiogenic, anti-proliferative, and pro-apoptotic activity in pre-clinical studies. Also, thalidomide was shown to down-regulate the expression of VEGF and TNF, which is believed to be the main driver of its anti-angiogenic activity. Clinical trials of Thalidomide have shown a significant efficacy against multiple myeloma, renal, and breast cancers [249]. Another example of a small molecule with anti-angiogenic ability is Nutlin-3, an MDM2 inhibitor which was found to suppress angiogenesis through inhibition of angiogenesis pathway-related gene expression [250]. Itraconazole, an anti-fungal agent, was also reported to have anti-angiogenic activity. Itraconazole blocked *in vitro* endothelial cell proliferation, migration and tube formation, in addition to inhibiting tumor growth and tumor vascularity in NSCLC xenograft models [251].

Potential New Anti-Angiogenic Agents

Some of the shortcomings that are associated with current anti-angiogenic treatments have prompted the scientists to develop more effective therapeutic options. In this context, novel therapeutic strategies targeting VEGF or its down-stream signaling pathways have been yielding promising results as new additions to the existing therapies. Anti-angiogenic agents can participate in cancer treatment by destroying the blood capillary networks, delaying delivery of oxygen and nutrients, and ultimately starving the tumor toward its extinction [252]. In this respect, some of the newly developed anti-angiogenic drugs, that are currently tested using *in vitro* and *in vivo* models with promising outcomes are discussed below.

F16

F16 is a novel molecule which was discovered through molecular modeling technique [253]. This novel compound has a unique chemical structure Fig. (**3**) which allows it to displace VEGF from binding to the VEGFR-2 receptors, eventually leading to diminished tyrosine kinase activity [254]. Interestingly, so far F16 has showed significant inhibition of VEGFR-2 activity, through competitive binding, with no direct effects on the kinase activity. Under *in vitro* conditions, F16 showed a remarkable inhibition of the critical angiogenesis steps such as, endothelial cell proliferation, migration, and tube formation Fig. (**3**). When tested using *in vivo* model, F16 exhibited tumor inhibition effects on highly aggressive xenograft models of human breast and colorectal cancers. This robust inhibition of tumor growth was combined with the reduction of tumor burden and with no observable toxicity to the experimental animals, which provided an advantage for F16 over the currently existing anti-angiogenic inhibitors [254]. Evaluation of tumor tissues from treated mice showed a significant reduction of CD31, a biomarker for endothelial cells, in F16 treated mice compared to untreated control. The reduction in CD31 was indicative of the anti-angiogenic and subsequent anti-tumor activity of F16. The pharmacokinetic (PK) evaluation of F16 on mice revealed a high-level distribution to different body organs with high accumulation to brain regions. Such elevation would open the possibility to target brain tumors, which is one of the deadliest cancers, afflicting mankind. Currently, efficacy studies in rodent model are underway, to confirm the efficacy of F16 against brain tumors. Remarkably, toxicity studies with F16 in mice revealed no significant changes in the hematological and physiological markers. On the other hand, existing anti-angiogenic drugs such as Sunitinib showed a significant elevation in serum Alanine Transaminase (ALT) and Amylase levels in experimental mice [255]. In conclusion, F16 is a promising molecule showing target specificity against VEGFR-2 leading to suppression of angiogenesis and tumor reduction with minimal toxicity.

JFD

Continued design, screening and testing for new anti-angiogenic drugs inhibitor has led to the development of another novel VEGFR-2 inhibitor named JFD, which also differs from some of the existing anti-angiogenic drugs in many aspects [253, 256]. JFD belongs to a class of organic compound that is analogous to the purine moiety (7-[2-hydroxy-3-(4-methoxyanilino) propyl]-1,3-dimeth-1-3,7-dihydro-1H-purine-2,6-dione). This unique purine based molecule is specific in its binding to the VEGFR-2 and therefore can decrease the levels of VEGFR-2 phosphorylation [256]. As a result of VEGFR-2 specific antagonism, that is shown in Fig. (**3**), JFD inhibits angiogenesis and some of the related events that include endothelial cell survival, proliferation, migration, and vascular network formation [256]. Subsequently, the original form of JFD was modified into a water-soluble form (JFD-WS) to increase its bioavailability while preserving its pharmacological activities. In addition to the confirmation of the anti-angiogenic properties, both the JFD original and JFD-WS were shown to have anti-tumorigenic effects in a patient-derived xenograft (PDX) implanted animal models [257]. Consequent to the onset of anti-angiogenic effects by JFD-WS, it appears that there was induction of apoptosis also Fig. (**3**) in the PDX tumors, which was confirmed by DNA fragmentation [258]. Treatment with JFD-WS also increased the expression of tumor suppressor protein p53 in the xenograft tumors. There was a significant increase in the expression of pro-apoptotic protein Bax, which typically decreases the levels of the anti-apoptotic protein Bcl-2 to cause cell death [258]. In addition to the increase in the expression of Bax, a significant increase in the levels of APAF-1 with a concomitant increase in the release of cytochrome *c* into the cytoplasm was also observed in the tumor tissues of JFD-WS-treated animals. These changes clearly indicated activation of pro-apoptotic mechanisms as a consequence of the anti-angiogenic effects in JFD-WS treated animals. Elevating p53 levels and inducing apoptosis is a unique property, and is not typically seen with other anti-angiogenic drugs. Furthermore, the preliminary PK studies in mice have confirmed that JFD-WS is distributed to various tissues within a shorter duration of time after intra-peritoneal (i.p.) injection, validating JFD-WS as a safer and effective anti-angiogenic compound. Therefore, our JFD-WS may be one of the unique types of anti-angiogenic agents with dual abilities [258].

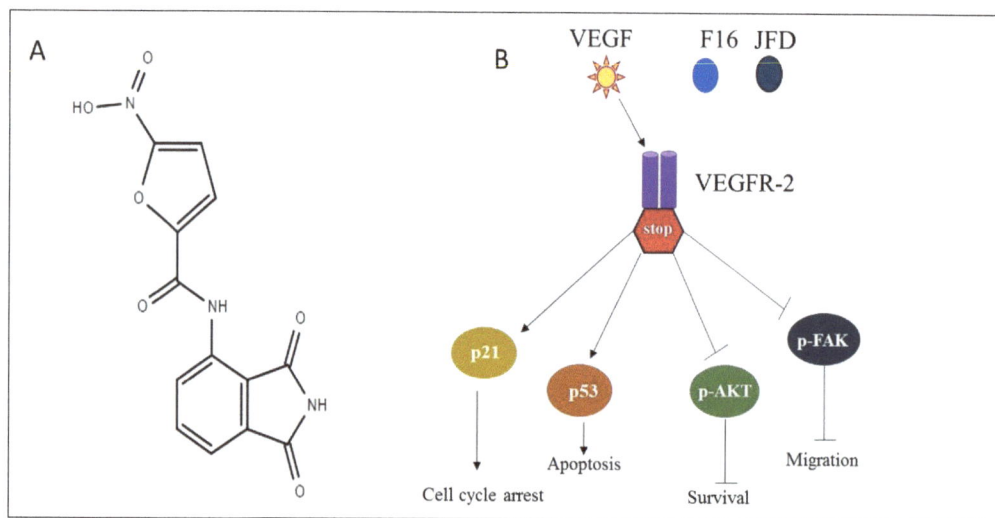

Fig. (3). Inhibitions of VEGFR2 by F16 and JFD. **A** Molecular structure of VEGFR2 inhibitor (F16). **B** Our *in vitro* studies revealed that F16 and JFD could interfere with multiple pathways involved in cancer development such as cell cycle, apoptosis, survival, and migration.

CONCLUSION

Thus far, several anti-angiogenic agents have been tested and approved for clinical use. Despite the modest clinical outcome exploited by tumor angiogenesis inhibitors, limited side effects observed with these agents made the field of tumor angiogenesis attractive and is still under careful scientific investigation. A decade after the advent of the first group of FDA approved antiangiogenic therapeutic agents, and more than five decades of the extensive angiogenesis research have produced unpreceded knowledge and complicated comprehension of the angiogenesis process. Cutting off blood the supplies typically provided to the tumor sites was initially perceived to be a direct forward mechanism that triggers tumor starvation and destruction. Some of the clinical trials with less impressive clinical outcome suggest that the initial strategy to target cancer progression through undernourishment approach is an underestimation of the complexity of angiogenesis process. The failure to target the tumor angiogenesis process attributed to significant challenges including development of resistance, which can be widely seen in other cancer treatments also. This arguably suggested that combination or multi-target therapeutic approach could serve and yield better clinical outcomes with anti-angiogenic agents [259, 260]. The resistance issue could be further explained and linked to another element, where preventing one source of blood supply to tumor can be substituted by various modes of vascularization confined in the same subset of the tumor [260, 261]. Other elements which can explain the failure of anti-angiogenic strategy are diverse and ranges from vascularization signals originating at the at molecular level, mediated by pro-angiogenic mediators, to the role of microRNAs, and unconventional angiogenesis mechanisms such as vasculogenic mimicry and endothelial cell metabolism [260]. Multiple lines of evidence pointing towards the detrimental effects caused undesirably by hypoxia during anti-angiogenic treatment makes hypoxia as an essential element that is tightly associated with the failure of anti-angiogenic drugs [99, 262]. Along with the unfavorable hypoxia development, targeting angiogenic mechanisms was suspected to deteriorate the delivery of chemotherapeutic agents. In conclusion, a comprehensive understanding of angiogenesis process at the transcriptional, translational and cellular levels, with extensive characterization of histological features of angiogenesis, could lead to development of strategies with better clinical outcomes. In addition, combination of anti-angiogenic and cytotoxic agents that are carefully balanced with precise multi-targeted approach would offer better therapeutic consequences.

CONSENT FOR PUBLICATION

Not applicable.

CONFLICT OF INTEREST

The authors confirm that no conflict of interest to declare for this publication.

ACKNOWLEDGEMENTS

Declared none.

REFERENCES

[1]   Weinberg RA. In Retrospect: The chromosome trail. Nature 2008; 453(7196): 725.
       [http://dx.doi.org/10.1038/453725a]

[2]   Diaz-Cano SJ. Tumor heterogeneity: mechanisms and bases for a reliable application of molecular
       marker design. Int J Mol Sci 2012; 13(2): 1951-2011.
       [http://dx.doi.org/10.3390/ijms13021951] [PMID: 22408433]

[3]   Hanahan D, Weinberg RA. The hallmarks of cancer. Cell 2000; 100(1): 57-70.
       [http://dx.doi.org/10.1016/S0092-8674(00)81683-9] [PMID: 10647931]

[4]   Natale G, Bocci G, Lenzi P. Looking for the Word "Angiogenesis" in the History of Health Sciences:
       From Ancient Times to the First Decades of the Twentieth Century. World J Surg 2017; 41(6): 1625-
       34.
       [http://dx.doi.org/10.1007/s00268-016-3680-1] [PMID: 27491322]

[5]   Ribatti D, Nico B, Crivellato E, Vacca A. Macrophages and tumor angiogenesis. Leukemia 2007;
       21(10): 2085-9.
       [http://dx.doi.org/10.1038/sj.leu.2404900] [PMID: 17878921]

[6]   Hori K, Suzuki M, Tanda S, Saito S. Characterization of heterogeneous distribution of tumor blood
       flow in the rat. Jpn J Cancer Res 1991; 82(1): 109-17.
       [http://dx.doi.org/10.1111/j.1349-7006.1991.tb01753.x] [PMID: 1705537]

[7]   Folkman J. Tumor angiogenesis: therapeutic implications. N Engl J Med 1971; 285(21): 1182-6.
       [http://dx.doi.org/10.1056/NEJM197111182852108] [PMID: 4938153]

[8]   Folkman J, Merler E, Abernathy C, Williams G. Isolation of a tumor factor responsible for
       angiogenesis. J Exp Med 1971; 133(2): 275-88.
       [http://dx.doi.org/10.1084/jem.133.2.275] [PMID: 4332371]

[9]   Gimbrone MA Jr, Leapman SB, Cotran RS, Folkman J. Tumor dormancy *in vivo* by prevention of
       neovascularization. J Exp Med 1972; 136(2): 261-76.
       [http://dx.doi.org/10.1084/jem.136.2.261] [PMID: 5043412]

[10]   Folkman J, Haudenschild CC, Zetter BR. Long-term culture of capillary endothelial cells. Proc Natl
       Acad Sci USA 1979; 76(10): 5217-21.
       [http://dx.doi.org/10.1073/pnas.76.10.5217] [PMID: 291937]

[11]   Senger DR, Galli SJ, Dvorak AM, Perruzzi CA, Harvey VS, Dvorak HF. Tumor cells secrete a
       vascular permeability factor that promotes accumulation of ascites fluid. Science 1983; 219(4587):
       983-5.
       [http://dx.doi.org/10.1126/science.6823562] [PMID: 6823562]

[12]   Ferrara N, Henzel WJ. Pituitary follicular cells secrete a novel heparin-binding growth factor specific
       for vascular endothelial cells. Biochem Biophys Res Commun 1989; 161(2): 851-8.
       [http://dx.doi.org/10.1016/0006-291X(89)92678-8] [PMID: 2735925]

[13]   Connolly DT, Heuvelman DM, Nelson R, *et al.* Tumor vascular permeability factor stimulates
       endothelial cell growth and angiogenesis. J Clin Invest 1989; 84(5): 1470-8.
       [http://dx.doi.org/10.1172/JCI114322] [PMID: 2478587]

[14]   Leung DW, Cachianes G, Kuang WJ, Goeddel DV, Ferrara N. Vascular endothelial growth factor is a
       secreted angiogenic mitogen. Science 1989; 246(4935): 1306-9.
       [http://dx.doi.org/10.1126/science.2479986] [PMID: 2479986]

[15]   Terman BI, Dougher-Vermazen M, Carrion ME, *et al.* Identification of the KDR tyrosine kinase as a
       receptor for vascular endothelial cell growth factor. Biochem Biophys Res Commun 1992; 187(3):
       1579-86.
       [http://dx.doi.org/10.1016/0006-291X(92)90483-2] [PMID: 1417831]

[16]   Majesky MW. Developmental biology in the vasculature--review series. Arterioscler Thromb Vasc

Biol 2009; 29(5): 622.
[http://dx.doi.org/10.1161/ATVBAHA.109.187112] [PMID: 19369655]

[17]   Bielenberg DR, Zetter BR. The Contribution of Angiogenesis to the Process of Metastasis. Cancer J 2015; 21(4): 267-73.
[http://dx.doi.org/10.1097/PPO.0000000000000138] [PMID: 26222078]

[18]   Jakobsson L, Franco CA, Bentley K, *et al.* Endothelial cells dynamically compete for the tip cell position during angiogenic sprouting. Nat Cell Biol 2010; 12(10): 943-53.
[http://dx.doi.org/10.1038/ncb2103] [PMID: 20871601]

[19]   Dimova I, Popivanov G, Djonov V. Angiogenesis in cancer - general pathways and their therapeutic implications. J BUON 2014; 19(1): 15-21.
[PMID: 24659637]

[20]   Bisacchi D, Benelli R, Vanzetto C, Ferrari N, Tosetti F, Albini A. Anti-angiogenesis and angioprevention: mechanisms, problems and perspectives. Cancer Detect Prev 2003; 27(3): 229-38.
[http://dx.doi.org/10.1016/S0361-090X(03)00030-8] [PMID: 12787731]

[21]   Greene HS. Heterologous Transplantation of Mammalian Tumors: Ii. The Transfer of Human Tumors to Alien Species. J Exp Med 1941; 73(4): 475-86.
[http://dx.doi.org/10.1084/jem.73.4.475] [PMID: 19871091]

[22]   Brem S, Brem H, Folkman J, Finkelstein D, Patz A. Prolonged tumor dormancy by prevention of neovascularization in the vitreous. Cancer Res 1976; 36(8): 2807-12.
[PMID: 1277191]

[23]   Nguyen M. Angiogenic factors as tumor markers. Invest New Drugs 1997; 15(1): 29-37.
[http://dx.doi.org/10.1023/A:1005766511385] [PMID: 9195287]

[24]   Carmeliet P, Jain RK. Angiogenesis in cancer and other diseases. Nature 2000; 407(6801): 249-57.
[http://dx.doi.org/10.1038/35025220] [PMID: 11001068]

[25]   Vempati P, Popel AS, Mac Gabhann F. Extracellular regulation of VEGF: isoforms, proteolysis, and vascular patterning. Cytokine Growth Factor Rev 2014; 25(1): 1-19.
[http://dx.doi.org/10.1016/j.cytogfr.2013.11.002] [PMID: 24332926]

[26]   Nowak DG, Woolard J, Amin EM, *et al.* Expression of pro- and anti-angiogenic isoforms of VEGF is differentially regulated by splicing and growth factors. J Cell Sci 2008; 121(Pt 20): 3487-95.
[http://dx.doi.org/10.1242/jcs.016410] [PMID: 18843117]

[27]   Park JE, Keller GA, Ferrara N. The vascular endothelial growth factor (VEGF) isoforms: differential deposition into the subepithelial extracellular matrix and bioactivity of extracellular matrix-bound VEGF. Mol Biol Cell 1993; 4(12): 1317-26.
[http://dx.doi.org/10.1091/mbc.4.12.1317] [PMID: 8167412]

[28]   Krilleke D, DeErkenez A, Schubert W, *et al.* Molecular mapping and functional characterization of the VEGF164 heparin-binding domain. J Biol Chem 2007; 282(38): 28045-56.
[http://dx.doi.org/10.1074/jbc.M700319200] [PMID: 17626017]

[29]   Gerhardt H, Golding M, Fruttiger M, *et al.* VEGF guides angiogenic sprouting utilizing endothelial tip cell filopodia. J Cell Biol 2003; 161(6): 1163-77.
[http://dx.doi.org/10.1083/jcb.200302047] [PMID: 12810700]

[30]   Ruhrberg C, Gerhardt H, Golding M, *et al.* Spatially restricted patterning cues provided by heparin-binding VEGF-A control blood vessel branching morphogenesis. Genes Dev 2002; 16(20): 2684-98.
[http://dx.doi.org/10.1101/gad.242002] [PMID: 12381667]

[31]   Grunstein J, Masbad JJ, Hickey R, Giordano F, Johnson RS. Isoforms of vascular endothelial growth factor act in a coordinate fashion To recruit and expand tumor vasculature. Mol Cell Biol 2000; 20(19): 7282-91.
[http://dx.doi.org/10.1128/MCB.20.19.7282-7291.2000] [PMID: 10982845]

[32] Ruiz de Almodovar C, Coulon C, Salin PA, *et al.* Matrix-binding vascular endothelial growth factor (VEGF) isoforms guide granule cell migration in the cerebellum via VEGF receptor Flk1. J Neurosci 2010; 30(45): 15052-66.
[http://dx.doi.org/10.1523/JNEUROSCI.0477-10.2010] [PMID: 21068311]

[33] Ng YS, Rohan R, Sunday ME, Demello DE, D'Amore PA. Differential expression of VEGF isoforms in mouse during development and in the adult. Dev Dyn 2001; 220(2): 112-21.
[http://dx.doi.org/10.1002/1097-0177(2000)9999:9999<::AID-DVDY1093>3.0.CO;2-D] [PMID: 11169844]

[34] Perrin RM, Konopatskaya O, Qiu Y, Harper S, Bates DO, Churchill AJ. Diabetic retinopathy is associated with a switch in splicing from anti- to pro-angiogenic isoforms of vascular endothelial growth factor. Diabetologia 2005; 48(11): 2422-7.
[http://dx.doi.org/10.1007/s00125-005-1951-8] [PMID: 16193288]

[35] Harper SJ, Bates DO. VEGF-A splicing: the key to anti-angiogenic therapeutics? Nat Rev Cancer 2008; 8(11): 880-7.
[http://dx.doi.org/10.1038/nrc2505] [PMID: 18923433]

[36] Bevan HS, van den Akker NM, Qiu Y, *et al.* The alternatively spliced anti-angiogenic family of VEGF isoforms VEGFxxxb in human kidney development. Nephron, Physiol 2008; 110(4): 57-67.
[http://dx.doi.org/10.1159/000177614] [PMID: 19039247]

[37] Chen DB, Zheng J. Regulation of placental angiogenesis. Microcirculation 2014; 21(1): 15-25.
[http://dx.doi.org/10.1111/micc.12093] [PMID: 23981199]

[38] Bates DO, Cui TG, Doughty JM, *et al.* VEGF165b, an inhibitory splice variant of vascular endothelial growth factor, is down-regulated in renal cell carcinoma. Cancer Res 2002; 62(14): 4123-31.
[PMID: 12124351]

[39] Woolard J, Wang WY, Bevan HS, *et al.* VEGF165b, an inhibitory vascular endothelial growth factor splice variant: mechanism of action, *in vivo* effect on angiogenesis and endogenous protein expression. Cancer Res 2004; 64(21): 7822-35.
[http://dx.doi.org/10.1158/0008-5472.CAN-04-0934] [PMID: 15520188]

[40] Rennel E, Waine E, Guan H, *et al.* The endogenous anti-angiogenic VEGF isoform, VEGF165b inhibits human tumour growth in mice. Br J Cancer 2008; 98(7): 1250-7.
[http://dx.doi.org/10.1038/sj.bjc.6604309] [PMID: 18349828]

[41] Rennel ES, Hamdollah-Zadeh MA, Wheatley ER, *et al.* Recombinant human VEGF165b protein is an effective anti-cancer agent in mice. Eur J Cancer 2008; 44(13): 1883-94.
[http://dx.doi.org/10.1016/j.ejca.2008.05.027] [PMID: 18657413]

[42] Simons M, Gordon E, Claesson-Welsh L. Mechanisms and regulation of endothelial VEGF receptor signalling. Nat Rev Mol Cell Biol 2016; 17(10): 611-25.
[http://dx.doi.org/10.1038/nrm.2016.87] [PMID: 27461391]

[43] Ivy SP, Wick JY, Kaufman BM. An overview of small-molecule inhibitors of VEGFR signaling. Nat Rev Clin Oncol 2009; 6(10): 569-79.
[http://dx.doi.org/10.1038/nrclinonc.2009.130] [PMID: 19736552]

[44] Ahmed Z, Bicknell R. Angiogenic signalling pathways. Methods Mol Biol 2009; 467: 3-24.
[http://dx.doi.org/10.1007/978-1-59745-241-0_1] [PMID: 19301662]

[45] Deryugina EI, Quigley JP. Tumor angiogenesis: MMP-mediated induction of intravasation- and metastasis-sustaining neovasculature. Matrix Biol 2015; 44-46: 94-112.
[http://dx.doi.org/10.1016/j.matbio.2015.04.004] [PMID: 25912949]

[46] Kerbel RS. Tumor angiogenesis. N Engl J Med 2008; 358(19): 2039-49.
[http://dx.doi.org/10.1056/NEJMra0706596] [PMID: 18463380]

[47] Soni S, Padwad YS. HIF-1 in cancer therapy: two decade long story of a transcription factor. Acta

Oncol 2017; 56(4): 503-15.
[http://dx.doi.org/10.1080/0284186X.2017.1301680] [PMID: 28358664]

[48]   Des Guetz G, Uzzan B, Nicolas P, *et al.* Microvessel density and VEGF expression are prognostic factors in colorectal cancer. Meta-analysis of the literature. Br J Cancer 2006; 94(12): 1823-32.
[http://dx.doi.org/10.1038/sj.bjc.6603176] [PMID: 16773076]

[49]   Yu L, Deng L, Li J, Zhang Y, Hu L. The prognostic value of vascular endothelial growth factor in ovarian cancer: a systematic review and meta-analysis. Gynecol Oncol 2013; 128(2): 391-6.
[http://dx.doi.org/10.1016/j.ygyno.2012.11.002] [PMID: 23142075]

[50]   Zhan P, Ji Y-N, Yu L-K. VEGF is associated with the poor survival of patients with prostate cancer: a meta-analysis. Transl Androl Urol 2013; 2(2): 99-105.
[PMID: 26816732]

[51]   Sa-Nguanraksa D, Chuangsuwanich T, Pongpruttipan T, O-Charoenrat P. High vascular endothelial growth factor gene expression predicts poor outcome in patients with non-luminal A breast cancer. Mol Clin Oncol 2015; 3(5): 1103-8.
[http://dx.doi.org/10.3892/mco.2015.574] [PMID: 26623059]

[52]   Cascone T, Heymach JV. Targeting the angiopoietin/Tie2 pathway: cutting tumor vessels with a double-edged sword? J Clin Oncol 2012; 30(4): 441-4.
[http://dx.doi.org/10.1200/JCO.2011.38.7621] [PMID: 22184396]

[53]   Huang H, Bhat A, Woodnutt G, Lappe R. Targeting the ANGPT-TIE2 pathway in malignancy. Nat Rev Cancer 2010; 10(8): 575-85.
[http://dx.doi.org/10.1038/nrc2894] [PMID: 20651738]

[54]   Folkman J. Angiogenesis: an organizing principle for drug discovery? Nat Rev Drug Discov 2007; 6(4): 273-86.
[http://dx.doi.org/10.1038/nrd2115] [PMID: 17396134]

[55]   Yuan HT, Khankin EV, Karumanchi SA, Parikh SM. Angiopoietin 2 is a partial agonist/antagonist of Tie2 signaling in the endothelium. Mol Cell Biol 2009; 29(8): 2011-22.
[http://dx.doi.org/10.1128/MCB.01472-08] [PMID: 19223473]

[56]   Raica M, Cimpean AM. Platelet-Derived Growth Factor (PDGF)/PDGF Receptors (PDGFR) Axis as Target for Antitumor and Antiangiogenic Therapy. Pharmaceuticals (Basel) 2010; 3(3): 572-99.
[http://dx.doi.org/10.3390/ph3030572] [PMID: 27713269]

[57]   Andrae J, Gallini R, Betsholtz C. Role of platelet-derived growth factors in physiology and medicine. Genes Dev 2008; 22(10): 1276-312.
[http://dx.doi.org/10.1101/gad.1653708] [PMID: 18483217]

[58]   Hellström M, Gerhardt H, Kalén M, *et al.* Lack of pericytes leads to endothelial hyperplasia and abnormal vascular morphogenesis. J Cell Biol 2001; 153(3): 543-53.
[http://dx.doi.org/10.1083/jcb.153.3.543] [PMID: 11331305]

[59]   Battegay EJ, Rupp J, Iruela-Arispe L, Sage EH, Pech M. PDGF-BB modulates endothelial proliferation and angiogenesis *in vitro via* PDGF beta-receptors. J Cell Biol 1994; 125(4): 917-28.
[http://dx.doi.org/10.1083/jcb.125.4.917] [PMID: 7514607]

[60]   Betsholtz C. Biology of platelet-derived growth factors in development. Birth Defects Res C Embryo Today 2003; 69(4): 272-85.
[http://dx.doi.org/10.1002/bdrc.10030] [PMID: 14745969]

[61]   Klinghoffer RA, Hamilton TG, Hoch R, Soriano P. An allelic series at the PDGFalphaR locus indicates unequal contributions of distinct signaling pathways during development. Dev Cell 2002; 2(1): 103-13.
[http://dx.doi.org/10.1016/S1534-5807(01)00103-4] [PMID: 11782318]

[62]   Babina IS, Turner NC. Advances and challenges in targeting FGFR signalling in cancer. Nat Rev Cancer 2017; 17(5): 318-32.

[http://dx.doi.org/10.1038/nrc.2017.8] [PMID: 28303906]

[63] Dienstmann R, Rodon J, Prat A, *et al.* Genomic aberrations in the FGFR pathway: opportunities for targeted therapies in solid tumors. Ann Oncol 2014; 25(3): 552-63.
[http://dx.doi.org/10.1093/annonc/mdt419] [PMID: 24265351]

[64] Murakami M, Nguyen LT, Hatanaka K, *et al.* FGF-dependent regulation of VEGF receptor 2 expression in mice. J Clin Invest 2011; 121(7): 2668-78.
[http://dx.doi.org/10.1172/JCI44762] [PMID: 21633168]

[65] Beenken A, Mohammadi M. The FGF family: biology, pathophysiology and therapy. Nat Rev Drug Discov 2009; 8(3): 235-53.
[http://dx.doi.org/10.1038/nrd2792] [PMID: 19247306]

[66] Bray SJ. Notch signalling in context. Nat Rev Mol Cell Biol 2016; 17(11): 722-35.
[http://dx.doi.org/10.1038/nrm.2016.94] [PMID: 27507209]

[67] Shutter JR, Scully S, Fan W, *et al.* Dll4, a novel Notch ligand expressed in arterial endothelium. Genes Dev 2000; 14(11): 1313-8.
[PMID: 10837024]

[68] Claxton S, Fruttiger M. Periodic Delta-like 4 expression in developing retinal arteries. Gene Expr Patterns 2004; 5(1): 123-7.
[http://dx.doi.org/10.1016/j.modgep.2004.05.004] [PMID: 15533827]

[69] Dudley AC. Tumor endothelial cells. Cold Spring Harb Perspect Med 2012; 2(3): a006536.
[http://dx.doi.org/10.1101/cshperspect.a006536] [PMID: 22393533]

[70] Gialeli C, Theocharis AD, Karamanos NK. Roles of matrix metalloproteinases in cancer progression and their pharmacological targeting. FEBS J 2011; 278(1): 16-27.
[http://dx.doi.org/10.1111/j.1742-4658.2010.07919.x] [PMID: 21087457]

[71] Kalluri R. Basement membranes: structure, assembly and role in tumour angiogenesis. Nat Rev Cancer 2003; 3(6): 422-33.
[http://dx.doi.org/10.1038/nrc1094] [PMID: 12778132]

[72] Bergers G, Brekken R, McMahon G, *et al.* Matrix metalloproteinase-9 triggers the angiogenic switch during carcinogenesis. Nat Cell Biol 2000; 2(10): 737-44.
[http://dx.doi.org/10.1038/35036374] [PMID: 11025665]

[73] Jones SN, Hancock AR, Vogel H, Donehower LA, Bradley A. Overexpression of Mdm2 in mice reveals a p53-independent role for Mdm2 in tumorigenesis. Proc Natl Acad Sci USA 1998; 95(26): 15608-12.
[http://dx.doi.org/10.1073/pnas.95.26.15608] [PMID: 9861017]

[74] Venkatesan T, Alaseem A, Chinnaiyan A, *et al.* MDM2 Overexpression Modulates the Angiogenesis-Related Gene Expression Profile of Prostate Cancer Cells. Cells 2018; 7(5): E41.
[http://dx.doi.org/10.3390/cells7050041] [PMID: 29748481]

[75] Ramakrishnan R, Zell JA, Malavé A, Rathinavelu A. Expression of vascular endothelial growth factor mRNA in GI-101A and HL-60 cell lines. Biochem Biophys Res Commun 2000; 270(3): 709-13.
[http://dx.doi.org/10.1006/bbrc.2000.2493] [PMID: 10772888]

[76] Narasimhan M, Rose R, Ramakrishnan R, Zell JA, Rathinavelu A. Identification of HDM2 as a regulator of VEGF expression in cancer cells. Life Sci 2008; 82(25-26): 1231-41.
[http://dx.doi.org/10.1016/j.lfs.2008.04.004] [PMID: 18504050]

[77] Narasimhan M, Rose R, Karthikeyan M, Rathinavelu A. Detection of HDM2 and VEGF co-expression in cancer cell lines: novel effect of HDM2 antisense treatment on VEGF expression. Life Sci 2007; 81(17-18): 1362-72.
[http://dx.doi.org/10.1016/j.lfs.2007.08.029] [PMID: 17931661]

[78] Rathinavelu A, Narasimhan M, Muthumani P. A novel regulation of VEGF expression by HIF-1α and

STAT3 in HDM2 transfected prostate cancer cells. J Cell Mol Med 2012; 16(8): 1750-7.
[http://dx.doi.org/10.1111/j.1582-4934.2011.01472.x] [PMID: 22004076]

[79]   Patterson DM, Gao D, Trahan DN, *et al.* Effect of MDM2 and vascular endothelial growth factor inhibition on tumor angiogenesis and metastasis in neuroblastoma. Angiogenesis 2011; 14(3): 255-66.
[http://dx.doi.org/10.1007/s10456-011-9210-8] [PMID: 21484514]

[80]   Zhou S, Gu L, He J, Zhang H, Zhou M. MDM2 regulates vascular endothelial growth factor mRNA stabilization in hypoxia. Mol Cell Biol 2011; 31(24): 4928-37.
[http://dx.doi.org/10.1128/MCB.06085-11] [PMID: 21986500]

[81]   Chen X, Qiu J, Yang D, *et al.* MDM2 promotes invasion and metastasis in invasive ductal breast carcinoma by inducing matrix metalloproteinase-9. PLoS One 2013; 8(11): e78794.
[http://dx.doi.org/10.1371/journal.pone.0078794] [PMID: 24236052]

[82]   Hanahan D, Folkman J. Patterns and emerging mechanisms of the angiogenic switch during tumorigenesis. Cell 1996; 86(3): 353-64.
[http://dx.doi.org/10.1016/S0092-8674(00)80108-7] [PMID: 8756718]

[83]   O'Reilly MS, Holmgren L, Shing Y, *et al.* Angiostatin: a novel angiogenesis inhibitor that mediates the suppression of metastases by a Lewis lung carcinoma. Cell 1994; 79(2): 315-28.
[http://dx.doi.org/10.1016/0092-8674(94)90200-3] [PMID: 7525077]

[84]   Eskens FALM. Angiogenesis inhibitors in clinical development; where are we now and where are we going? Br J Cancer 2004; 90(1): 1-7.
[http://dx.doi.org/10.1038/sj.bjc.6601401] [PMID: 14710197]

[85]   Jain RK. Antiangiogenesis strategies revisited: from starving tumors to alleviating hypoxia. Cancer Cell 2014; 26(5): 605-22.
[http://dx.doi.org/10.1016/j.ccell.2014.10.006] [PMID: 25517747]

[86]   Folkman J. Anti-angiogenesis: new concept for therapy of solid tumors. Ann Surg 1972; 175(3): 409-16.
[http://dx.doi.org/10.1097/00000658-197203000-00014] [PMID: 5077799]

[87]   Van der Veldt AAM, Lubberink M, Bahce I, *et al.* Rapid decrease in delivery of chemotherapy to tumors after anti-VEGF therapy: implications for scheduling of anti-angiogenic drugs. Cancer Cell 2012; 21(1): 82-91.
[http://dx.doi.org/10.1016/j.ccr.2011.11.023] [PMID: 22264790]

[88]   Robinson SP, Boult JKR, Vasudev NS, Reynolds AR. Monitoring the Vascular Response and Resistance to Sunitinib in Renal Cell Carcinoma *In Vivo* with Susceptibility Contrast MRI. Cancer Res 2017; 77(15): 4127-34.
[http://dx.doi.org/10.1158/0008-5472.CAN-17-0248] [PMID: 28566330]

[89]   Milosevic MF, Townsley CA, Chaudary N, *et al.* Sorafenib Increases Tumor Hypoxia in Cervical Cancer Patients Treated With Radiation Therapy: Results of a Phase 1 Clinical Study. Int J Radiat Oncol Biol Phys 2016; 94(1): 111-7.
[http://dx.doi.org/10.1016/j.ijrobp.2015.09.009] [PMID: 26547383]

[90]   Zhou J, Zhang H, Wang H, *et al.* Early prediction of tumor response to bevacizumab treatment in murine colon cancer models using three-dimensional dynamic contrast-enhanced ultrasound imaging. Angiogenesis 2017; 20(4): 547-55.
[http://dx.doi.org/10.1007/s10456-017-9566-5] [PMID: 28721500]

[91]   Jain RK. Normalizing tumor vasculature with anti-angiogenic therapy: a new paradigm for combination therapy. Nat Med 2001; 7(9): 987-9.
[http://dx.doi.org/10.1038/nm0901-987] [PMID: 11533692]

[92]   Kamoun WS, Ley CD, Farrar CT, *et al.* Edema control by cediranib, a vascular endothelial growth factor receptor-targeted kinase inhibitor, prolongs survival despite persistent brain tumor growth in mice. J Clin Oncol 2009; 27(15): 2542-52.

[http://dx.doi.org/10.1200/JCO.2008.19.9356] [PMID: 19332720]

[93] Batchelor TT, Sorensen AG, di Tomaso E, *et al.* AZD2171, a pan-VEGF receptor tyrosine kinase inhibitor, normalizes tumor vasculature and alleviates edema in glioblastoma patients. Cancer Cell 2007; 11(1): 83-95.
[http://dx.doi.org/10.1016/j.ccr.2006.11.021] [PMID: 17222792]

[94] Batchelor TT, Gerstner ER, Emblem KE, *et al.* Improved tumor oxygenation and survival in glioblastoma patients who show increased blood perfusion after cediranib and chemoradiation. Proc Natl Acad Sci USA 2013; 110(47): 19059-64.
[http://dx.doi.org/10.1073/pnas.1318022110] [PMID: 24190997]

[95] Winkler F, Kozin SV, Tong RT, *et al.* Kinetics of vascular normalization by VEGFR2 blockade governs brain tumor response to radiation: role of oxygenation, angiopoietin-1, and matrix metalloproteinases. Cancer Cell 2004; 6(6): 553-63.
[PMID: 15607960]

[96] Luqmani YA. Mechanisms of drug resistance in cancer chemotherapy. Med Princ Pract 2005; 14 (Suppl. 1): 35-48.
[http://dx.doi.org/10.1159/000086183] [PMID: 16103712]

[97] Pàez-Ribes M, Allen E, Hudock J, *et al.* Antiangiogenic therapy elicits malignant progression of tumors to increased local invasion and distant metastasis. Cancer Cell 2009; 15(3): 220-31.
[http://dx.doi.org/10.1016/j.ccr.2009.01.027] [PMID: 19249680]

[98] Ebos JM, Lee CR, Cruz-Munoz W, Bjarnason GA, Christensen JG, Kerbel RS. Accelerated metastasis after short-term treatment with a potent inhibitor of tumor angiogenesis. Cancer Cell 2009; 15(3): 232-9.
[http://dx.doi.org/10.1016/j.ccr.2009.01.021] [PMID: 19249681]

[99] Loges S, Mazzone M, Hohensinner P, Carmeliet P. Silencing or fueling metastasis with VEGF inhibitors: antiangiogenesis revisited. Cancer Cell 2009; 15(3): 167-70.
[http://dx.doi.org/10.1016/j.ccr.2009.02.007] [PMID: 19249675]

[100] Keshet E, Ben-Sasson SA. Anticancer drug targets: approaching angiogenesis. J Clin Invest 1999; 104(11): 1497-501.
[http://dx.doi.org/10.1172/JCI8849] [PMID: 10587512]

[101] Ton NC, Jayson GC. Resistance to anti-VEGF agents. Curr Pharm Des 2004; 10(1): 51-64.
[http://dx.doi.org/10.2174/1381612043453603] [PMID: 14754405]

[102] Bergers G, Hanahan D. Modes of resistance to anti-angiogenic therapy. Nat Rev Cancer 2008; 8(8): 592-603.
[http://dx.doi.org/10.1038/nrc2442] [PMID: 18650835]

[103] Kopetz S, Hoff PM, Morris JS, *et al.* Phase II trial of infusional fluorouracil, irinotecan, and bevacizumab for metastatic colorectal cancer: efficacy and circulating angiogenic biomarkers associated with therapeutic resistance. J Clin Oncol 2010; 28(3): 453-9.
[http://dx.doi.org/10.1200/JCO.2009.24.8252] [PMID: 20008624]

[104] Cidon EU, Alonso P, Masters B. Markers of Response to Antiangiogenic Therapies in Colorectal Cancer: Where Are We Now and What Should Be Next? Clin Med Insights Oncol 2016; 10 (Suppl. 1): 41-55.
[PMID: 27147901]

[105] Drevs J, Zirrgiebel U, Schmidt-Gersbach CIM, *et al.* Soluble markers for the assessment of biological activity with PTK787/ZK 222584 (PTK/ZK), a vascular endothelial growth factor receptor (VEGFR) tyrosine kinase inhibitor in patients with advanced colorectal cancer from two phase I trials. Ann Oncol 2005; 16(4): 558-65.
[http://dx.doi.org/10.1093/annonc/mdi118] [PMID: 15705616]

[106] Cao Y. Off-tumor target--beneficial site for antiangiogenic cancer therapy? Nat Rev Clin Oncol 2010;

7(10): 604-8.
[http://dx.doi.org/10.1038/nrclinonc.2010.118] [PMID: 20683436]

[107]   Kreisl TN, Kim L, Moore K, *et al.* Phase II trial of single-agent bevacizumab followed by bevacizumab plus irinotecan at tumor progression in recurrent glioblastoma. J Clin Oncol 2009; 27(5): 740-5.
[http://dx.doi.org/10.1200/JCO.2008.16.3055] [PMID: 19114704]

[108]   Vanneman M, Dranoff G. Combining immunotherapy and targeted therapies in cancer treatment. Nat Rev Cancer 2012; 12(4): 237-51.
[http://dx.doi.org/10.1038/nrc3237] [PMID: 22437869]

[109]   Huber V, Camisaschi C, Berzi A, *et al.* Cancer acidity: An ultimate frontier of tumor immune escape and a novel target of immunomodulation. Semin Cancer Biol 2017; 43: 74-89.
[http://dx.doi.org/10.1016/j.semcancer.2017.03.001] [PMID: 28267587]

[110]   Huang X, Raskovalova T, Lokshin A, *et al.* Combined antiangiogenic and immune therapy of prostate cancer. Angiogenesis 2005; 8(1): 13-23.
[http://dx.doi.org/10.1007/s10456-005-2893-y] [PMID: 16132614]

[111]   Amin A, Plimack ER, Infante JR, *et al.* 1052pdnivolumab (N) (Anti-Pd-1; Bms-936558, Ono-4538) in Combination with Sunitinib (S) or Pazopanib (P) in Patients (Pts) with Metastatic Renal Cell Carcinoma (Mrcc) Annals of Oncology 2014; 25 (4): iv362-.

[112]   Sporn MB. Approaches to prevention of epithelial cancer during the preneoplastic period. Cancer Res 1976; 36(7 PT 2): 2699-702.
[PMID: 1277177]

[113]   Rothwell PM, Wilson M, Elwin C-E, *et al.* Long-term effect of aspirin on colorectal cancer incidence and mortality: 20-year follow-up of five randomised trials. Lancet 2010; 376(9754): 1741-50.
[http://dx.doi.org/10.1016/S0140-6736(10)61543-7] [PMID: 20970847]

[114]   Arber N, Eagle CJ, Spicak J, *et al.* PreSAP Trial Investigators. Celecoxib for the prevention of colorectal adenomatous polyps. N Engl J Med 2006; 355(9): 885-95.
[http://dx.doi.org/10.1056/NEJMoa061652] [PMID: 16943401]

[115]   Yoshiji H, Noguchi R, Namisaki T, *et al.* Branched-chain amino acids suppress the cumulative recurrence of hepatocellular carcinoma under conditions of insulin-resistance. Oncol Rep 2013; 30(2): 545-52.
[http://dx.doi.org/10.3892/or.2013.2497] [PMID: 23708326]

[116]   Online Label Repository FDA. 2017. [cited 2017 Nov 20]; Available fromhttps://labels.fda.gov/

[117]   Ferrara N, Hillan KJ, Gerber HP, Novotny W. Discovery and development of bevacizumab, an anti-VEGF antibody for treating cancer. Nat Rev Drug Discov 2004; 3(5): 391-400.
[http://dx.doi.org/10.1038/nrd1381] [PMID: 15136787]

[118]   Gerber H-P, Ferrara N. Pharmacology and pharmacodynamics of bevacizumab as monotherapy or in combination with cytotoxic therapy in preclinical studies. Cancer Res 2005; 65(3): 671-80.
[PMID: 15705858]

[119]   Ilhan-Mutlu A, Osswald M, Liao Y, *et al.* Bevacizumab Prevents Brain Metastases Formation in Lung Adenocarcinoma. Mol Cancer Ther 2016; 15(4): 702-10.
[http://dx.doi.org/10.1158/1535-7163.MCT-15-0582] [PMID: 26809491]

[120]   Hurwitz H, Fehrenbacher L, Novotny W, *et al.* Bevacizumab plus irinotecan, fluorouracil, and leucovorin for metastatic colorectal cancer. N Engl J Med 2004; 350(23): 2335-42.
[http://dx.doi.org/10.1056/NEJMoa032691] [PMID: 15175435]

[121]   Rosen LS, Jacobs IA, Burkes RL. Bevacizumab in Colorectal Cancer: Current Role in Treatment and the Potential of Biosimilars. Target Oncol 2017; 12(5): 599-610.
[http://dx.doi.org/10.1007/s11523-017-0518-1] [PMID: 28801849]

[122] Fuchs CS, Tomasek J, Yong CJ, *et al.* REGARD Trial Investigators. Ramucirumab monotherapy for previously treated advanced gastric or gastro-oesophageal junction adenocarcinoma (REGARD): an international, randomised, multicentre, placebo-controlled, phase 3 trial. Lancet 2014; 383(9911): 31-9.
[http://dx.doi.org/10.1016/S0140-6736(13)61719-5] [PMID: 24094768]

[123] Wilke H, Muro K, Van Cutsem E, *et al.* RAINBOW Study Group. Ramucirumab plus paclitaxel *versus* placebo plus paclitaxel in patients with previously treated advanced gastric or gastro-oesophageal junction adenocarcinoma (RAINBOW): a double-blind, randomised phase 3 trial. Lancet Oncol 2014; 15(11): 1224-35.
[http://dx.doi.org/10.1016/S1470-2045(14)70420-6] [PMID: 25240821]

[124] Garon EB, Ciuleanu T-E, Arrieta O, *et al.* Ramucirumab plus docetaxel *versus* placebo plus docetaxel for second-line treatment of stage IV non-small-cell lung cancer after disease progression on platinum-based therapy (REVEL): a multicentre, double-blind, randomised phase 3 trial. Lancet 2014; 384(9944): 665-73.
[http://dx.doi.org/10.1016/S0140-6736(14)60845-X] [PMID: 24933332]

[125] Tabernero J, Yoshino T, Cohn AL, *et al.* RAISE Study Investigators. Ramucirumab versus placebo in combination with second-line FOLFIRI in patients with metastatic colorectal carcinoma that progressed during or after first-line therapy with bevacizumab, oxaliplatin, and a fluoropyrimidine (RAISE): a randomised, double-blind, multicentre, phase 3 study. Lancet Oncol 2015; 16(5): 499-508.
[http://dx.doi.org/10.1016/S1470-2045(15)70127-0] [PMID: 25877855]

[126] Petrylak DP, Tagawa ST, Kohli M, *et al.* Docetaxel As Monotherapy or Combined With Ramucirumab or Icrucumab in Second-Line Treatment for Locally Advanced or Metastatic Urothelial Carcinoma: An Open-Label, Three-Arm, Randomized Controlled Phase II Trial. J Clin Oncol 2016; 34(13): 1500-9.
[http://dx.doi.org/10.1200/JCO.2015.65.0218] [PMID: 26926681]

[127] Saif MW, Knost JA, Chiorean EG, *et al.* Phase 1 study of the anti-vascular endothelial growth factor receptor 3 monoclonal antibody LY3022856/IMC-3C5 in patients with advanced and refractory solid tumors and advanced colorectal cancer. Cancer Chemother Pharmacol 2016; 78(4): 815-24.
[http://dx.doi.org/10.1007/s00280-016-3134-3] [PMID: 27566701]

[128] Pytowski B, Goldman J, Persaud K, *et al.* Complete and specific inhibition of adult lymphatic regeneration by a novel VEGFR-3 neutralizing antibody. J Natl Cancer Inst 2005; 97(1): 14-21.
[http://dx.doi.org/10.1093/jnci/dji003] [PMID: 15632376]

[129] Roberts N, Kloos B, Cassella M, *et al.* Inhibition of VEGFR-3 activation with the antagonistic antibody more potently suppresses lymph node and distant metastases than inactivation of VEGFR-2. Cancer Res 2006; 66(5): 2650-7.
[http://dx.doi.org/10.1158/0008-5472.CAN-05-1843] [PMID: 16510584]

[130] Wu Y, Zhong Z, Huber J, *et al.* Anti-vascular endothelial growth factor receptor-1 antagonist antibody as a therapeutic agent for cancer. Clin Cancer Res 2006; 12(21): 6573-84.
[http://dx.doi.org/10.1158/1078-0432.CCR-06-0831] [PMID: 17085673]

[131] LoRusso PM, Krishnamurthi S, Youssoufian H, *et al.* Icrucumab, a fully human monoclonal antibody against the vascular endothelial growth factor receptor-1, in the treatment of patients with advanced solid malignancies: a Phase 1 study. Invest New Drugs 2014; 32(2): 303-11.
[http://dx.doi.org/10.1007/s10637-013-9998-8] [PMID: 23903897]

[132] Moore M, Gill S, Asmis T, *et al.* Randomized phase II study of modified FOLFOX-6 in combination with ramucirumab or icrucumab as second-line therapy in patients with metastatic colorectal cancer after disease progression on first-line irinotecan-based therapy. Ann Oncol 2016; 27(12): 2216-24.
[http://dx.doi.org/10.1093/annonc/mdw412] [PMID: 27733377]

[133] Vahdat LT, Layman R, Yardley DA, *et al.* Randomized Phase II Study of Ramucirumab or Icrucumab in Combination with Capecitabine in Patients with Previously Treated Locally Advanced or Metastatic

Breast Cancer. Oncologist 2017; 22(3): 245-54.
[http://dx.doi.org/10.1634/theoncologist.2016-0265] [PMID: 28220020]

[134] Fong TA, Shawver LK, Sun L, *et al.* SU5416 is a potent and selective inhibitor of the vascular endothelial growth factor receptor (Flk-1/KDR) that inhibits tyrosine kinase catalysis, tumor vascularization, and growth of multiple tumor types. Cancer Res 1999; 59(1): 99-106.
[PMID: 9892193]

[135] Stopeck A, Sheldon M, Vahedian M, Cropp G, Gosalia R, Hannah A. Results of a Phase I dose-escalating study of the antiangiogenic agent, SU5416, in patients with advanced malignancies. Clin Cancer Res 2002; 8(9): 2798-805.
[PMID: 12231519]

[136] Smolich BD, Yuen HA, West KA, Giles FJ, Albitar M, Cherrington JM. The antiangiogenic protein kinase inhibitors SU5416 and SU6668 inhibit the SCF receptor (c-kit) in a human myeloid leukemia cell line and in acute myeloid leukemia blasts. Blood 2001; 97(5): 1413-21.
[http://dx.doi.org/10.1182/blood.V97.5.1413] [PMID: 11222388]

[137] Laird AD, Vajkoczy P, Shawver LK, *et al.* SU6668 is a potent antiangiogenic and antitumor agent that induces regression of established tumors. Cancer Res 2000; 60(15): 4152-60.
[PMID: 10945623]

[138] Sessa C, Viganò L, Grasselli G, *et al.* Phase I clinical and pharmacological evaluation of the multi-tyrosine kinase inhibitor SU006668 by chronic oral dosing. Eur J Cancer 2006; 42(2): 171-8.
[http://dx.doi.org/10.1016/j.ejca.2005.09.033] [PMID: 16406576]

[139] Sun L, Liang C, Shirazian S, *et al.* Discovery of 5-[5-fluoro-2-oxo-1,2- dihydroindol-(3Z--ylidenemethyl]-2,4- dimethyl-1H-pyrrole-3-carboxylic acid (2-diethylaminoethyl)amide, a novel tyrosine kinase inhibitor targeting vascular endothelial and platelet-derived growth factor receptor tyrosine kinase. J Med Chem 2003; 46(7): 1116-9.
[http://dx.doi.org/10.1021/jm0204183] [PMID: 12646019]

[140] Mendel DB, Laird AD, Xin X, *et al. In vivo* antitumor activity of SU11248, a novel tyrosine kinase inhibitor targeting vascular endothelial growth factor and platelet-derived growth factor receptors: determination of a pharmacokinetic/pharmacodynamic relationship. Clin Cancer Res 2003; 9(1): 327-37.
[PMID: 12538485]

[141] Motzer RJ, Hutson TE, Tomczak P, *et al.* Sunitinib *versus* interferon alfa in metastatic renal-cell carcinoma. N Engl J Med 2007; 356(2): 115-24.
[http://dx.doi.org/10.1056/NEJMoa065044] [PMID: 17215529]

[142] Motzer RJ, Hutson TE, Tomczak P, *et al.* Overall survival and updated results for sunitinib compared with interferon alfa in patients with metastatic renal cell carcinoma. J Clin Oncol 2009; 27(22): 3584-90.
[http://dx.doi.org/10.1200/JCO.2008.20.1293] [PMID: 19487381]

[143] Demetri GD, van Oosterom AT, Garrett CR, *et al.* Efficacy and safety of sunitinib in patients with advanced gastrointestinal stromal tumour after failure of imatinib: a randomised controlled trial. Lancet 2006; 368(9544): 1329-38.
[http://dx.doi.org/10.1016/S0140-6736(06)69446-4] [PMID: 17046465]

[144] Raymond E, Dahan L, Raoul J-L, *et al.* Sunitinib malate for the treatment of pancreatic neuroendocrine tumors. N Engl J Med 2011; 364(6): 501-13.
[http://dx.doi.org/10.1056/NEJMoa1003825] [PMID: 21306237]

[145] Mackey JR, Kerbel RS, Gelmon KA, *et al.* Controlling angiogenesis in breast cancer: a systematic review of anti-angiogenic trials. Cancer Treat Rev 2012; 38(6): 673-88.
[http://dx.doi.org/10.1016/j.ctrv.2011.12.002] [PMID: 22365657]

[146] Sehdev S. Sunitinib toxicity management - a practical approach Can Urol Assoc J 2012; 10 (11–12Suppl7): S248-51.

[147] Ravaud A, de la Fouchardière C, Caron P, *et al.* A multicenter phase II study of sunitinib in patients with locally advanced or metastatic differentiated, anaplastic or medullary thyroid carcinomas: mature data from the THYSU study. Eur J Cancer 2017; 76: 110-7.
[http://dx.doi.org/10.1016/j.ejca.2017.01.029] [PMID: 28301826]

[148] Wilhelm SM, Carter C, Tang L, *et al.* BAY 43-9006 exhibits broad spectrum oral antitumor activity and targets the RAF/MEK/ERK pathway and receptor tyrosine kinases involved in tumor progression and angiogenesis. Cancer Res 2004; 64(19): 7099-109.
[http://dx.doi.org/10.1158/0008-5472.CAN-04-1443] [PMID: 15466206]

[149] Wilhelm S, Adnane L, Hirth-Dietrich C, Ehrlich P, Lynch M. Preclinical characterization of BAY 73-4506: A kinase inhibitor with broad spectrum antitumor activity targeting oncogenic and angiogenic kinases. Mol Cancer Ther 2007; 6(11) (Suppl.): B260.

[150] Brose MS, Nutting CM, Jarzab B, *et al.* DECISION investigators. Sorafenib in radioactive iodine-refractory, locally advanced or metastatic differentiated thyroid cancer: a randomised, double-blind, phase 3 trial. Lancet 2014; 384(9940): 319-28.
[http://dx.doi.org/10.1016/S0140-6736(14)60421-9] [PMID: 24768112]

[151] Bruix J, Raoul JL, Sherman M, *et al.* Efficacy and safety of sorafenib in patients with advanced hepatocellular carcinoma: subanalyses of a phase III trial. J Hepatol 2012; 57(4): 821-9.
[http://dx.doi.org/10.1016/j.jhep.2012.06.014] [PMID: 22727733]

[152] Wilhelm SM, Dumas J, Adnane L, *et al.* Regorafenib (BAY 73-4506): a new oral multikinase inhibitor of angiogenic, stromal and oncogenic receptor tyrosine kinases with potent preclinical antitumor activity. Int J Cancer 2011; 129(1): 245-55.
[http://dx.doi.org/10.1002/ijc.25864] [PMID: 21170960]

[153] Cabanillas ME, Brose MS, Holland J, Ferguson KC, Sherman SI. A phase I study of cabozantinib (XL184) in patients with differentiated thyroid cancer. Thyroid 2014; 24(10): 1508-14.
[http://dx.doi.org/10.1089/thy.2014.0125] [PMID: 25102375]

[154] Harris PA, Boloor A, Cheung M, *et al.* Discovery of 5-[[4-[(2,3-dimethyl-2H-ind-zol-6-yl)methylamino]-2-pyrimidinyl]amino]-2-methyl-benzenesulfonamide (Pazopanib), a novel and potent vascular endothelial growth factor receptor inhibitor. J Med Chem 2008; 51(15): 4632-40.
[http://dx.doi.org/10.1021/jm800566m] [PMID: 18620382]

[155] Hosaka S, Horiuchi K, Yoda M, *et al.* A novel multi-kinase inhibitor pazopanib suppresses growth of synovial sarcoma cells through inhibition of the PI3K-AKT pathway. J Orthop Res 2012; 30(9): 1493-8.
[http://dx.doi.org/10.1002/jor.22091] [PMID: 22359392]

[156] Olaussen KA, Commo F, Tailler M, *et al.* Synergistic proapoptotic effects of the two tyrosine kinase inhibitors pazopanib and lapatinib on multiple carcinoma cell lines. Oncogene 2009; 28(48): 4249-60.
[http://dx.doi.org/10.1038/onc.2009.277] [PMID: 19749798]

[157] Paesler J, Gehrke I, Gandhirajan RK, *et al.* The vascular endothelial growth factor receptor tyrosine kinase inhibitors vatalanib and pazopanib potently induce apoptosis in chronic lymphocytic leukemia cells *in vitro* and *in vivo*. Clin Cancer Res 2010; 16(13): 3390-8.
[http://dx.doi.org/10.1158/1078-0432.CCR-10-0232] [PMID: 20570929]

[158] Sternberg CN, Davis ID, Mardiak J, *et al.* Pazopanib in locally advanced or metastatic renal cell carcinoma: results of a randomized phase III trial. J Clin Oncol 2010; 28(6): 1061-8.
[http://dx.doi.org/10.1200/JCO.2009.23.9764] [PMID: 20100962]

[159] van der Graaf WTA, Blay J-Y, Chawla SP, *et al.* EORTC Soft Tissue and Bone Sarcoma Group; PALETTE study group. Pazopanib for metastatic soft-tissue sarcoma (PALETTE): a randomised, double-blind, placebo-controlled phase 3 trial. Lancet 2012; 379(9829): 1879-86.
[http://dx.doi.org/10.1016/S0140-6736(12)60651-5] [PMID: 22595799]

[160] Sternberg CN, Hawkins RE, Wagstaff J, *et al.* A randomised, double-blind phase III study of

pazopanib in patients with advanced and/or metastatic renal cell carcinoma: final overall survival results and safety update. Eur J Cancer 2013; 49(6): 1287-96.
[http://dx.doi.org/10.1016/j.ejca.2012.12.010] [PMID: 23321547]

[161] Dinkic C, Eichbaum M, Schmidt M, *et al.* Pazopanib (GW786034) and cyclophosphamide in patients with platinum-resistant, recurrent, pre-treated ovarian cancer - Results of the PACOVAR-trial. Gynecol Oncol 2017; 146(2): 279-84.
[http://dx.doi.org/10.1016/j.ygyno.2017.05.013] [PMID: 28528917]

[162] Wedge SR, Ogilvie DJ, Dukes M, *et al.* ZD6474 inhibits vascular endothelial growth factor signaling, angiogenesis, and tumor growth following oral administration. Cancer Res 2002; 62(16): 4645-55.
[PMID: 12183421]

[163] Thornton K, Kim G, Maher VE, *et al.* Vandetanib for the treatment of symptomatic or progressive medullary thyroid cancer in patients with unresectable locally advanced or metastatic disease: U.S. Food and Drug Administration drug approval summary. Clin Cancer Res 2012; 18(14): 3722-30.
[http://dx.doi.org/10.1158/1078-0432.CCR-12-0411] [PMID: 22665903]

[164] Fallahi P, Di Bari F, Ferrari SM, *et al.* Selective use of vandetanib in the treatment of thyroid cancer. Drug Des Devel Ther 2015; 9: 3459-70.
[PMID: 26170630]

[165] Yakes FM, Chen J, Tan J, *et al.* Cabozantinib (XL184), a novel MET and VEGFR2 inhibitor, simultaneously suppresses metastasis, angiogenesis, and tumor growth. Mol Cancer Ther 2011; 10(12): 2298-308.
[http://dx.doi.org/10.1158/1535-7163.MCT-11-0264] [PMID: 21926191]

[166] Zhou L, Liu X-D, Sun M, *et al.* Targeting MET and AXL overcomes resistance to sunitinib therapy in renal cell carcinoma. Oncogene 2016; 35(21): 2687-97.
[http://dx.doi.org/10.1038/onc.2015.343] [PMID: 26364599]

[167] Choueiri TK, Pal SK, McDermott DF, *et al.* A phase I study of cabozantinib (XL184) in patients with renal cell cancer. Ann Oncol 2014; 25(8): 1603-8.
[http://dx.doi.org/10.1093/annonc/mdu184] [PMID: 24827131]

[168] Schiff D, Desjardins A, Cloughesy T, *et al.* Phase 1 dose escalation trial of the safety and pharmacokinetics of cabozantinib concurrent with temozolomide and radiotherapy or temozolomide after radiotherapy in newly diagnosed patients with high-grade gliomas. Cancer 2016; 122(4): 582-7.
[http://dx.doi.org/10.1002/cncr.29798] [PMID: 26588662]

[169] Elisei R, Schlumberger MJ, Müller SP, *et al.* Cabozantinib in progressive medullary thyroid cancer. J Clin Oncol 2013; 31(29): 3639-46.
[http://dx.doi.org/10.1200/JCO.2012.48.4659] [PMID: 24002501]

[170] Choueiri TK, Escudier B, Powles T, *et al.* METEOR investigators. Cabozantinib *versus* everolimus in advanced renal cell carcinoma (METEOR): final results from a randomised, open-label, phase 3 trial. Lancet Oncol 2016; 17(7): 917-27.
[http://dx.doi.org/10.1016/S1470-2045(16)30107-3] [PMID: 27279544]

[171] Choueiri TK, Halabi S, Sanford BL, *et al.* Cabozantinib *Versus* Sunitinib As Initial Targeted Therapy for Patients With Metastatic Renal Cell Carcinoma of Poor or Intermediate Risk: The Alliance A031203 CABOSUN Trial. J Clin Oncol 2017; 35(6): 591-7.
[http://dx.doi.org/10.1200/JCO.2016.70.7398] [PMID: 28199818]

[172] Smith M, De Bono J, Sternberg C, *et al.* Phase III Study of Cabozantinib in Previously Treated Metastatic Castration-Resistant Prostate Cancer: COMET-1. J Clin Oncol 2016; 34(25): 3005-13.
[http://dx.doi.org/10.1200/JCO.2015.65.5597] [PMID: 27400947]

[173] Wedge SR, Kendrew J, Hennequin LF, *et al.* AZD2171: a highly potent, orally bioavailable, vascular endothelial growth factor receptor-2 tyrosine kinase inhibitor for the treatment of cancer. Cancer Res 2005; 65(10): 4389-400.
[http://dx.doi.org/10.1158/0008-5472.CAN-04-4409] [PMID: 15899831]

[174] Curwen JO, Musgrove HL, Kendrew J, Richmond GHP, Ogilvie DJ, Wedge SR. Inhibition of vascular endothelial growth factor-a signaling induces hypertension: examining the effect of cediranib (recentin; AZD2171) treatment on blood pressure in rat and the use of concomitant antihypertensive therapy. Clin Cancer Res 2008; 14(10): 3124-31.
[http://dx.doi.org/10.1158/1078-0432.CCR-07-4783] [PMID: 18483380]

[175] Fox E, Aplenc R, Bagatell R, *et al.* A phase 1 trial and pharmacokinetic study of cediranib, an orally bioavailable pan-vascular endothelial growth factor receptor inhibitor, in children and adolescents with refractory solid tumors. J Clin Oncol 2010; 28(35): 5174-81.
[http://dx.doi.org/10.1200/JCO.2010.30.9674] [PMID: 21060028]

[176] Liu JF, Barry WT, Birrer M, *et al.* Combination cediranib and olaparib *versus* olaparib alone for women with recurrent platinum-sensitive ovarian cancer: a randomised phase 2 study. Lancet Oncol 2014; 15(11): 1207-14.
[http://dx.doi.org/10.1016/S1470-2045(14)70391-2] [PMID: 25218906]

[177] Hoff PM, Hochhaus A, Pestalozzi BC, *et al.* Cediranib plus FOLFOX/CAPOX *versus* placebo plus FOLFOX/CAPOX in patients with previously untreated metastatic colorectal cancer: a randomized, double-blind, phase III study (HORIZON II). J Clin Oncol 2012; 30(29): 3596-603.
[http://dx.doi.org/10.1200/JCO.2012.42.6031] [PMID: 22965965]

[178] Brown N, McBain C, Nash S, *et al.* Multi-Center Randomized Phase II Study Comparing Cediranib plus Gefitinib with Cediranib plus Placebo in Subjects with Recurrent/Progressive Glioblastoma. PLoS One 2016; 11(5): e0156369.
[http://dx.doi.org/10.1371/journal.pone.0156369] [PMID: 27232884]

[179] Wood JM, Bold G, Buchdunger E, *et al.* PTK787/ZK 222584, a novel and potent inhibitor of vascular endothelial growth factor receptor tyrosine kinases, impairs vascular endothelial growth factor-induced responses and tumor growth after oral administration. Cancer Res 2000; 60(8): 2178-89.
[PMID: 10786682]

[180] Banerjee S, A'Hern R, Detre S, *et al.* Biological evidence for dual antiangiogenic-antiaromatase activity of the VEGFR inhibitor PTK787/ZK222584 *in vivo*. Clin Cancer Res 2010; 16(16): 4178-87.
[http://dx.doi.org/10.1158/1078-0432.CCR-10-0456] [PMID: 20682704]

[181] Katsura Y, Wada H, Murakami M, *et al.* PTK787/ZK222584 combined with interferon alpha and 5-fluorouracil synergistically inhibits VEGF signaling pathway in hepatocellular carcinoma. Ann Surg Oncol 2013; 20 (Suppl. 3): S517-26.
[http://dx.doi.org/10.1245/s10434-013-2948-z] [PMID: 23508585]

[182] de Bazelaire C, Alsop DC, George D, *et al.* Magnetic resonance imaging-measured blood flow change after antiangiogenic therapy with PTK787/ZK 222584 correlates with clinical outcome in metastatic renal cell carcinoma. Clin Cancer Res 2008; 14(17): 5548-54.
[http://dx.doi.org/10.1158/1078-0432.CCR-08-0417] [PMID: 18765547]

[183] Hecht JR, Trarbach T, Hainsworth JD, *et al.* Randomized, placebo-controlled, phase III study of first-line oxaliplatin-based chemotherapy plus PTK787/ZK 222584, an oral vascular endothelial growth factor receptor inhibitor, in patients with metastatic colorectal adenocarcinoma. J Clin Oncol 2011; 29(15): 1997-2003.
[http://dx.doi.org/10.1200/JCO.2010.29.4496] [PMID: 21464406]

[184] Brandes AA, Stupp R, Hau P, *et al.* EORTC study 26041-22041: phase I/II study on concomitant and adjuvant temozolomide (TMZ) and radiotherapy (RT) with PTK787/ZK222584 (PTK/ZK) in newly diagnosed glioblastoma. Eur J Cancer 2010; 46(2): 348-54.
[http://dx.doi.org/10.1016/j.ejca.2009.10.029] [PMID: 19945857]

[185] Cully M. Cancer: Tumour vessel normalization takes centre stage. Nat Rev Drug Discov 2017; 16(2): 87.
[http://dx.doi.org/10.1038/nrd.2017.4] [PMID: 28148936]

[186] Thurston G, Rudge JS, Ioffe E, *et al.* Angiopoietin-1 protects the adult vasculature against plasma

leakage. Nat Med 2000; 6(4): 460-3.
[http://dx.doi.org/10.1038/74725] [PMID: 10742156]

[187] Daly C, Eichten A, Castanaro C, *et al.* Angiopoietin-2 functions as a Tie2 agonist in tumor models, where it limits the effects of VEGF inhibition. Cancer Res 2013; 73(1): 108-18.
[http://dx.doi.org/10.1158/0008-5472.CAN-12-2064] [PMID: 23149917]

[188] Papadopoulos KP, Kelley RK, Tolcher AW, *et al.* A Phase I First-in-Human Study of Nesvacumab (REGN910), a Fully Human Anti-Angiopoietin-2 (Ang2) Monoclonal Antibody, in Patients with Advanced Solid Tumors. Clin Cancer Res 2016; 22(6): 1348-55.
[http://dx.doi.org/10.1158/1078-0432.CCR-15-1221] [PMID: 26490310]

[189] Buchanan A, Clementel V, Woods R, *et al.* Engineering a therapeutic IgG molecule to address cysteinylation, aggregation and enhance thermal stability and expression. MAbs 2013; 5(2): 255-62.
[http://dx.doi.org/10.4161/mabs.23392] [PMID: 23412563]

[190] Pili R, Carducci M, Brown P, Hurwitz H. An open-label study to determine the maximum tolerated dose of the multitargeted tyrosine kinase inhibitor CEP-11981 in patients with advanced cancer. Invest New Drugs 2014; 32(6): 1258-68.
[http://dx.doi.org/10.1007/s10637-014-0147-9] [PMID: 25152243]

[191] Arnett SO, Teillaud J-L, Wurch T, Reichert JM, Dunlop C, Huber M. IBC's 21st Annual Antibody Engineering and 8th Annual Antibody Therapeutics International Conferences and 2010 Annual Meeting of the Antibody Society. December 5-9, 2010, San Diego, CA USA. MAbs 2011; 3(2): 133-52.
[http://dx.doi.org/10.4161/mabs.3.2.14939] [PMID: 21304271]

[192] Nogova L, Sequist LV, Perez Garcia JM, *et al.* Evaluation of BGJ398, a Fibroblast Growth Factor Receptor 1-3 Kinase Inhibitor, in Patients With Advanced Solid Tumors Harboring Genetic Alterations in Fibroblast Growth Factor Receptors: Results of a Global Phase I, Dose-Escalation and Dose-Expansion Study. J Clin Oncol 2017; 35(2): 157-65.
[http://dx.doi.org/10.1200/JCO.2016.67.2048] [PMID: 27870574]

[193] Gavine PR, Mooney L, Kilgour E, *et al.* AZD4547: an orally bioavailable, potent, and selective inhibitor of the fibroblast growth factor receptor tyrosine kinase family. Cancer Res 2012; 72(8): 2045-56.
[http://dx.doi.org/10.1158/0008-5472.CAN-11-3034] [PMID: 22369928]

[194] Paik PK, Shen R, Berger MF, *et al.* A Phase Ib Open-Label Multicenter Study of AZD4547 in Patients with Advanced Squamous Cell Lung Cancers. Clin Cancer Res 2017; 23(18): 5366-73.
[http://dx.doi.org/10.1158/1078-0432.CCR-17-0645] [PMID: 28615371]

[195] Guagnano V, Furet P, Spanka C, *et al.* Discovery of 3-(2,6-dichloro-3,5-dimethoxy-phenyl)-1-{6-[4-(4-ethyl-piperazin-1-yl)-phenylamino]-pyrimidin-4-yl}-1-methyl-urea (NVP-BGJ398), a potent and selective inhibitor of the fibroblast growth factor receptor family of receptor tyrosine kinase. J Med Chem 2011; 54(20): 7066-83.
[http://dx.doi.org/10.1021/jm2006222] [PMID: 21936542]

[196] Guagnano V, Kauffmann A, Wöhrle S, *et al.* FGFR genetic alterations predict for sensitivity to NVP-BGJ398, a selective pan-FGFR inhibitor. Cancer Discov 2012; 2(12): 1118-33.
[http://dx.doi.org/10.1158/2159-8290.CD-12-0210] [PMID: 23002168]

[197] Sequist L V, Cassier P, Varga A, *et al.* Abstract CT326: Phase I study of BGJ398, a selective pan-FGFR inhibitor in genetically preselected advanced solid tumors Cancer Res 2014 Sep; 74 (19): CT326-6.

[198] Laing N, McDermott B, Wen S, *et al.* Inhibition of platelet-derived growth factor receptor α by MEDI-575 reduces tumor growth and stromal fibroblast content in a model of non-small cell lung cancer. Mol Pharmacol 2013; 83(6): 1247-56.
[http://dx.doi.org/10.1124/mol.112.084079] [PMID: 23558446]

[199] Higuchi A, Oshima T, Yoshihara K, *et al.* Clinical significance of platelet-derived growth factor

receptor-β gene expression in stage II/III gastric cancer with S-1 adjuvant chemotherapy. Oncol Lett 2017; 13(2): 905-11.
[http://dx.doi.org/10.3892/ol.2016.5494] [PMID: 28356977]

[200] Liu J, Liu C, Qiu L, Li J, Zhang P, Sun Y. Overexpression of both platelet-derived growth factor-BB and vascular endothelial growth factor-C and its association with lymphangiogenesis in primary human non-small cell lung cancer. Diagn Pathol 2014; 9: 128.
[http://dx.doi.org/10.1186/1746-1596-9-128] [PMID: 24972450]

[201] Jayson GC, Parker GJM, Mullamitha S, *et al.* Blockade of platelet-derived growth factor receptor-beta by CDP860, a humanized, PEGylated di-Fab', leads to fluid accumulation and is associated with increased tumor vascularized volume. J Clin Oncol 2005; 23(5): 973-81.
[http://dx.doi.org/10.1200/JCO.2005.01.032] [PMID: 15466784]

[202] Iqbal N, Iqbal N. Imatinib: a breakthrough of targeted therapy in cancer. Chemother Res Pract 2014; 2014: 357027.
[http://dx.doi.org/10.1155/2014/357027] [PMID: 24963404]

[203] Waller CF. Imatinib mesylate. Recent Results Cancer Res 2014; 201: 1-25.
[http://dx.doi.org/10.1007/978-3-642-54490-3_1] [PMID: 24756783]

[204] Takimoto CH, Calvo E. Principles of Oncologic Pharmacotherapy.Cancer Management: A Multidisciplinary Approach. 11th ed., 2008.

[205] Peng B, Dutreix C, Mehring G, *et al.* Absolute bioavailability of imatinib (Glivec) orally *versus* intravenous infusion. J Clin Pharmacol 2004; 44(2): 158-62.
[http://dx.doi.org/10.1177/0091270003262101] [PMID: 14747424]

[206] Hensley ML, Ford JM. Imatinib treatment: specific issues related to safety, fertility, and pregnancy. Semin Hematol 2003; 40(2) (Suppl. 2): 21-5.
[http://dx.doi.org/10.1053/shem.2003.50038] [PMID: 12783371]

[207] Murakami H, Ikeda M, Okusaka T, *et al.* A Phase I study of MEDI-575, a PDGFRα monoclonal antibody, in Japanese patients with advanced solid tumors. Cancer Chemother Pharmacol 2015; 76(3): 631-9.
[http://dx.doi.org/10.1007/s00280-015-2832-6] [PMID: 26223436]

[208] Phuphanich S, Raizer J, Chamberlain M, *et al.* Phase II study of MEDI-575, an anti-platelet-derived growth factor-α antibody, in patients with recurrent glioblastoma. J Neurooncol 2017; 131(1): 185-91.
[http://dx.doi.org/10.1007/s11060-016-2287-6] [PMID: 27844311]

[209] Williams R. Discontinued in 2013: oncology drugs. Expert Opin Investig Drugs 2015; 24(1): 95-110.
[http://dx.doi.org/10.1517/13543784.2015.971154] [PMID: 25315907]

[210] Loizos N, Xu Y, Huber J, *et al.* Targeting the platelet-derived growth factor receptor alpha with a neutralizing human monoclonal antibody inhibits the growth of tumor xenografts: implications as a potential therapeutic target. Mol Cancer Ther 2005; 4(3): 369-79.
[PMID: 15767546]

[211] Chiorean EG, Sweeney C, Youssoufian H, *et al.* A phase I study of olaratumab, an anti-platele--derived growth factor receptor alpha (PDGFRα) monoclonal antibody, in patients with advanced solid tumors. Cancer Chemother Pharmacol 2014; 73(3): 595-604.
[http://dx.doi.org/10.1007/s00280-014-2389-9] [PMID: 24452395]

[212] Deshpande HA, Cecchini M, Ni Choileain S, Jones R. Olaratumab for the treatment of soft tissue sarcoma. Drugs Today (Barc) 2017; 53(4): 247-55.
[http://dx.doi.org/10.1358/dot.2017.53.4.2560077] [PMID: 28492292]

[213] Heinrich MC, Griffith D, McKinley A, *et al.* Crenolanib inhibits the drug-resistant PDGFRA D842V mutation associated with imatinib-resistant gastrointestinal stromal tumors. Clin Cancer Res 2012; 18(16): 4375-84.
[http://dx.doi.org/10.1158/1078-0432.CCR-12-0625] [PMID: 22745105]

[214] Zimmerman EI, Turner DC, Buaboonnam J, *et al.* Crenolanib is active against models of drug-resistant FLT3-ITD-positive acute myeloid leukemia. Blood 2013; 122(22): 3607-15.
[http://dx.doi.org/10.1182/blood-2013-07-513044] [PMID: 24046014]

[215] Galanis A, Ma H, Rajkhowa T, *et al.* Crenolanib is a potent inhibitor of FLT3 with activity against resistance-conferring point mutants. Blood 2014; 123(1): 94-100.
[http://dx.doi.org/10.1182/blood-2013-10-529313] [PMID: 24227820]

[216] Lewis NL, Lewis LD, Eder JP, *et al.* Phase I study of the safety, tolerability, and pharmacokinetics of oral CP-868,596, a highly specific platelet-derived growth factor receptor tyrosine kinase inhibitor in patients with advanced cancers. J Clin Oncol 2009; 27(31): 5262-9.
[http://dx.doi.org/10.1200/JCO.2009.21.8487] [PMID: 19738123]

[217] Janku F, George S, Razak A, *et al.* DCC-2618, a pan KIT and PDGFR switch control inhibitor, achieves proof-of-concept in a first-in-human study. Eur J Cancer 2016; 69: S4.
[http://dx.doi.org/10.1016/S0959-8049(16)32613-2]

[218] Smith BD, Hood MM, Wise SC, *et al.* Abstract 2690: DCC-2618 is a potent inhibitor of wild-type and mutant KIT, including refractory Exon 17 D816 KIT mutations, and exhibits efficacy in refractory GIST and AML xenograft models Cancer Res 2015 Aug; 75 (15): 2690-0.

[219] Schneeweiss MA, Peter B, Blatt K, *et al.* The Multi-Kinase Inhibitor DCC-2618 Inhibits Proliferation and Survival of Neoplastic Mast Cells and Other Cell Types Involved in Systemic Mastocytosis Blood 2016 Dec; 128(22): 1965-5.

[220] Janku F, Razak A, Gordon M, *et al.* Abstract LB-039: Translational research in a phase I proof-o--concept study supports that DCC-2618 is a pan-KIT inhibitor Cancer Res 2017 Jul; 77 (13): LB-03--9.

[221] Evans EK, Hodous BL, Gardino A, *et al.* First Selective KIT D816V Inhibitor for Patients with Systemic Mastocytosis Blood 2014 Dec; 124(21): 3217-7.

[222] Evans EK, Hodous BL, Gardino AK, *et al.* Abstract 791: BLU-285, the first selective inhibitor of PDGFRα D842V and KIT Exon 17 mutants Cancer Res 2015 Aug; 75 (15): 791-1.

[223] Evans E, Gardino A, Hodous B, *et al.* Blu-285, a Potent and Selective Inhibitor for Hematologic Malignancies with KIT Exon 17 Mutations Blood 2015 Dec; 126(23): 568-8.

[224] Gebreyohannes YK, Wozniak A, Zhai M-E, *et al.* Abstract 2081: Robust activity of BLU-285, a potent and highly selective inhibitor of mutant KIT and PDGFRα, in patient-derived xenograft (PDX) models of gastrointestinal stromal tumor (GIST) Cancer Res 2017 Jul; 77 (13): 2081-1.

[225] Wu Y, Cain-Hom C, Choy L, *et al.* Therapeutic antibody targeting of individual Notch receptors. Nature 2010; 464(7291): 1052-7.
[http://dx.doi.org/10.1038/nature08878] [PMID: 20393564]

[226] Grego-Bessa J, Díez J, Timmerman L, de la Pompa JL. Notch and epithelial-mesenchyme transition in development and tumor progression: another turn of the screw. Cell Cycle 2004; 3(6): 718-21.
[http://dx.doi.org/10.4161/cc.3.6.949] [PMID: 15197341]

[227] Thurston G, Noguera-Troise I, Yancopoulos GD. The Delta paradox: DLL4 blockade leads to more tumour vessels but less tumour growth. Nat Rev Cancer 2007; 7(5): 327-31.
[http://dx.doi.org/10.1038/nrc2130] [PMID: 17457300]

[228] Takebe N, Nguyen D, Yang SX. Targeting notch signaling pathway in cancer: clinical development advances and challenges. Pharmacol Ther 2014; 141(2): 140-9.
[http://dx.doi.org/10.1016/j.pharmthera.2013.09.005] [PMID: 24076266]

[229] Weng AP, Ferrando AA, Lee W, *et al.* Activating mutations of NOTCH1 in human T cell acute lymphoblastic leukemia. Science 2004; 306(5694): 269-71.
[http://dx.doi.org/10.1126/science.1102160] [PMID: 15472075]

[230] Yabuuchi S, Pai SG, Campbell NR, *et al.* Notch signaling pathway targeted therapy suppresses tumor

progression and metastatic spread in pancreatic cancer. Cancer Lett 2013; 335(1): 41-51.
[http://dx.doi.org/10.1016/j.canlet.2013.01.054] [PMID: 23402814]

[231] Ferrarotto R, Mitani Y, Diao L, *et al.* Activating NOTCH1 Mutations Define a Distinct Subgroup of Patients With Adenoid Cystic Carcinoma Who Have Poor Prognosis, Propensity to Bone and Liver Metastasis, and Potential Responsiveness to Notch1 Inhibitors. J Clin Oncol 2017; 35(3): 352-60.
[http://dx.doi.org/10.1200/JCO.2016.67.5264] [PMID: 27870570]

[232] Munster P, Eckhardt SG, Patnaik A, *et al.* Abstract C42: Safety and preliminary efficacy results of a first-in-human phase I study of the novel cancer stem cell (CSC) targeting antibody brontictuzumab (OMP-52M51, anti-Notch1) administered intravenously to patients with certain advanced solid tumor Mol Cancer Ther 2016 Jan; 14(12) (2): C42-2.

[233] Gavai AV, Quesnelle C, Norris D, *et al.* Discovery of Clinical Candidate BMS-906024: A Potent Pan-Notch Inhibitor for the Treatment of Leukemia and Solid Tumors. ACS Med Chem Lett 2015; 6(5): 523-7.
[http://dx.doi.org/10.1021/acsmedchemlett.5b00001] [PMID: 26005526]

[234] Zweidler-McKay PA, DeAngelo DJ, Douer D, *et al.* The Safety and Activity of BMS-906024, a Gamma Secretase Inhibitor (GSI) with Anti-Notch Activity, in Patients with Relapsed T-Cell Acute Lymphoblastic Leukemia (T-ALL): Initial Results of a Phase 1 Trial Blood 2014 Dec; 124(21): 968-8.

[235] Knoechel B, Bhatt A, Pan L, *et al.* Complete hematologic response of early T-cell progenitor acute lymphoblastic leukemia to the γ-secretase inhibitor BMS-906024: genetic and epigenetic findings in an outlier case. Cold Spring Harb Mol Case Stud 2015; 1(1): a000539.
[http://dx.doi.org/10.1101/mcs.a000539] [PMID: 27148573]

[236] Chen X, Gong L, Ou R, *et al.* Sequential combination therapy of ovarian cancer with cisplatin and γ-secretase inhibitor MK-0752. Gynecol Oncol 2016; 140(3): 537-44.
[http://dx.doi.org/10.1016/j.ygyno.2015.12.011] [PMID: 26704638]

[237] Krop I, Demuth T, Guthrie T, *et al.* Phase I pharmacologic and pharmacodynamic study of the gamma secretase (Notch) inhibitor MK-0752 in adult patients with advanced solid tumors. J Clin Oncol 2012; 30(19): 2307-13.
[http://dx.doi.org/10.1200/JCO.2011.39.1540] [PMID: 22547604]

[238] Wolfe MS. Secretase targets for Alzheimer's disease: identification and therapeutic potential. J Med Chem 2001; 44(13): 2039-60.
[http://dx.doi.org/10.1021/jm0004897] [PMID: 11405641]

[239] Cook JJ, Wildsmith KR, Gilberto DB, *et al.* Acute gamma-secretase inhibition of nonhuman primate CNS shifts amyloid precursor protein (APP) metabolism from amyloid-beta production to alternative APP fragments without amyloid-beta rebound. J Neurosci 2010; 30(19): 6743-50.
[http://dx.doi.org/10.1523/JNEUROSCI.1381-10.2010] [PMID: 20463236]

[240] Niva C, Parkinson J, Olsson F, van Schaick E, Lundkvist J, Visser SAG. Has inhibition of Aβ production adequately been tested as therapeutic approach in mild AD? A model-based meta-analysis of γ-secretase inhibitor data. Eur J Clin Pharmacol 2013; 69(6): 1247-60.
[http://dx.doi.org/10.1007/s00228-012-1459-3] [PMID: 23288352]

[241] Yen W-C, Fischer MM, Axelrod F, *et al.* Targeting Notch signaling with a Notch2/Notch3 antagonist (tarextumab) inhibits tumor growth and decreases tumor-initiating cell frequency. Clin Cancer Res 2015; 21(9): 2084-95.
[http://dx.doi.org/10.1158/1078-0432.CCR-14-2808] [PMID: 25934888]

[242] Oettle H, Seufferlein T, Luger T, *et al.* Final results of a phase I/II study in patients with pancreatic cancer, malignant melanoma, and colorectal carcinoma with trabedersen J Clin Oncol 2012 May; 30 (15)

[243] Luistro L, He W, Smith M, *et al.* Preclinical profile of a potent gamma-secretase inhibitor targeting notch signaling with *in vivo* efficacy and pharmacodynamic properties. Cancer Res 2009; 69(19): 7672-80.

[http://dx.doi.org/10.1158/0008-5472.CAN-09-1843] [PMID: 19773430]

[244]   Huynh C, Poliseno L, Segura MF, *et al.* The novel gamma secretase inhibitor RO4929097 reduces the tumor initiating potential of melanoma. PLoS One 2011; 6(9): e25264.
[http://dx.doi.org/10.1371/journal.pone.0025264] [PMID: 21980408]

[245]   Tolcher AW, Messersmith WA, Mikulski SM, *et al.* Phase I study of RO4929097, a gamma secretase inhibitor of Notch signaling, in patients with refractory metastatic or locally advanced solid tumors. J Clin Oncol 2012; 30(19): 2348-53.
[http://dx.doi.org/10.1200/JCO.2011.36.8282] [PMID: 22529266]

[246]   Strosberg JR, Yeatman T, Weber J, *et al.* A phase II study of RO4929097 in metastatic colorectal cancer. Eur J Cancer 2012; 48(7): 997-1003.
[http://dx.doi.org/10.1016/j.ejca.2012.02.056] [PMID: 22445247]

[247]   Diaz-Padilla I, Wilson MK, Clarke BA, *et al.* A phase II study of single-agent RO4929097, a gamma-secretase inhibitor of Notch signaling, in patients with recurrent platinum-resistant epithelial ovarian cancer: A study of the Princess Margaret, Chicago and California phase II consortia. Gynecol Oncol 2015; 137(2): 216-22.
[http://dx.doi.org/10.1016/j.ygyno.2015.03.005] [PMID: 25769658]

[248]   De Jesus-Acosta A, Laheru D, Maitra A, *et al.* A phase II study of the gamma secretase inhibitor RO4929097 in patients with previously treated metastatic pancreatic adenocarcinoma. Invest New Drugs 2014; 32(4): 739-45.
[http://dx.doi.org/10.1007/s10637-014-0083-8] [PMID: 24668033]

[249]   Mercurio A, Adriani G, Catalano A, *et al.* A Mini-Review on Thalidomide: Chemistry, Mechanisms of Action, Therapeutic Potential and Anti-Angiogenic Properties in Multiple Myeloma Curr Med Chem 2009 May;

[250]   Alaseem A, Venkatesan T, Alhazzani K, Rathinavelu A. Analysis of the regulation of angiogenesis pathway by inhibiting MDM2 function in LNCaP-MST prostate cancer cells using PCR array. Cancer Research 2015; 75(15) Abstract 80.
[http://dx.doi.org/10.1158/1538-7445.AM2015-80]

[251]   Aftab BT, Dobromilskaya I, Liu JO, Rudin CM. Itraconazole inhibits angiogenesis and tumor growth in non-small cell lung cancer. Cancer Res 2011; 71(21): 6764-72.
[http://dx.doi.org/10.1158/0008-5472.CAN-11-0691] [PMID: 21896639]

[252]   Gerstner ER, Duda DG, di Tomaso E, *et al.* VEGF inhibitors in the treatment of cerebral edema in patients with brain cancer. Nat Rev Clin Oncol 2009; 6(4): 229-36.
[http://dx.doi.org/10.1038/nrclinonc.2009.14] [PMID: 19333229]

[253]   Sridhar J, Akula N, Sivanesan D, Narasimhan M, Rathinavelu A, Pattabiraman N. Identification of novel angiogenesis inhibitors. Bioorg Med Chem Lett 2005; 15(18): 4125-9.
[http://dx.doi.org/10.1016/j.bmcl.2005.06.001] [PMID: 15993586]

[254]   Rathinavelu A, Alhazzani K, Dhandayuthapani S, Kanagasabai T. Anti-cancer effects of F16: A novel vascular endothelial growth factor receptor-specific inhibitor. Tumour Biol 2017; 39(11): 1010428317726841.
[http://dx.doi.org/10.1177/1010428317726841] [PMID: 29130389]

[255]   Alhazzani K, Dhandayuthapani S, Cheema K, *et al.* Pharmacokinetic and Safety Profile of a Novel Anti-angiogenic Agent F16 with High Levels of Distribution to the Brain. American Association for Pharmaceutical Scientists (AAPS) 2016 Nov; Abstract - 3312

[256]   Dhandayuthapani S, Rathinavelu A. JFD, a novel small molecule for inhibiting vascular endothelial growth factor receptor-mediated angiogenesis. Cancer Research 2014 Apr; 74 (19) Abstract - 1021 - 1,
[http://dx.doi.org/10.1158/1538-7445.AM2015-1380]

[257]   Kanagasabai T, Alvarez J, Bhalani M, Dhandayuthapani S, Rathinavelu A. The *in vivo* activity of a novel anti-angiogenic compound, JFD-WS, in human breast adenocarcinoma xenograft implanted

athymic nude mice. Cancer Research 2015 Apr; 75 (15) Abstract - 1380 - 0, [http://dx.doi.org/10.1158/1538-7445.AM2015-1380]

[258] Rathinavelu A, Kanagasabai T, Dhandayuthapani S, Alhazzani K. Anti-angiogenic and pro-apoptotic effects of a small-molecule JFD-WS in *in vitro* and breast cancer xenograft mouse models. Oncol Rep 2018; 39(4): 1711-24.
[PMID: 29436685]

[259] Lin Z, Zhang Q, Luo W. Angiogenesis inhibitors as therapeutic agents in cancer: Challenges and future directions. Eur J Pharmacol 2016; 793: 76-81.
[http://dx.doi.org/10.1016/j.ejphar.2016.10.039] [PMID: 27840192]

[260] Ronca R, Benkheil M, Mitola S, Struyf S, Liekens S. Tumor angiogenesis revisited: Regulators and clinical implications. Med Res Rev 2017; 37(6): 1231-74.
[http://dx.doi.org/10.1002/med.21452] [PMID: 28643862]

[261] Hillen F, Griffioen AW. Tumour vascularization: sprouting angiogenesis and beyond. Cancer Metastasis Rev 2007; 26(3-4): 489-502.
[http://dx.doi.org/10.1007/s10555-007-9094-7] [PMID: 17717633]

[262] Pàez-Ribes M, Allen E, Hudock J, *et al.* Antiangiogenic therapy elicits malignant progression of tumors to increased local invasion and distant metastasis. Cancer Cell 2009; 15(3): 220-31.
[http://dx.doi.org/10.1016/j.ccr.2009.01.027] [PMID: 19249680]

CHAPTER 4

Anti-Angiogenesis Drugs: Hopes and Disappointments in Certain Cancers

Georgios M. Iatrakis[*]

Technological Educational Institute of Athens, Agiou Spyridonos, 12210 Egaleo, Athens, Greece

Abstract: In cancer, neovascularization seems necessary for tumor progression and metastasis. The hypothesis that cancer progression is angiogenesis-dependent has repeatedly been confirmed by experimental inhibition of tumor growth with angiogenesis inhibitors. Receptors for VEGF (VEGFRs) are expressed on tumor endothelium and tumor cells and, as expected, VEGF-A overexpression is associated with poor prognosis (reduced survival). There are both positive and negative angiogenesis regulators and, as such, two strategies for inhibiting pathologic angiogenesis can be adopted: the inhibition of positively-acting agents (*e.g.*, VEGFR inhibitors) and the administration of negatively-acting agents (*e.g.*, angiostatin (from the Greek words "angio" and "stasis" meaning stopping)).

Keywords: Angiogenesis, Anti-angiogenesis drugs, Cancer, Growth factors, Negative angiogenesis regulators, Positive angiogenesis regulators.

INTRODUCTION

Fetal liver and spleen carry the burden of hemopoiesis until birth [1, 2]. Blood vessels constitute the first organ in the embryo and form the largest network in the body [3]. After birth, the cardiovascular system ensures the delivery of blood with oxygen, nutrients and immune cells to all organs, and the removal of waste tissue metabolites. The word "angiogenesis" derives from the Greek words "angio" (vase) and "genesis" (creation) and it means the formation of new blood vessels (which contributes to numerous malignant disorders). Angiogenesis is active under specific physiological conditions in healthy adults but the vasculature can also be abnormally activated to generate new blood vessels during pathological conditions such as cancer and chronic inflammation [4]. Angiogenesis is a complex (normal or pathologic) process expressing under positive or negative control of natural growth factors (which are endogenous molecules that mainly

---
[*] **Corresponding author Georgios M. Iatrakis:** Technological Educational Institute of Athens, Athens, Greece; Tel/Fax: 0030-210-6611178; E-mail: giatrakis@teiath.gr

Atta-ur-Rahman & Mohammad Iqbal Choudhary (Eds.)

promote cell proliferation). Furthermore, hyaluronic acid (hyaluronan) is a glycosaminoglycan (normally present in the extracellular matrix of tissues in continuous remodeling as in wound healing processes), that acts as a significant modulator of cell behavior by angiogenesis and other mechanisms. Hyaluronic acid (a polymer of disaccharides) is widely distributed throughout connective, epithelial, and neural tissues. Its molecular weight is very high (>3 millions Da). As in wound healing, it contributes significantly to cell proliferation and migration. However, cell proliferation and migration are also cancer tissues "characteristics" and, as such, hyaluronic acid may also be involved in the progression of some malignant tumors. Hyaluronic acid is degraded by a family of enzymes (hyaluronidases), which are tumor suppressors. The degradation products of hyaluronan (oligosaccharides) and very low-molecular-weight hyaluronan exhibit pro-angiogenic properties and can induce inflammatory responses (perhaps another "component" of carcinogenesis).

The relationship between the immune system and angiogenesis has been described both in physiological (pregnancy) and pathological (cancer) conditions. Actually, different types of immune cells (myeloid, macrophages and denditric cells) are able to modulate tumor neovascularization [5]. Considering that the immune system seems to be an important component in tumoural angiogenesis, immune modulation could be used as a new therapeutic strategy in combination with other cancer treatments.

The growth (and metastasis) of solid tumors mainly depends on their ability for angiogenesis to ensure their own blood supply. Taking into account that tumor tissue's vasculature is different from normal vasculature, molecular insights into angiogenesis process could offer new therapeutic opportunities. Over the past fifteen years, much work has been performed to understand and modify the process of angiogenesis for successful therapeutic interventions against a broad spectrum of cancers. Actually, there are both positive and negative angiogenesis regulators. As the tumor grows and cells in the center of the tumor become hypoxic, the tumor initiates recruitment of its own blood supply, by shifting the balance between angiogenesis inhibitors (negative angiogenesis regulators) and stimulators (positive angiogenesis regulators) towards the latter [6].

Growth factors induce neovascularization by stimulating endothelial cell proliferation. Vascular Endothelial Growth Factor-A (VEGF-A) is the main growth factor controlling angiogenesis. It belongs to a broader family of growth factors, including VEGF-B, VEGF-C, VEGF-D, VEGF-E and Placental GF (PLGF). In general, VEGF is considered the key driver of tumour angiogenesis. VEGF-A, acting *via* its receptors (which are expressed on endothelial cells), stimulates endothelial mitogenesis and promotes endothelial survival. In cancer, neovascularization seems necessary for tumor growth (not initially) and metastasis. The hypothesis that cancer progression is angiogenesis-dependent has repeatedly been confirmed by experimental inhibition of tumor growth with angiogenesis inhibitors. Receptors for VEGF (VEGFRs) are expressed on tumor endothelium and tumor cells and, as expected, VEGF-A overexpression is associated with poor prognosis (reduced survival). As mentioned above, there are both positive and negative angiogenesis regulators and, as such, two strategies for inhibiting pathologic angiogenesis can be adopted: the inhibition of positively-acting agents (*e.g.*, VEGFR inhibitors) and the administration of negatively-acting agents (*e.g.*, angiostatin (from the Greek words "angio" and "stasis" meaning stopping)). Some agents are, probably, more efficient when combined with chemotherapy than as monotherapy. Main examples of anti-angiogenesis drugs are listed below.

Anti-Angiogenesis Drugs

Antibodies that Bind to and Neutralize VEGF

Antibodies that bind to and neutralize VEGF have been employed to decrease VEGF signaling in patients with malignancy [7]. The most information for these antibodies is available on **bevacizumab** (Avastin (Roche)), a VEGF-blocking monoclonal humanised antibody that inhibits angiogenesis [8] and that was designed to normalize tumor vasculature and reduce intratumoral pressure [9]. After IV infusion, its circulating half-life is 17 to 21 days. "As expected", plasma VEGF-A (and VEGFR-2) is included in the potential predictive markers for **bevacizumab** efficacy [10]. More than 450 clinical trials investigated the use of **bevacizumab** in various tumour types (including colorectal, breast, gastric, non small cell lung, brain, ovarian and prostate cancer) in advanced and early stage disease. So far, over 500,000 patients have been treated with **bevacizumab**.

Hopes: Bevacizumab improved progression-free survival in many solid malignancies when combined with cytotoxic chemotherapy. Actually, **bevacizumab** improved progression-free survival and the proportion of patients achieving a response compared to those who received chemotherapy alone [11]. As such, it is on the World Health Organization's List of Essential Medicines (most important medications needed in a basic health system) and it was the best-selling cancer drug in the world. It became the first angiogenesis inhibitor approved for treatment of cancer in the United States, based on its efficacy in advanced colorectal cancer [12]. Similarly, it had been approved for breast cancer and, recently, limited data showed (again) some efficacy in the treatment of metastatic breast cancers [9, 13]. Taking into account that almost one in three breast cancer cases are metastatic at diagnosis, **bevacizumab** (among similar drugs) was considered a major innovation. In the past, E2100, a randomized, phase III trial (>700 patients with previously untreated locally recurrent or metastatic breast cancer), showed that after the addition of **bevacizumab** to the weekly administered paclitaxel, the risk of progression was reduced by more than half and the overall response rate had more than doubled, confirming a substantial and robust **bevacizumab** treatment effect [14]. Similarly, **bevacizumab** plus docetaxel (AVADO trial), showed efficacy in women with breast cancer including elderly patients [15]. In more detail, docetaxel plus **bevacizumab** (15 mg/kg administered every three weeks) resulted in significantly increased progression free survival compared to docetaxel therapy alone. Although the study was not designed to compare different doses, the 15mg/kg every 3 weeks dose consistently showed a tendency towards greater efficacy, with limited impact on the known safety profile of docetaxel. Today, some investigators believe that **bevacizumab** is beneficial in a subset of breast cancer patients when sufficient numbers of vessels (increased pretreatment microvascular density) are initially present [16]. Although the FDA revoked metastatic breast cancer from **bevacizumab** indication in 2011 (see below), **bevacizumab** combined with paclitaxel has been written in the breast cancer National Comprehensive Cancer Network (NCCN) guidelines [17] and this combination was used successfully in case reports [18]. There are strong beliefs among cancer survivors that the medicine is effective and potential harm is manageable [19]. Furthermore, recent data showed an improved overall survival with **bevacizumab** in breast cancer patients which contradicts the findings of other studies [20].

Disappointments: Biomarkers that reliably predict for the clinical efficacy of **bevacizumab** in cancer patients have not yet been identified. Furthermore, tumours show emerging resistance to regimens that include **bevacizumab** and, as such, **bevacizumab** has little effect on overall survival [21]. In general, **bevacizumab** failed to demonstrate superiority to placebo (in terms of disease progression and mortality rates) in breast cancer; with similar findings in colorectal, renal and pancreatic cancer. When several studies showed no evidence of effectiveness, in December 2011, the approval of FDA for **bevacizumab** in breast cancer was withdrawn [19]. The specific indication that was withdrawn was for the use of bevacizumab in metastatic breast cancer, with paclitaxel for the treatment of patients who have not received chemotherapy for metastatic HER2-negative breast cancer [22]. According to the previous studies, **bevacizumab** does not prolong overall or disease-free survival or improve sufficiently the quality of life to outweigh the risk of its side-effects, including hypertension and proteinuria according to recent data [23]. The next year of withdrawal (2011), an FDA panel rejected an appeal by Roche. Similarly, another panel of cancer experts ruled that **bevacizumab** should no longer be used in breast cancer patients, although preoperative **bevacizumab** and chemotherapy may benefit a subset of breast cancer patients [16]. However, the above decisions were met with a hostile reaction from many clinicians and cancer survivors [19]. Recently, it was suggested that **bevacizumab** may enhance invasion and penetration ability of breast cancer cells under serum starvation conditions [24]. Furthermore, the addition of **bevacizumab** to endocrine therapy in first-line treatment failed to produce a statistically significant increase in progression free survival or overall survival in women with HER2-negative/hormone receptor-positive advanced breast cancer [25]. Because of the risk of impaired wound healing, at least four weeks (and preferably six to eight weeks) should elapse between major surgery and administration of **bevacizumab**. Finally, venous thrombosis is frequent in patients who receive **bevacizumab**-containing chemotherapy [26].

Soluble "Decoy" Receptors for VEGF

Aflibercept is an intravenously administered recombinant protein that functions as a soluble "decoy" receptor for VEGF. It inactivates multiple members of the VEGF family (including VEGF-A, VEGF-B and PLGF) by preventing binding to their receptors. **Aflibercept** is approved in the United States for use in combination with FOL-F-IRI (FOL – folinic acid [leucovorin]), F – fluorouracil (5-FU), IRI – irinotecan) for the treatment of patients with metastatic colorectal cancer (that is resistant to or has progressed following an oxaliplatin-containing regimen).

Hopes: Compared with anti-VEGF monoclonal antibodies, **aflibercept** has potentially higher affinity for VEGF-A.

Disappointments: As most anticancer drugs, side effects of **aflibercept** include gastrointestinal disorders (diarrhoea, abdominal pain) and fatigue. Its bone marrow toxicity (myelosuppression) can cause some common serious side effects (of most anticancer drugs) such as leukopenia (neutropenia), thrombocytopenia and impaired wound healing. Because of the risk for the latter side effect, in general (except in emergency situations), six to eight weeks (at least four weeks) should elapse between major surgery and administration of **aflibercept**. A common side-effect of **aflibercept** is hypertension.

Anti-VEGF Receptor Antibodies

These antibodies target the cell surface receptor for VEGF (VEGFR).

Ramucirumab is a promising monoclonal antibody directed against the VEGF receptor 2 (blocking receptor activation), that has being tested in colorectal cancer. **Ramucirumab** can be used in combination with FOL-F-IRI (FOL – folinic acid (leucovorin)), F – fluorouracil (5-FU), IRI – irinotecan) for the treatment of patients with metastatic colorectal cancer (that is resistant to or has progressed following an oxaliplatin-containing regimen or bevacizumab (see above)).

Hopes: Median survival and median progression-free survival are modestly but significantly increased with **ramucirumab**. In contrast to similar agents, the risk of arterial and venous thromboembolism is not increased [27].

Disappointments: Ramucirumab increases the risk of hemorrhage, which may be severe or fatal.

Antiangiogenic (Small Molecule) Tyrosine Kinases Inhibitors

Tyrosine kinases (TKs) belong to the broader family of protein kinases and function as an "on" or "off" switch in many cellular activities. If mutated, and stuck in the "on" position, can cause unregulated growth of the cell and cancer development. TKs inhibitors (TKIs) have demonstrated promising anticancer activity in a variety of malignancies and have the advantage of oral bioavailability (unlike monoclonal antibodies). Examples of TKs inhibited by the antiangiogenic TKIs include the following, although the complete functional spectrum of TKs is not always known:

- c-kit receptor; implicated in cell proliferation, survival, and migration
- Epidermal growth factor receptor (EGFR); implicated in angiogenic and mitogenic functions
- Fibroblast growth factor receptor (FGFR/FGFR1, FGFR2, FGFR3); implicated in mitogenic activity
- Platelet derived growth factor receptor (PDGFR/PDGFR-alpha, PDGFR-beta).
    Examples of antiangiogenic TKs inhibitors (in clinical use) and the above receptor tyrosine kinases they target include the following:
    - For c-kit receptor:
      -Pazopanib
      -Regorafenib
      -Sunitinib

    - For EGFR
      -Vandetanib
    - For FGFR/FGFR1, FGFR2, FGFR3:
      -Sorafenib inhibits FGFR1
      -Regorafenib inhibits FGFR1 and FGFR2
      -Pazopanib inhibits FGFR1 and FGFR3
      -Lenvatinib inhibits FGFR

- PDGFR/PDGFR-alpha, PDGFR-beta
  - Pazopanib inhibits PDGFR-alpha and PDGFR-beta
  - Regorafenib inhibits PDGFR-alpha and PDGFR-beta
  - Sunitinib inhibits PDGFR-alpha and PDGFR-beta
  - Sorafenib inhibits PDGFR

Hopes: TKs inhibitors showed some efficacy in a broad spectrum of cancers, including advanced renal cell carcinoma, differentiated thyroid carcinoma, gastrointestinal stromal tumor, hepatocellular carcinoma, pancreatic neuro-endocrine tumors, and small cell lung cancer.

Disappointments: TKs inhibitors, compared with monoclonal antibodies, have low target affinity, require daily dosing (due to short circulating half-lives), and are responsible for some (serious) side effects, including thrombotic events [28]. Furthermore, the administration of **TKs inhibitors** has been shown to generate tumor hypoxia which might accelerate tumor progression and metastasis by increasing cancer stem cells population. This could explain axillary lymph node progression during sunitinib treatment [29].

Vascular Disrupting Agents

(Low-molecular-weight) **vascular disrupting agents (VDAs)** directly damage tumor blood vessels and, thus, influence tumor integrity and growth. VDAs selectively disrupt the endothelial linings of tumor vessels, stopping blood flow to the tumor (while blood flow to normal tissues remains relatively intact). Among others, modified adenoviral vectors, adeno-associated viral vectors, retroviral vectors, lentiviral vectors, and herpes simplex viral vectors probably could be used as a tumor vascular targeting therapy. However, potential barriers to this effort could be toxicities to normal tissues (as other anti-cancer therapies), neutralizing antibodies and poor access to extravascular tumor tissue (probably "expected"!).

Immunomodulatory Drugs

Thalidomide was shown to exhibit clinical activity in several malignant disorders (although some years ago, marketed as a sedative, it was taken off the market because of severe teratogenicity). Its clinical activity have been linked to abnormal angiogenesis but its primary function is related to immunomodulation. Recently, thalidomide, combined with chemotherapy, was safe and mildly effective in treating patients with advanced colorectal cancer [30]. Moreover, by modifying the original thalidomide structure, some potent **immunomodulatory drugs** were synthesized including lenalidomide and pomalidomide.

Hopes: In multiple myeloma, which generally carries a poor prognosis, lenalidomide (compared to placebo) induces a complete or almost excellent partial response and it improves progression-free survival and overall survival.

Disappointments: The data are still limited and further studies should be conducted to clarify the effectiveness of thalidomide combination with chemotherapy. Furthermore, similarly to thalidomide, lenalidomide is probably teratogenic in humans (pregnancy category X) and cannot be prescribed for women who might be conceiving. As most anticancer drugs, lenalidomide can cause some common serious side effects such as myelosuppression resulting in leukopenia (neutropenia) and thrombocytopenia. Other serious side effects of lenalidomide include thrombosis, pulmonary embolus, and hepatotoxicity. However, bone marrow toxicity is its major dose-limiting toxicity.

CONCLUDING REMARKS

It seems that most tumors begin as non-angiogenic neoplasms and one critical mechanism behind tumor aggressiveness or dormancy is the ability of the tumor cell population to induce angiogenesis [31]. Thus, neovascularization is necessary for cancer growth and metastasis. Considering that cancer progression is angiogenesis-dependent, the inhibition of tumor growth with angiogenesis inhibitors is crucial in certain cancers. There are both positive and negative angiogenesis regulators and, as such, two main strategies for inhibiting pathologic angiogenesis can be adopted: the inhibition of positively-acting agents and the administration of negatively-acting agents. Among others, these agents could contribute to cancer inactivity by providing an environment of cellular and angiogenic dormancy. However, serious side effects and reduced efficacy have been shown for certain of these agents. Furthermore, to improve the efficacy of certain antiangiogenic agents, the concurrent use of cancer stem cells-targeting agents will be required.

CONFLICT OF INTEREST

The author confirms that he has no conflict of interest to declare for this publication.

ACKNOWLEDGEMENTS

Declared none.

REFERENCES

[1]   Tavassoli M. Embryonic and fetal hemopoiesis: an overview. Blood Cells 1991; 17(2): 269-81. [PMID: 1912596]

[2]　Martin MA, Bhatia M. Analysis of the human fetal liver hematopoietic microenvironment. Stem Cells Dev 2005; 14(5): 493-504.
[http://dx.doi.org/10.1089/scd.2005.14.493] [PMID: 16305335]

[3]　Carmeliet P. Angiogenesis in health and disease. Nat Med 2003; 9(6): 653-60.
[http://dx.doi.org/10.1038/nm0603-653] [PMID: 12778163]

[4]　Chung AS, Lee J, Ferrara N. Targeting the tumour vasculature: insights from physiological angiogenesis. Nat Rev Cancer 2010; 10(7): 505-14.
[http://dx.doi.org/10.1038/nrc2868] [PMID: 20574450]

[5]　Spinelli FM, Vitale DL, Demarchi G, Cristina C, Alaniz L. The immunological effect of hyaluronan in tumor angiogenesis. Clin Transl Immunology 2015; 4(12): e52.
[http://dx.doi.org/10.1038/cti.2015.35] [PMID: 26719798]

[6]　Hanahan D, Folkman J. Patterns and emerging mechanisms of the angiogenic switch during tumorigenesis. Cell 1996; 86(3): 353-64.
[http://dx.doi.org/10.1016/S0092-8674(00)80108-7] [PMID: 8756718]

[7]　Grothey A, Galanis E. Targeting angiogenesis: progress with anti-VEGF treatment with large molecules. Nat Rev Clin Oncol 2009; 6(9): 507-18.
[http://dx.doi.org/10.1038/nrclinonc.2009.110] [PMID: 19636328]

[8]　Suzuki S, Sakurai K, Adachi K, *et al.* Examination of the response rate of paclitaxel and bevacizumab therapy for metastatic advanced breast cancer according to the lymphopenia grade. Gan To Kagaku Ryoho 2015; 42(10): 1249-51.
[PMID: 26489562]

[9]　Chen DR, Lin C, Wang YF. Window of opportunity: A new insight into sequential bevacizumab and paclitaxel in two cases of metastatic triple-negative breast cancer. Exp Ther Med 2015; 10(3): 885-8.
[PMID: 26622409]

[10]　Miles DW, de Haas SL, Dirix LY, *et al.* Biomarker results from the AVADO phase 3 trial of first-line bevacizumab plus docetaxel for HER2-negative metastatic breast cancer. Br J Cancer 2013; 108(5): 1052-60.
[http://dx.doi.org/10.1038/bjc.2013.69] [PMID: 23422754]

[11]　Bartsch R, Gnant M, Steger GG. Bevacizumab: no comeback in early breast cancer? Lancet Oncol 2015; 16(9): 1001-3.; Carmeliet P. Angiogenesis in health and disease. Nat Med 2003; 9: 653.

[12]　Kuo CJ. Overview of angiogenesis inhibitors 2015. UpToDate.

[13]　Sengupta S, Rojas R, Mahadevan A, Kasper E, Jeyapalan S. CPT-11/bevacizumab for the treatment of refractory brain metastases in patients with HER2-neu-positive breast cancer. Oxf Med Case Reports 2015; 2015(4): 254-7.

[14]　Gray R, Bhattacharya S, Bowden C, Miller K, Comis RL. Independent review of E2100: a phase III trial of bevacizumab plus paclitaxel versus paclitaxel in women with metastatic breast cancer. J Clin Oncol 2009; 27(30): 4966-72.
[http://dx.doi.org/10.1200/JCO.2008.21.6630] [PMID: 19720913]

[15]　Pivot X, Schneeweiss A, Verma S, *et al.* Efficacy and safety of bevacizumab in combination with docetaxel for the first-line treatment of elderly patients with locally recurrent or metastatic breast cancer: results from AVADO. Eur J Cancer 2011; 47(16): 2387-95.
[http://dx.doi.org/10.1016/j.ejca.2011.06.018] [PMID: 21757334]

[16]　Tolaney SM, Boucher Y, Duda DG, *et al.* Role of vascular density and normalization in response to neoadjuvant bevacizumab and chemotherapy in breast cancer patients. Proc Natl Acad Sci USA 2015; 112(46): 14325-30.
[http://dx.doi.org/10.1073/pnas.1518808112] [PMID: 26578779]

[17]　Li Q, Yan H, Zhao P, Yang Y, Cao B. Efficacy and safety of bevacizumab combined with

chemotherapy for managing metastatic breast cancer: A meta-analysis of randomized controlled trials. Sci Rep 2015; 5: 15746.
[http://dx.doi.org/10.1038/srep15746] [PMID: 26503902]

[18] Ogata H, Kikuchi Y, Natori K, *et al.* Liver Metastasis of a Triple-Negative Breast Cancer and Complete Remission for 5 Years After Treatment With Combined Bevaci-zumab/Paclitaxel/Carboplatin: Case Report and Review of the Literature. Medicine (Baltimore) 2015; 94(42): e1756.
[http://dx.doi.org/10.1097/MD.0000000000001756]

[19] Vitry A, Nguyen T, Entwistle V, Roughead E. Regulatory withdrawal of medicines marketed with uncertain benefits: the bevacizumab case study. J Pharm Policy Pract 2015; 8: 25. eCollection 2015.
[http://dx.doi.org/10.1186/s40545-015-0046-2]

[20] Bear HD, Tang G, Rastogi P, *et al.* Neoadjuvant plus adjuvant bevacizumab in early breast cancer (NSABP B-40 [NRG Oncology]): secondary outcomes of a phase 3, randomised controlled trial. Lancet Oncol 2015; 16(9): 1037-48.
[http://dx.doi.org/10.1016/S1470-2045(15)00041-8] [PMID: 26272770]

[21] Jubb AM, Harris AL. Biomarkers to predict the clinical efficacy of bevacizumab in cancer. Lancet Oncol 2010; 11(12): 1172-83.
[http://dx.doi.org/10.1016/S1470-2045(10)70232-1] [PMID: 21126687]

[22] Sasich LD, Sukkari SR. The US FDAs withdrawal of the breast cancer indication for Avastin (bevacizumab). Saudi Pharm J 2012; 20(4): 381-5.
[http://dx.doi.org/10.1016/j.jsps.2011.12.001] [PMID: 23960813]

[23] Launay-Vacher V, Janus N, Beuzeboc P, *et al.* Renovascular safety of bevacizumab in breast cancer patients. The prognostic value of hypertension and proteinuria. Bull Cancer 2012; pii: S0007-4551(15): 00273-8. (Epub ahead of print).
[http://dx.doi.org/10.1016/j.bulcan.2015.09.001]

[24] Wei L, Cuicui Z, Jing W, Kai L. Antiangiogenic drugs enhance the ability of invasion and metastasis of breast cancer cells under serum starvation and hypoxia. Zhonghua Zhong Liu Za Zhi 2015; 37(4): 244-50.
[PMID: 26462887]

[25] Martín M, Loibl S, von Minckwitz G, *et al.* Phase III trial evaluating the addition of bevacizumab to endocrine therapy as first-line treatment for advanced breast cancer: the letrozole/fulvestrant and avastin (LEA) study. J Clin Oncol 2015; 33(9): 1045-52.
[http://dx.doi.org/10.1200/JCO.2014.57.2388] [PMID: 25691671]

[26] Shirakawa T, Nakano M, Nio K, *et al.* Retrospective analysis of cardiovascular diseases related to chemotherapies for advanced solid tumor patients. Anticancer Drugs 2016. [Epub ahead of print].
[http://dx.doi.org/10.1097/CAD.0000000000000392] [PMID: 27272413]

[27] Abdel-Rahman O, ElHalawani H. Risk of cardiovascular adverse events in patients with solid tumors treated with ramucirumab: A meta analysis and summary of other VEGF targeted agents. Crit Rev Oncol Hematol 2016; 102: 89-100.
[http://dx.doi.org/10.1016/j.critrevonc.2016.04.003] [PMID: 27129437]

[28] Giles FJ, Stopeck AT, Silverman LR, *et al.* SU5416, a small molecule tyrosine kinase receptor inhibitor, has biologic activity in patients with refractory acute myeloid leukemia or myelodysplastic syndromes. Blood 2003; 102(3): 795-801.
[http://dx.doi.org/10.1182/blood-2002-10-3023] [PMID: 12649163]

[29] Conley SJ, Gheordunescu E, Kakarala P, *et al.* Antiangiogenic agents increase breast cancer stem cells *via* the generation of tumor hypoxia. Proc Natl Acad Sci USA 2012; 109(8): 2784-9.
[http://dx.doi.org/10.1073/pnas.1018866109] [PMID: 22308314]

[30] Huang XE, Yan XC, Wang L, *et al.* Thalidomide combined with chemotherapy in treating patients with advanced colorectal cancer. Asian Pac J Cancer Prev 2015; 16(17): 7867-9.

[http://dx.doi.org/10.7314/APJCP.2015.16.17.7867] [PMID: 26625812]

[31] Almog N. Molecular mechanisms underlying tumor dormancy. Cancer Lett 2010; 294(2): 139-46.
[http://dx.doi.org/10.1016/j.canlet.2010.03.004] [PMID: 20363069]

CHAPTER 5

Anti-Angiogenic Therapy for Retinal Diseases

Mitzy E. Torres Soriano[1,3,*], **Jesica Dimattia**[1] and **Maximiliano Gordon**[1,2]

[1] *Retina Department, Ophthalmology Service, Hospital Provincial del Centenario, Rosario, Argentina*

[2] *Centro de la Visión Gordon-Manavella, Rosario, Argentina*

[3] *Clínica de Ojos "Dr. Carlos Ferroni", Rosario, Argentina*

Abstract: Ocular angiogenesis is a major cause of disease and permanent blindness. The introduction of anti-vascular endothelial growth factor (anti-VEGF) agents has revolutionized the treatment of retinal vasogenic conditions. These drugs are now commonly employed for the treatment of a group of ocular pathologies, including exudative macular degeneration, diabetic macular edema, and retinal vein occlusion.

The most common anti-VEGF therapies for retinal diseases are bevacizumab (Avastin®), ranibizumab (Lucentis®) and aflibercept (Eylea®).

Multicenter, randomized, controlled clinical trials have been designed to study the efficacy of anti-VEGF therapy in common retinal angiogenic diseases. However, when it comes to extremely rare or uncommon retinal diseases, we must often rely on case studies or small series to elucidate a potential beneficial effect of anti-VEGF treatment. Continued experience with the use of anti-VEGF pharmacotherapy may offer additional treatment modalities for these conditions that have limited therapeutic options, and may also provide insight into their molecular pathophysiology.

In this chapter, we will describe the role of angiogenesis in retinal diseases, anti-angiogenic therapies that are available at the moment, evidence based on clinical trials and new researches on ocular anti-VEGF therapy.

Keywords: Antiangiogenesis, Vasculogenesis, Vascular endothelial growth factor (VEGF), Ischemia, Anti-VEGF therapy, Anti-platelet-derived growth factor (anti-PDGF), Bevacizumab, Ranibizumab, Aflibercept, Retinal disease, Clinical trials.

VASCULOGENESIS AND ANGIOGENESIS

The vasculogenesis process is the *de novo* formation of blood vessels during embryonic development by migration and differentiation of endothelial progenitor

---
[*] **Corresponding author Mitzy E. Torres Soriano:** Centro de la Visión Gordon - Manavella, Montevideo 763, CP 2000, Rosario - Santa Fe, Argentina; Tel/Fax: +54 (341) 4400239/4244850; E-mail: mitzytorres@yahoo.com

Atta-ur-Rahman & Mohammad Iqbal Choudhary (Eds.)

cells called angioblasts, while the blood formation process in adults is known as angiogenesis or neovascularization, and implies the formation of new blood vessels from the existing vasculature [1 - 5]. Angiogenesis is limited to sites of abnormal vascular surface. An activated vascular endothelium can be induced by tissue injury or wound healing, by hormonal cycling such as in pregnancy and ovulation, or by tumor-induced vessel growth. In all of these circumstances, platelets act as the initial responder to vascular change and provide a flexible delivery system for angiogenesis- related molecules. The process of postnatal angiogenesis is regulated by a continuous interplay of stimuli and inhibitors of angiogenesis, and their imbalance contributes to numerous inflammatory, malignant, ischemic, and immune disorders [6].

Recent work has demonstrated that angiogenesis also occurs through the recruitment of endothelial progenitor cells (EPC) from the bone marrow [1 - 5].

Angiogenesis plays an important role in chronic inflammation and fibrosis, tumor growth and vascularization of ischemic tissue. This is why there has been a great interest in understanding cell and molecular mechanisms of neovascularization and the therapeutic effects of angiogenic and antiangiogenic factors [1, 4, 5, 7].

Both mechanisms take place during retinal vasculogenesis. Development of retinal vasculature begins at the 14th week of gestation with the formation of major blood vessels in the central retina, and it is mediated by the vasculogenesis process. It implies the migration, sprouting and differentiation of a great number of spindle-shaped mesenchymal precursor cells from the optic disk to the peripheral retina, reaching the nasal edge between the 32nd and 36th weeks of gestation and the temporal edge by the time of birth. Then, during the second phase, the angiogenesis process will increase vascular density and extend vascularization to the peripheral inner retina. For this phase to take place, all of the following processes are necessary: the stimulation, sprouting and migration of endothelial cells, the proteolysis of the endothelial basement membrane, the adjacent extracellular matrix (ECM) degradation, the recruitment of supporting cells (pericytes) and, finally, the completion of the vascular circuit [2 - 5, 8, 9].

The development of the outer retinal plexus and the radial peripapillary capillaries (RPCs) is only determined by angiogenesis [2 - 4].

GROWTH FACTORS AND OTHER MEDIATORS INVOLVED IN ANGIOGENESIS

Multiple growth factors mediate angiogenic activity, but the most relevant ones are the vascular endothelial growth factor (VEGF) and angiopoietins in the embryonic vasculogenesis and adult angiogenesis [1, 4, 5, 7, 10, 11].

The vascular endothelial growth factor (VEGF) was initially named as vascular permeability factor, and it is secreted by many mesenchymal and stromal cells. Within this family, we can mention VEGF-A, VEGF-B, VEGF-C, VEGF-D and PlGF (placental growth factor). The major mediator of tumoral angiogenesis is VEGF-A. Although VEGFR-1 is a high-affinity VEGF receptor, the major transducer is VEGFR-2, receptor tyrosine kinase (RTK), restricted to endothelial cells and their precursors [1, 4, 5, 7, 10, 11].

Hypoxic tumor cells also begin to make a plethora of other growth factors and cytokines, which have the capacity to replace VEGF and stimulate new blood vessels growth, included among these are FGF (fibroblast growth factor), PDGFB (platelet-derived growth factor subunit B protein), HGF (hepatocyte growth factor protein), EGF (epidermal growth factor), IL-8 (interleukin-8 protein), IL-6 (interleukin-6 protein), Ang-2 (angiopoietin 2), SDF1α (stromal cell-derived factor 1 α protein), PDGF-C (platelet-derived growth factor C), CXCL6 (C-X-C motif chemokine 6 protein), *etc.*, as well as their receptors [12].

In angiogenesis promoted by endothelial cell precursors, VEGF acts through VEGFR-2, stimulating the mobilization of endothelial cell precursors from the bone marrow and advancing their proliferation and differentiation at the site of angiogenesis. In genesis promoted by preexisting local vessels, VEGF stimulates both proliferation and mobilization of endothelial cells, thus starting the sprout of new capillaries. Proliferation, differentiation and migration of endothelial cells can also be promoted by the basic fibroblast growth factor (FGF-2) [1, 4, 5, 11].

Induction of VEGF is the result of hypoxia through hypoxia-inducible factor 1 (HIF-1), low pH, inflammatory cytokines (IL-6), growth factors (basic fibroblast growth factor), sex hormones (androgens and estrogens), chemokines, oncogene activation and decreased tumor suppressor gene activity [1, 3 - 5, 7] (Fig. **1**).

Newly-formed blood vessels are fragile and need to be stabilized. Perycytes, smooth muscle cells and the deposit of proteins of the extracellular matrix (ECM) are necessary for stabilization. Angiopoietins 1 and 2 (Ang-1 and Ang-2), the platelet-derived growth factor (PDGF) and the transforming growth factor-beta (TGF-β) stabilize newly-formed vessels by promoting the production of ECM proteins [1, 4, 7].

ECM proteins are key components of angiogenesis, because they favor motility and direct migration of endothelial cells required for the formation of new blood vessels. These processes are controlled by various types of proteins, including: in the first place, integrins, a large family of cell surface receptor that participates in cell-cell and cell-extracellular matrix interactions; second, matricellular proteins, which destabilize cell-matrix interactions, thus promoting angiogenesis; and third, proteinases, such as plasminogen activating proteinases and matrix metallo-proteinases, which are important for the tissue remodeling during endothelial invasion. Also, these proteinases split extracellular proteins, releasing growth factors bound to the matrix, like VEGF and FGF-2, which stimulate angiogenesis. In turn, proteinases can release inhibitors like endostatin [1, 4, 7].

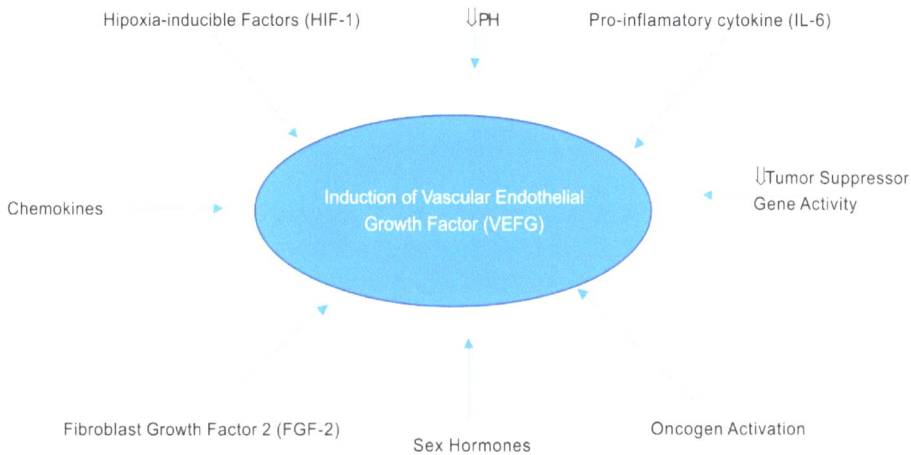

Fig. (1). Induction of VEGF.

Pigment epithelium-derived factor (PEDF), a glycoprotein from the serine protease inhibitor superfamily, is the most powerful inhibitor of angiogenesis known and has anti-inflammatory and antioxidant properties. It inhibits growth and migration of retinal endothelial cells and suppresses ischemia-induced retinal neovascularization. In cases of hypoxia, PEDF concentration decreases [1, 13].

OCULAR ANGIOGENESIS

Living organisms can keep a dynamic balance through mechanisms of self-regulation. In natural conditions, there is a balance between angiogenic and antiangiogenic molecules. When these conditions are altered, for instance, because of hypoxia or inflammatory processes, imbalance leads to the formation of abnormal vessels [1, 5, 10, 11].

Ocular angiogenesis is a major cause of disease and permanent blindness. It affects all age groups and it is an important factor in diabetic retinopathy, exudative age-related macular degeneration, corneal neovascularization, retinopathy of prematurity (ROP), retinal vein occlusion, neovascular glaucoma and sickle cell retinopathy, among others [1, 5, 7, 10].

At the level of the cornea, inflammation, hypoxia and limbal stem cell deficiency are the main factors that stimulate neovascularization. There are various causes for corneal inflammation [10].

Neovascularization of the iris, rubeosis iridis, is mainly secondary to retinal ischemia. The main causes include retinal vein occlusion, advanced diabetic retinopathy, ocular ischemic syndrome and intraocular tumors [10].

Retinal neovascularization originates from the retinal circulation. These neovessels are histologically different from normal retinal vessels: they don't maintain the blood-retinal barrier, and their development is usually nourished by fibrous tissue with contractile capability into the avascular vitreous gel. These features are responsible for extravascular leakage, preretinal or vitreous hemorrhages and tractional retinal detachment. New intraretinal vessels are dilated and tortuous vascular segments, known as intraretinal microvascular abnormalities (IRMAs). They occur in response to focal ischemia and are generally located around or adjacent to areas of arterial or capillary non perfusion. They are abnormally permeable to plasmatic proteins. Hypoxia is believed to be the initial stimulus for upregulation of growth factors, integrins and proteinases, which allow for proliferation and migration of endothelial cells [1].

At the level of the choroid, the new vessels grow from the choroidal vasculature, through Bruch's membrane, and into the retinal pigment epithelium (RPE) and the subretinal space. Due to unknown reasons, neovascularization occurs almost exclusively in the central macular region and in perimacular regions. Vessels are friable or can leak, so there is an accumulation of fluid, lipids and blood that results in death of central photoreceptors. This is observed most frequently in wet age-related macular degeneration (AMD), and is the main cause of severe vision loss in elderly people. Other common causes are high myopia, choroidal rupture, angioid streaks, ocular histoplasmosis syndrome, multifocal choroiditis and punctate inner choroidopathy. Oxidative damage, inflammation and hypoxia, to a lesser extent, are considered to have an influence on the balance of pro-angiogenic and antiangiogenic factors, promoting angiogenesis [1].

ANGIOGENESIS INHIBITORS

Judah Folkman recognized that new blood vessel formation is important for tumor growth and proposed anti-angiogenesis as a novel approach to cancer therapy. Discovery of vascular permeability factor/ vascular endothelial growth factor (VEGF-A) as the primary tumor angiogenesis factor prompted the development of a number of drugs that targeted it or its receptors [12]. Antiangiogenic therapy heralded a new era on the treatment of ocular neovascularization and associated pathologies. It mainly consists in inhibiting the production of VEGF, or its biological effects, because of its role in endothelial cell proliferation, vascular permeability increased and ocular inflammation [5, 6, 11, 14].

Antiangiogenic agents can act by means of three main mechanisms: directly inhibiting VEGF bonding, suppressing its synthesis or blocking VEGF signaling [6, 11].

Some direct VEGF inhibitors are bevacizumab, ranibizumab, pegaptanib, and aflibercept.

Bevacizumab (Avastin/Genentech): It is a humanized monoclonal full-length antibody of 150 kDa. It can block all forms of VEGF-A. It was approved by the Food and Drug Administration (FDA) in 2004 for systemic therapy for metastatic colorectal cancer. It is intended for intraocular administration and it is used off-label [5, 14 - 17] (Fig. **2**).

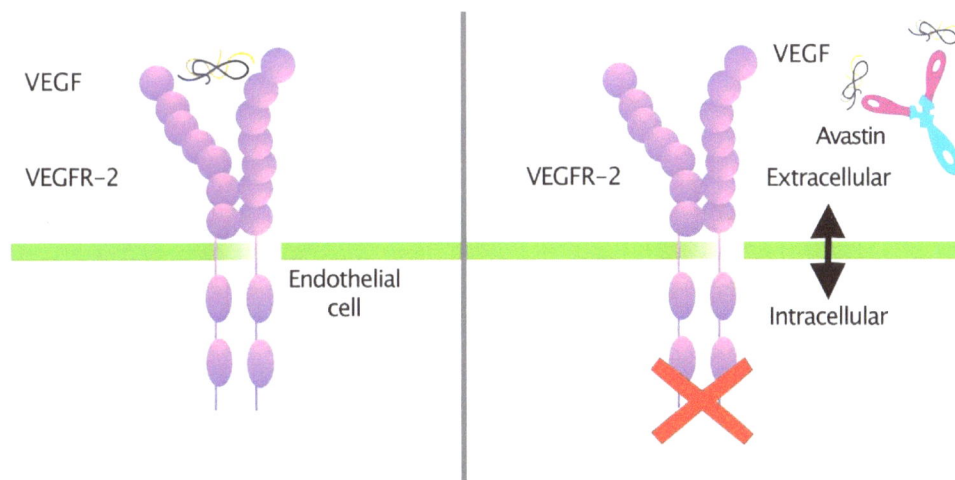

Fig. (2). Angiogenesis is mediated primarily through the interaction between VEGF and VEGFR-2. Avastin inhibits VEGF extracellularly and therefore, may inhibit angiogenesis without disrupting targets outside the VEGF pathway.

Ranibizumab (Lucentis, Genentech/Novartis): It is a humanized monoclonal antibody fragment of very low molecular weight: 48 kDa. This fragment can penetrate the retinal layer more easily than the full-length antibody. Therefore, it can bind to VEGF-A with higher affinity and, as a result, it can block the cascade reaction caused by the combination of VEFG-A and VEGF R1 and R2 receptors in the vascular endothelium. Its estimated vitreous half-life elimination is 9 days and the systemic one is 2 days. It blocks endothelial cell proliferation, neovascularization and capillary permeability. It received approval for the treatment of neovascularization in AMD in 2006, of macular edema associated to retinal vein occlusion (RVO) in 2010, and of diabetic macular edema in 2012. Ranibizumab approved dose is 0.5 mg and it is administered by intravitreal injection [5, 14, 16, 17].

Pegaptanib (Macugen, Eyetech, Pharmaceuticals/Pfizer): It is an RNA aptamer directed against the VEGF-165 isoform. It was the first aptamer to be approved by the FDA for use in humans, in 2004, for the treatment of all types of age-related macular degeneration [5, 14, 16, 17].

Aflibercept or VEGF Trap (Eylea, Regeneron Pharmaceuticals): It is a 115-kDa recombinant fusion protein comprising the critical VEGF binding domain of human VEGF receptors 1 and 2 fused to the Fc region of human IgG1. This molecule acts as soluble decoy receptor that binds to VEGF-A, VEGF-B and PlGF to inhibit the binding and activation of these VEGF receptors (Fig. **3**). It has a longer half-life and higher binding affinity to VEGF-A. Aflibercept was approved by the FDA in 2011 for wet AMD and in 2014 for diabetic macular edema [5, 14, 16, 17].

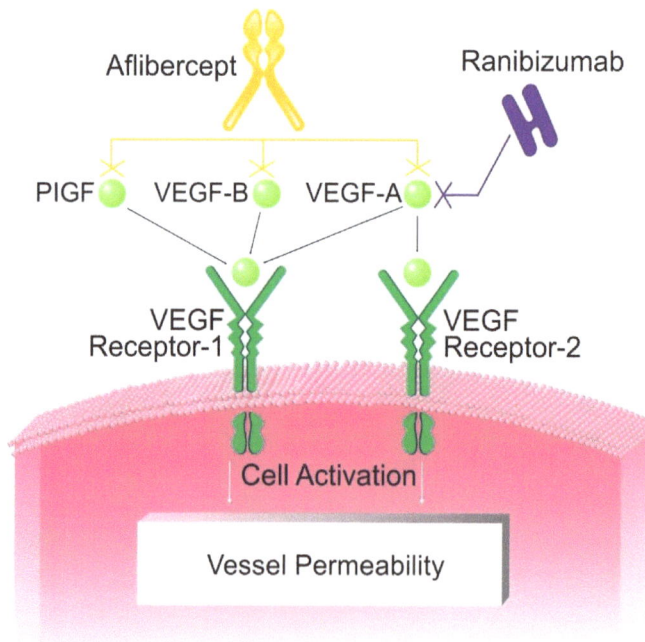

Fig. (3). Mechanism of action of Aflibercept and Ranibizumab.

THE USE OF ANGIOGENESIS INHIBITORS IN RETINAL DISEASE TREATMENT

Anti-VEGF therapy for wet AMD was first introduced in 2005 with the off-label use of bevacizumab (Avastin). Anti-VEGF agents specifically designed for intraocular use (pegaptanib [Macugen], ranibizumab [Lucentis] and aflibercept [Eylea]) were approved immediately afterwards. Intravitreal anti-VEGF therapy soon became popular for the treatment of other retinal diseases. It is approved for the treatment of wet AMD, diabetic macular edema (DME), myopic choroidal neovascularization and macular edema associated to RVO [7, 11, 18].

Age-related Macular Degeneration (AMD): It is the leading cause of blindness among people over 65 years old in the US, Europe and Australia. There are two main types: dry and wet AMD. Dry AMD is characterized by hard or soft drusen and RPE changes. In advanced cases, geographic atrophy can be observed. On the contrary, wet AMD is characterized by choroidal neovascular membrane (CNVM), which is often associated with subretinal fluid, hemorrhage, lipid exudation and, eventually, subretinal fibrosis (Fig. **4**). Risk factors include age, family history of AMD, race, smoking and high blood pressure.

Pathophysiology results from the combination of multiple mechanisms, some of which are still not known in full. It is believed that oxidative stress is a major predisposing factor. Inflammatory processes have also been implicated. Genetic variations of factor H gene, a major inhibitor of the complement pathway, has been associated to sustained complement activation, which results in atrophy of the photoreceptors and the RPE, and disruption of Bruch's membrane with resulting choroidal neovascularization. The cause for the development of choroidal neovascular membrane is thought to be the increase in angiogenic stimuli that overcome compensatory antiangiogenic mechanisms in the eye. This imbalance may be due to tissue hypoxia, inflammation or a combination of both. High concentration of VEGF is found in patients with wet AMD, while in contrast, PEDF is found to have lower concentrations in the vitreous in elderly patients [7, 9].

Laser photocoagulation of CNVM was first used in an attempt to preserve vision. It reduces the rate of severe vision loss. However, this type of treatment is not appropriate for patients with subfoveal lesions, and is associated with a high recurrence rate of up to 51%. Photodynamic therapy (PDT), which uses the combination of photosensitizing agents and low energy laser to achieve selective destruction of CNVM, is another treatment option. It was found to be effective for subfoveal lesions. However, in spite of the initial success in the prevention of immediate blindness, the rate of vision improvement remained low. A great advancement in the treatment of wet AMD was achieved thanks to the introduction of antiangiogenic drugs. Multiple randomized trials demonstrated the treatment with anti-VEGF agents was successful in reducing the incidence of vision loss, as well as in improving vision in more than 30% of patients [7, 9].

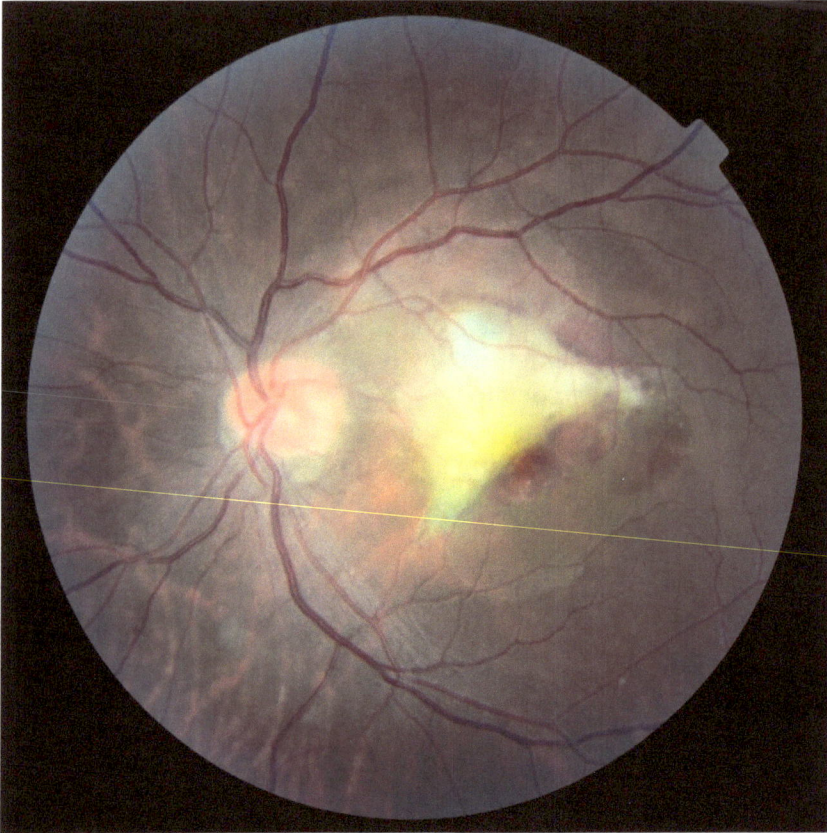

Fig. (4). Fundus photograph showing choroidal neovascular membrane associated with subretinal fluid, hemorrhage, lipid exudation and subretinal fibrosis.

In 2004, the FDA approved the first anti-VEGF treatment with the inclusion of pegaptanib sodium (Macugen; EyeTech, New York, NY).

The VISION study demonstrated pegaptanib efficacy over placebo for the treatment of wet AMD.

In 2006, ranibizumab was approved by the FDA for use in neovascular AMD. ANCHOR and MARINA are the reference studies that assessed ranibizumab efficacy in this pathology.

Clinical Trials

The MARINA [19] study was a randomized, double-blind, sham-controlled trial on patients with minimally-classic or occult neovascularization who were treated with ranibizumab, monthly injections of two different drug doses (0.3 and 0.5 mg) for 24 months. The outcomes showed that vision improved or was maintained in 95% of patients after 12 months in comparison with 62% of patients in the sham treatment group. Almost 40% of patients gained 15 or more ETDRS letters in comparison to the sham subgroup.

ANCHOR [20] study was a randomized, double-blind, sham-controlled trial on patients with predominantly classic neovascularization who were treated with ranibizumab and sham photodynamic therapy or with sham injections and photodynamic therapy. Ninety five percent (95%) of patients treated with ranibizumab improved or maintained visual acuity (VA) in comparison to 64% of patients treated with photodynamic therapy. Similar results were reported at 24 months: 90% vs. 65.7%. Mean improvement was 11 letters and almost 80% of patients maintained visual acuity after 24 months. Due to all these factors, the FDA approved ranibizumab in July 2006.

The PIER [21] study assessed the efficacy and safety of ranibizumab in doses of 0.3 mg and 0.5 mg administered monthly for 3 months and every 3 months thereafter. As in the two studies previously mentioned, VA improved during the first 3 months, reducing its effect in the quarterly treatment regimen groups.

The EXCITE [22] study evaluated the possibilities of treatment at regular intervals (same regimen as in PIER study) after the administration of 3 loading doses, but follow-up visits and evaluations were done on a monthly basis. As in the PIER study, the analysis of the subgroups showed an improvement after the third injection that remained stable until the end of the study period in around 40% of subjects.

The PrONTO [23] study demonstrated that good results could be achieved regarding VA without the need of monthly treatments. During this study, 3 loading injections of ranibizumab were administered to all patients, who were then followed-up and retreated if certain predefined criteria were met (this is called PRN or *pro re nata* regimen, "on-demand"): visual acuity reduction of at least 5 letters with fluid in the macula as per OCT, retinal thickness increase of 100 µm as per OCT, new-onset classic NVC, new hemorrhage or macular fluid as per OCT at least one month after injection.

Due to the limitations of the PrONTO study regarding sample size and lack of a control group, a new study was performed: the SUSTAIN [24] study, which consisted in the administration of 3 loading injections of ranibizumab and retreatment if similar criteria as in the PrONTO study were met. The improvement in visual acuity decreased after changing to PRN regimen.

The SAILOR [25] study, the largest trial to date, assessed the efficacy and safety of ranibizumab in 4300 patients during 12 months. This phase IIIb study had two cohorts. Subjects in the first cohort were randomized to receive either 0.3 mg or 0.5 mg of ranibizumab, with a loading injection and a PRN regimen from the second month on, following similar criteria to those of the PrONTO study. Patients were stratified by treatment history (whether they had received previous treatment or not). Patients in the second cohort (open-label study) received a 0.5 mg injection followed by a PRN regimen, and they were classified again based on their treatment history. The results supported the drug's safety and VA improvements were smaller than with the monthly treatment.

Taking all this into consideration, the most conservative strategy to bring the results of the trials closer to daily clinical practice is the administration of one single injection until a "dry" macula is achieved, followed by monthly follow-up and retreatment if fluid persists or recurs. The problem is that, in doing this, we are treating the disease after its onset, *i.e.* we fall behind.

In 2007, Spaide [26] suggested the "treat and extend" protocol, which consists in administering monthly injections to the patient until fluid disappears, and an additional injection in the macula showing no signs of activity. The patient was scheduled a new visit in 6-8 weeks; if there was evidence of fluid during this visit, the patient would be retreated and would return after 4 weeks. If there was no evidence of fluid in this visit, the patient would still be retreated but the next visit would be scheduled for 10-12 weeks afterwards. This was done in order to maintain the benefits and reduce the number of injections to a minimum while anticipating any potential recurrence of the disease.

The LUCAS Study [27] compared the efficacy and safety of treat and extend regimen of intravitreal bevacizumab versus intravitreal ranibizumab in wet AMD. The follow up was two years and concluded that the two drugs appear to have equivalent effects on visual acuity when administered according to the protocol.

The HORIZON [28, 29] study was an open-label phase III extension study on patients who had completed two years of monthly treatments under the MARINA and ANCHOR studies. Sixty one percent (61%) of patients who had participated in these studies received an additional one-year treatment with a PRN regimen at the ophthalmologist discretion, but they made visits on a quarterly basis.

The 600 patients who had been treated with ranibizumab and continued the treatment for one additional year under this PRN regimen lost 5.3 letters in a year, while those who had been treated with photodynamic therapy and those who had received no treatment lost another 2.4 and 3.1 letters, respectively.

The HORIZON study has demonstrated that monthly treatments would be accurate for a significant number of patients even beyond two years. This long-term study showed that reducing the frequency of injections during the third and fourth years was associated to loss of vision. Therefore, "on demand" treatments seem to be inadequate even beyond two years of treatment.

These studies prove that monthly treatments are more effective, but if another type of dosage regimen has to be chosen after the three loading doses, it is evident by these studies that tighter controls are needed by means of monthly OCTs as well as visual acuity tests, which become a necessary guide for treatment. When patients are followed up more frequently, fewer injections are needed; on the contrary, patients with a hope of longer follow-up intervals need more injections.

As regards bevacizumab, clinical trials were carried out to assess its efficacy and safety. Some of these were CATT (Comparison of AMD Treatment Trials) and IVAN (effectiveness of Lucentis and Avastin in the treatment of wet AMD).

The CATT (Comparison of Age-Related Macular Degeneration Treatments Trial) [30] was intended to compare the efficacy and safety of ranibizumab and bevacizumab, as well as to compare the efficacy of the monthly and "on demand" treatment regimens in terms of visual acuity. It is a multicenter, randomized two-year clinical trial that recruited 1208 patients from 44 medical centers in the US.

Inclusion criteria were being ≥50 years old, having previously untreated active choroidal neovascularization secondary to AMD, and visual acuity between 20/25 and 20/230. Active choroidal neovascularization had to be confirmed by leakage on fluorescein angiography and fluid on OCT.

Study groups were defined after the first injection, which was mandatory in all cases, based on drug and dosage regimen as follows: ranibizumab every 28 days (ranibizumab/monthly), bevacizumab every 28 days (bevacizumab/monthly), ranibizumab only if there were signs of active neovascularization (ranibizumab/on-demand) and bevacizumab only if there were signs of active neovascularization (bevacizumab/on-demand).

Doses of 0.5 mg (0.05 ml) of ranibizumab and 1.25 mg (0.05 ml) of bevacizumab were used. The primary objective of this non-inferiority study was to assess the mean change in visual acuity one year after the baseline visit by means of ETDRS testing. Secondary objectives were the proportion of patients with a change in visual acuity of ≥15 letters, the number of injections, the changes in fluid and foveal thickness as per OCT, the change in lesion size as per fluorescein angiography, the incidence of both ocular and systemic adverse events, and the analysis of annual cost for each drug.

The study revealed that the results for monthly administration of bevacizumab were equal to those for monthly administration of ranibizumab, with a letter gain of 8.0 and 8.5, respectively. "On demand" treatment regimen showed the same results for bevacizumab and ranibizumab, with a letter gain of 5.9 and 6.8, respectively. The results for "on-demand" ranibizumab regimen were equal to those for monthly ranibizumab regimen. However, the comparison between "on demand" and monthly treatment regimens with bevacizumab was not conclusive (it did not reach non-inferiority level), and the same happened with the comparison of "on demand" bevacizumab and monthly ranibizumab regimens [30].

TREX-AMD (Treat and Extend Protocol in Patients with Wet Age-Related Macular Degeneration) is a phase 3b, multicenter, randomized clinical trial. Sixty subjects were randomized to monthly or TREX cohorts with intravitreal ranibizumab. Two-year prospective trial results demonstrated that the treat and extend neovascular AMD management strategy resulted in visual anatomic gains comparable to those obtained with monthly dosing [31].

In 2011, the use of aflibercept (VEGF Trap-Eye) was approved by the FDA. This is a fusion protein that binds to all isoforms of VEGF with higher affinity than ranibizumab and bevacizumab.

This increase in VEGF binding activity was expected to reduce injection frequency. This advanced the VIEW 1 and 2 studies [11, 15, 17].

VIEW 1 and VIEW 2. The efficacy and safety of Eylea were assessed in two multicenter, randomized, double-blind active-controlled trials on patients with exudative AMD. A total of 2412 efficacy-evaluable patients were treated (1817 were treated with Eylea). Patients' age ranged between 49 and 99 (mean age = 76 years). In these clinical trials, approximately 89% of patients randomized to Eylea were ≥65 years old and approximately 63% were ≥75 years old. On each trial, patients were randomized to one of the following four dosage regimens: 1) 2 mg of Eylea every 8 weeks after the first 3 monthly doses (1 per month) (Eylea 2Q8); 2) 2 mg of Eylea every 4 weeks (Eylea 2Q4); 3) 0.5 mg of Eylea every 4 weeks (Eylea 0.5Q4); and 4) 0.5 mg of ranibizumab every 4 weeks (ranibizumab 0.5Q4).

During the second year, patients continued receiving the initially defined dose, but the dosage regimen was modified according to the results of visual and anatomical tests, with a maximum dosage interval of 12 weeks defined as per protocol.

On both trials, the primary efficacy endpoint was the rate of patients on the set per protocol who maintained visual acuity, *i.e.* who lost <15 letters from baseline at week 52.

At week 52 of the VIEW 1 study, 95.1% of patients in the Eylea 2Q8 group had maintained vision vs. 94.4% of patients in the ranibizumab 0.5Q4 group.

At week 52 of the VIEW 2 study, 95.6% of patients in the Eylea 2Q8 group had maintained vision vs. 94.4% of patients in the ranibizumab 0.5Q4 group. In both trials, Eylea treatment was proved to be non-inferior and clinically equivalent to the ranibizumab 0.5Q4 dosage regimen.

According to the analysis of combined data from VIEW 1 and VIEW 2 trials, Eylea showed clinically significant changes as regards the baseline value for the predefined secondary efficacy endpoint corresponding to NEI VFQ-25 (National Eye Institute Visual Function Questionnaire), while no clinically relevant differences were observed for ranibizumab. The scale of these changes was similar to that observed in published studies, which corresponds to a 15-letter gain in best-corrected visual acuity (BCVA).

During the second year, efficacy was generally maintained until the last assessment on week 96; 2-4% of patients required all injections on a monthly basis and a third part of patients required at least one injection on a monthly basis [32].

All study groups in both trials evidenced a marked decrease in the mean area of choroidal neovascularization (CNV).

Efficacy results for all evaluable subgroups of each trial (for example, age, sex, race, baseline visual acuity, type of lesion, size of the lesion) and in the analysis of combined data matched the results for global populations [32].

Diabetic Macular Edema (DME): It is the leading cause of moderate vision loss in diabetic patients and can present in any stage of retinopathy. It is defined as a clinical picture characterized by retinal thickening in the macular area that may or may not be accompanied by hard exudates (Fig. **5**). Its pathogenesis is complex and multifactorial. It results from the disruption of the inner blood-retinal barrier, although the incompetence of the RPE (the outer blood-retinal barrier) observed in diabetic patients or the presence of a mechanical traction factor can also contribute to this disease. VEGF is an important mediator of blood-retinal barrier disruption that leads to intravascular fluid leakage into the extravascular space and to the development of macular edema.

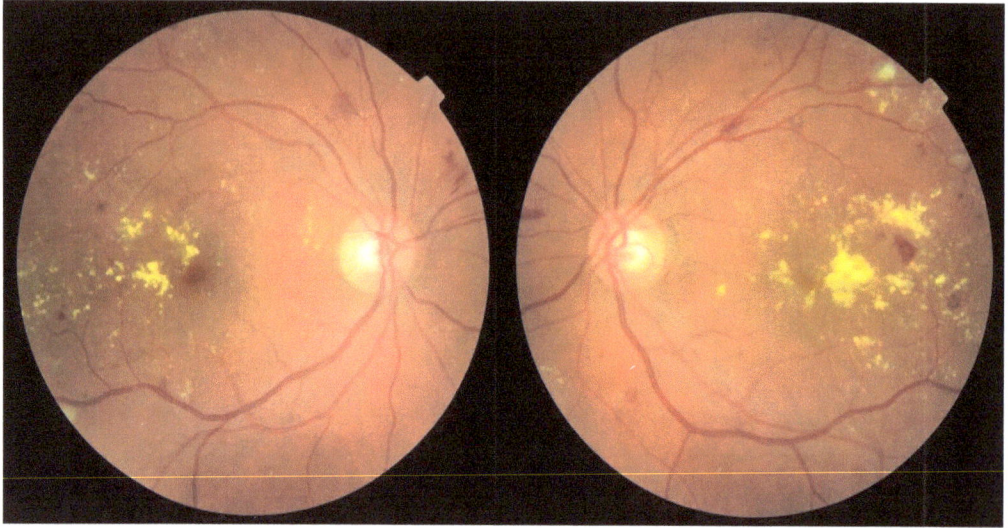

Fig. (5). Diabetic macula edema. Fundus photographs showing retinal hemorrhages and multiple hard exudates.

Among DME risk factors, we can mention systemic hypertension, hyperlipidemia and hyperglycemia. Other risk factors are cardiovascular diseases, kidney failure, advanced diabetic retinopathy, and vitreomacular traction syndrome.

The initial results of the Early Treatment Diabetic Retinopathy Study (ETDRS) on laser efficacy and safety for the treatment of DME have barely suffered changes three decades after its publication. Results are positive regarding focal edema, but the effectiveness decreases for diffuse edema. In general, it can be said that early laser treatment reduces the risk of moderate vision loss (loss of 15 or more letters) in 50% of patients with DME. On the other hand, it is worth mentioning that this is a destructive procedure and there is a risk for complications. Based on evidence of dysregulation of VEGF as an alternative to DME drug treatment [7, 17].

Ranibizumab (IVR, Lucentis; Genentech Inc./Novartis) belongs to a drug class that inhibits VEGF-A activity, which reduces edema and stabilizes or improves vision. It has European Medicines Agency (EMA) marketing authorization for the treatment of visual impairment due to diabetic macular edema in adults, and it has been recommended by the National Institute for Health Care and Excellence

(NICE) in April 2013 as an alternative treatment for patients with central retinal thickness of 400 microns or more at the beginning of treatment.

The following are the four randomized clinical trials carried out by the NICE as proof of clinical efficacy: RESTORE (ranibizumab monotherapy or combined with laser versus laser monotherapy for diabetic macular edema), RESOLVE (safety and efficacy of ranibizumab in diabetic macular edema), and READ-2 (ranibizumab for diabetic macular edema).

The FDA approved intravitreal ranibizumab for the treatment of DME based on Genentech, RISE and RIDE phase III clinical trials.

The NICE suggests the administration of up to 0.5 mg ranibizumab as intravitreal injection per month until maximum visual acuity is achieved; the "stability" criterion is defined as stable VA for three consecutive months. The FDA has approved the lowest dose of 0.3 mg per month for the treatment of DME.

The intraocular use of bevacizumab (IVB, Avastin, Genentech Inc.) has not been approved, but it is a much cheaper alternative. Several randomized clinical trials conclude that visual acuity improves (BCVA ETDRS ≥ 15 letters) with IVB in comparison to laser therapy, although the effect size is smaller as follow-up time is increased.

Aflibercept (IVA, Eylea; Regeneron/Bayer HealthCare) was recently added to the anti-VEGF class. The DA VINCI Study Group published the results corresponding to one year comparing different doses and dosing regimens of IVA against macular laser in DME patients, and demonstrated visual acuity showed a clinically significant improvement. Other two similar clinical trials (VISTA and VIVID) revealed equally encouraging results [7, 17, 19].

The DRCR Network (DRCR.net) is a collaborative network dedicated to facilitating multicenter clinical research of diabetic retinopathy, diabetic macular edema and other retinal diseases. Recently, results of Protocol I and T, conducted by DRCR.net were published.

PROTOCOL I: Intravitreal ranibizumab with prompt or deferred (≥ 24 weeks) focal/grid laser is more effective through 2 years in increasing visual acuity compared with focal/grid laser treatment alone for the treatment of DME involving the central macula.

Focal/grid laser treatment at the initiation of intravitreal ranibizumab is no better, and possibly worse, for vision outcomes than deferring laser treatment for 24 weeks or more in eyes with DME involving the fovea and with vision impairment [33].

PROTOCOL T: The 2-year clinical trial compared 3 drugs for diabetic macular edema (DME) and found that gains in vision were greater for participants receiving the drug aflibercept than for those receiving bevacizumab, but only among participants starting treatment with 20/50 or worse vision. At one year aflibercept had superior gains to ranibizumab in this vision subgroup, however a difference could not be identified at 2 years. The 3 drugs yielded similar gains in vision for patients with 20/32 or 20/40 vision at the start of treatment.

Two-year results of Protocol T study show that about half the number of anti-VEGF injections needed to treat diabetic macular edema in the first year of the study were needed in the second year, regardless of which study agent was used [34].

Retinal Vein Occlusion (RVO): After diabetic retinopathy, this is the second cause of retinal vascular disease leading to substantial vision loss. It is characterized by intravascular or extravascular occlusion resulting in hemorrhages (Fig. **6**), fluid exudation and ischemia with different levels of severity. Such vascular damage is accompanied by an inflammatory response cascade that makes it difficult for normal regulatory mechanisms to interact. Ischemia-induced production of diverse cytokines will lead to the formation of new blood vessels and the increase of capillary permeability, and therefore promote macular edema RVO patients present high VEGF and IL-6 values [35, 36].

Depending on the location of the occlusion, RVO can be categorized as central retinal vein occlusion (CRVO) or branch retinal vein occlusion (BRVO).

It can be divided in two types: ischemic and nonischemic, regardless of whether it is CRVO or BRVO. Ischemic RVO is associated with significant loss of visual acuity and a poor prognosis, since it entails complications like macular edema, retinal neovascularization and neovascular glaucoma. In 16% of cases, perfused RVO may progress to ischemia.

Macular edema is present in most cases of CRVO and it occurs in 5-15% of eyes with BRVO [35, 36].

The treatment for macular edema due to retinal vein occlusion has changed significantly over the past decade. According to the guidelines provided by the Central and Branch Vein Occlusion Study Groups, for many years, macular edema in CRVO was observed, while in BRVO grid laser photocoagulation was applied. Panphotocoagulation of the ischemic retina is indicated both for BRVO and CRVO when there is neovascularization in the iris, the retina or the optic disk. Intra- and extraocular administration of corticosteroids has been used to treat edema associated with RVO; the SCORE study results have validated this treatment for edema in CRVO and, at the same time, confirmed grid laser photocoagulation as a superior treatment for macular edema in BRVO.

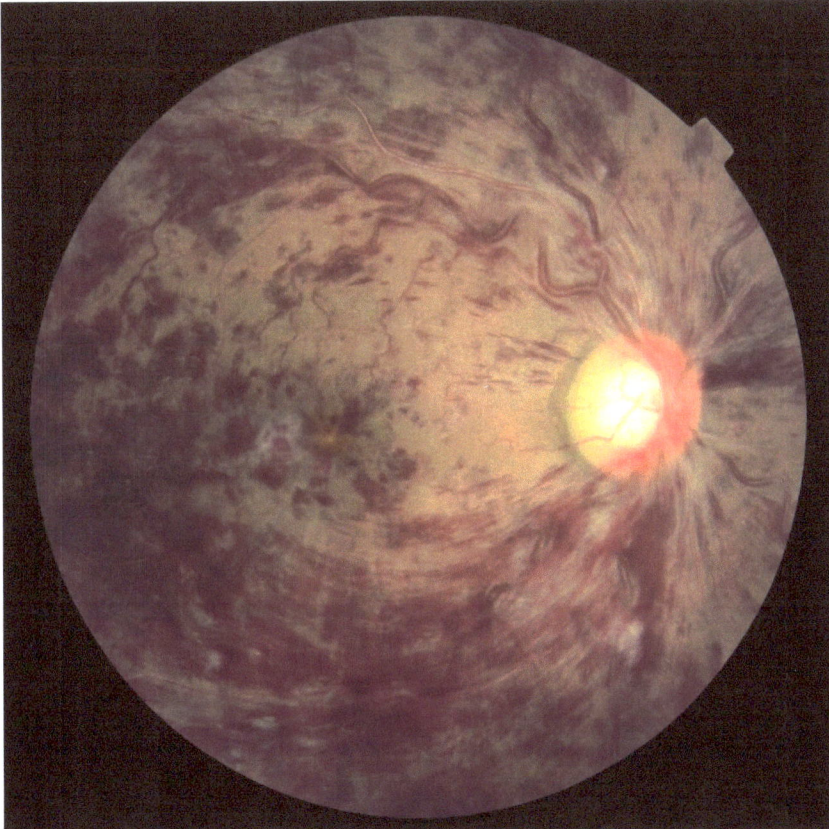

Fig. (6). Fundus photograph of Central Vein Occlusion. Multiples flamed and round retinal hemorrhages and tortuosity vascular vessels are showing.

More recently, longer-lasting results have been reported with dexamethasone intravitreal implant [35].

The anti-VEGF agents that are available nowadays (ranibizumab, aflibercept, and bevacizumab) have been used to reduce macular edema due to RVO and have been successful [11, 35].

In May 2013, the NICE recommended ranibizumab (Lucentis, Novartis) as a possible treatment for macular edema caused by retinal vein occlusion.

Indications include macular edema in CRVO or BRVO only in case of failure of grid laser photocoagulation or if this treatment is not appropriate due to the extension of the hemorrhage.

The CRUISE (central retinal vein occlusion) and BRAVO (branch retinal vein occlusion) multicenter studies, assessed the efficacy of ranibizumab in comparison to a sham procedure for the treatment of visual impairment caused by macular edema secondary to RVO. In brief, patients were randomized into three groups: 0.3 mg ranibizumab, 0.5 mg ranibizumab, and sham/0.5 mg ranibizumab. Patients were given a loading dose of 6 monthly injections and were then shifted to a PRN protocol. The study showed that after 12 months of follow-up there was a significant improvement in the VA in the ranibizumab-treated groups with a mean increase of 13.9 letters in both the 0.3 mg and the 0.5 mg dose compared with a mean of 7.3 letters in the sham/0.5 mg group. The visual gains achieved after the first 6 monthly doses could be maintained during the next 6 months using a PRN protocol [37].

An extension study for CRUISE was the HORIZON study which included 87% of patients who participated in the CRUISE trial. Follow-ups were set every 3 months and patients were injected if central foveal thickness (CFT) was >250 μm or there were signs of vision-threatening edema. At the end of the study VA gains in the sham/0.5 mg group were very similar to the 0.3 mg/0.5 mg group; however, this likely occurred because the 0.3/0.5 mg group had more loss in visual acuity compared to the sham/0.5 mg group over that period. Patients with CRVO had a mean number of 2.9, 3.8, and 3.5 injections in the sham/0.5 mg, the 0.3/0.5 mg, and 0.5 mg groups, respectively. The authors concluded that the loss in visual acuity was due to the longer 3-month follow-up period and the low number of injections. Perhaps a more suitable strategy would be monthly follow-up until patients reach stability and then extending follow-up periods gradually to ensure adequate treatment [38].

The RETAIN study was an extension trial for HORIZON. There were 32 patients who completed the HORIZON trial and were enrolled in the RETAIN study, out of which only 27 completed 2 years of follow-up, for a total of 4 years since the start of CRUISE. The patients gained an overall increase of 14 letters that was not statistically significant from the gains achieved at the end of CRUISE, suggesting most patients were able to maintain their gains throughout HORIZON and RETAIN [39].

In February 2014, the NICE recommended aflibercept (Eylea, Bayer) as a possible treatment for people with vision problems caused by macular edema due to central retinal vein occlusion. The use of aflibercept for the treatment of macular edema due to CRVO was particularly studied in COPERNICUS and GALILEO trials [7, 18, 35].

The CRAVE study compared efficacy of monthly treatment with bevacizumab or ranibizumab for macular edema due to retinal vein occlusion. The trial randomized 98 patients to treatment with bevacizumab or ranibizumab. At 6 months, there were no differences in change in central foveal thickness between groups. Both groups showed similar functional outcomes [40].

The SCORE 2 study investigated whether bevacizumab is noninferior to aflibercept for the treatment of macular edema secondary to central retinal or hemiretinal vein occlusion. This study demonstrated that intravitreal bevacizumab was noninferior to aflibercept with respect to visual acuity after 6 months of treatment [41].

Choroidal Neovascularization Secondary to Myopia: Myopia is a common multifactorial condition that affects 20-40% of world population. When the refractive error is over -6 diopters, myopia is considered high, and is usually associated with axial length of more than 26 mm. Its global prevalence is 0.5-5%. Systemic associations of high myopia include preterm birth and Down, Ehlers-Danlos, Knobloch, Marfan, Noonan, Pierre-Robin, and Stickler syndromes.

Pathologic myopia, also called degenerative myopia, is characterized by an excessive lengthening of the globe and pathological changes associated with the posterior pole, such as choroidal fundus, posterior staphyloma and myopic cone. It has a 0.9-3.1% prevalence and, according to studies, it is considered the main cause for blindness in 7% and 12-27% of European and Asian populations, respectively [42].

Choroidal neovascularization (CNV) is one of the complications of pathologic myopia and it occurs in 5.2-11.3% of patients with high myopia. Clinically, myopic CNV may be associated with underlying abnormalities, like focal chorioretinal atrophy or disruption of the RPE-Bruch's membrane-choriocapillaris complex, known as "lacker cracks". Patients usually present with reduced visual acuity, central scotoma or metamorphopsia.

Pathogenesis of myopic CNV is still not fully understood, but it is believed that it implies an imbalance of proangiogenic and antiangiogenic factors, caused by the mechanical stress of the progressively stretching retina.

Before the anti-VEGF therapy was implemented, the treatment for myopic CNV was mainly laser photocoagulation for extrafoveal CNV and verteporfin photodynamic therapy for subfoveal CNV [42].

In November 2013, the NICE approved Ranibizumab (Lucentis) for the treatment of choroidal neovascularization associated with pathologic myopia in the United Kingdom. Ranibizumab is the only anti-VEGF therapy that has been authorized for the treatment of myopic CNV, and it has proven to have a great potential for vision improvement and prevention of irreversible damage in the retina in phase II REPAIR and phase III RADIANCE clinical trials.

Intraocular use of Bevacizumab (Avastin) has not been approved and therefore lacks a safety and efficacy profile.

MYRROR, a phase III clinical trial, is currently trying to establish the role of aflibercept (Eylea) in the treatment of myopic CNV [18, 42].

Other Indications for Anti-VEGF Use

Since anti-VEGF agents were introduced in ophthalmology, they have been used to treat a wide variety of ocular pathologies, even without the corresponding license [11].

Choroidal Neovascularization (not AMD): A choroidal neovascular membrane may complicate any pathological process resulting in a defect in Bruch's membrane, and may represent a threat for vision through fluid leakage, hemorrhage and subretinal fibrosis. Anti-VEGF agents are now widely used for the treatment of CNV, regardless of its etiology. They have been successful in treating CNV related to angioid streaks, uveitis and trauma [7, 9].

Diabetic Retinopathy: According to the WHO, after the evolution of this disease over 15 years, 2% of diabetic patients are blind due to the development of diabetic retinopathy and another 10% suffers significant visual impairment as a consequence of macular edema.

Proliferative diabetic retinopathy (PDR) is the entity that is most commonly associated to retinal and optic disk neovascularization. Prolonged hyperglycemia induces oxidative stress in cells, which leads to the expression of altered genes and affects the normal metabolic pathways. It may cause glycosylation of proteins so their function is substantially altered and endothelial cells are damaged. Changes in retinal vasculature may eventually result in reduced perfusion of retinal tissue and retinal ischemia. This induces the activity of the hypoxia-inducible factor (HIF), which increases the expression of the VEGF and the transcription of several other angiogenic factors. Apart from the ischemic stimuli, the VEGF expression is also stimulated by other inflammatory mediators [9, 11].

Since the RPE-photoreceptor complex accounts for most of the oxygen consumption in the retina, laser photocoagulation therapy results in a reduced metabolic function of the retina, and a consequent decrease in the production of angiogenic factors. In spite of its benefits, it has adverse effects like loss of peripheral visual field, reduced night vision and exacerbation of macular edema.

Several anti-VEGF agents show a beneficial potential in PDR. Bevacizumab has shown some benefit as adjuvant therapy before vitrectomy in these patients, since it reduces the intraoperatory bleeding and postoperative vitreous hemorrhage. However, in cases of rapid regression and contraction of fibrovascular membranes after treatment with anti-VEGF agents, progressive tractional retinal detachments have been reported [11].

Protocol S conducted by DRCR.net involved 394 study eyes with PDR who were randomly assigned to panretinal photocoagulation (PRP) or intravitreous ranibizumab (0.5 mg). The two-year primary outcome results demonstrated that the eyes assigned to ranibizumab had visual acuity that was non-inferior to eyes managed with PRP [42].

Recently FDA approved Lucentis® intravitreal injection of 0.3 mg for the monthly treatment of all forms of diabetic retinopathy based on an analysis of the Diabetic Retinopathy Clinical Research Network's Protocol S study [44].

Retinopathy of Prematurity (ROP): It refers to neovascularization that occurs in the peripheral retina of preterm infants. It continues to be the leading cause of blindness in the pediatric population [11, 15].

In the normal development of the retina, relative ischemia of the peripheral retina encourages the migration of vasculogenic precursors from the optic nerve. In preterm infants, one the factors involved in ROP pathogenesis is supplemental oxygen therapy in high concentrations. This treatment eliminates normal hypoxia of the peripheral retina in this stage of development and reduces the stimulus for normal neovascularization. Therefore, when the oxygen therapy is stopped, the avascular retina upregulates VEGF production, which leads to peripheral neovascularization [2, 3, 8, 10, 11, 15].

Cryotherapy of peripheral ischemic retina and laser photocoagulation are some of the preventive treatment options. These treatments destroy most of the cells that produce VEGF in the retina.

The use of anti-VEGF for ROP is an emerging therapy, and the reason may be that a consistent production of VEGF has been demonstrated [8, 10, 15].

Series of cases in which intravitreal bevacizumab has been used, both as monotherapy and in combination with traditional laser therapy or vitrectomy, in patients with stage 3+, 4, and 5 ROP have revealed encouraging results in stage 3, but not so in stages 4 and 5 since membrane contraction may worsen retinal detachment [10].

Sickle Cell Retinopathy: Sickle cell anemia (Hb SS) is a homozygous recessive disorder. It is the result of the substitution of a hemoglobin aminoacid, glutamic acid for valine substitution, which causes polymerization of deoxygenated hemoglobin and the formation of sickle red blood cells. It is believed that rigid, extended, sickle-shaped red blood cells cause mechanical microvascular occlusions, leading to retinal ischemia. Neovascularization happens in the boundaries of ischemic and nonischemic tissue of the peripheral retina, and is generally described as having a sea-fan shape, but this is not pathognomonic.

In many cases, proliferative sickle cell retinopathy regresses naturally due to auto-infarction of the neovasculature, and therefore the need for therapeutic intervention can be avoided.

The goal of the available treatment options is to prevent advanced lesions from the development of vitreous hemorrhages or retinal detachments. Laser photocoagulation of the ischemic retina and tissue around the sea fan may favor regression of neovascularization and may reduce angiogenic factors, thus preventing complications in the late stage of the disease. Cryotherapy is used to treat the peripheral ischemic retina when it is not possible to use laser therapy due to poor visualization caused by media opacity.

Large-scale clinical trials to assess the benefits of antiangiogenic agents in proliferative sickle cell retinopathy have not been carried out yet [3, 7].

Central Serous Chorioretinopathy: Central serous chorioretinopathy (CSC) is a well-characterized disorder leading to serous neurosensory elevation of the central macula. The acute form of the disease is associated with focal leakage at the level of the retinal pigment epithelium (RPE) demonstrated with fluorescein angiography (Fig. **7**). Fortunately, the disorder is self-limited in the majority of patients, who also regain excellent vision. Occasionally, the neurosensory detachment persists and leads to pigment epithelial and photoreceptor damage with visual impairment [45]. When the signs and symptoms become chronic, treatment is necessary. Laser selective photocoagulation, photodynamic therapy and anti-VEGF treatment are options of treatment for these cases.

Iijima H. *et al.* hypothesized that the choroidal circulatory disturbance in CSC is caused by impaired fibrinolysis and the resulting thrombotic occlusion in the choroidal veins [45]. Although VEGF levels are not elevated in aqueous samples from CSC eyes, some have hypothesized that hypoxic conditions in the choroid or RPE could lead to compartmentalized VEGF expression not detected in aqueous samples. Given this hypothesis and the remarkable success of these drugs in other disorders, numerous small trials have been undertaken.

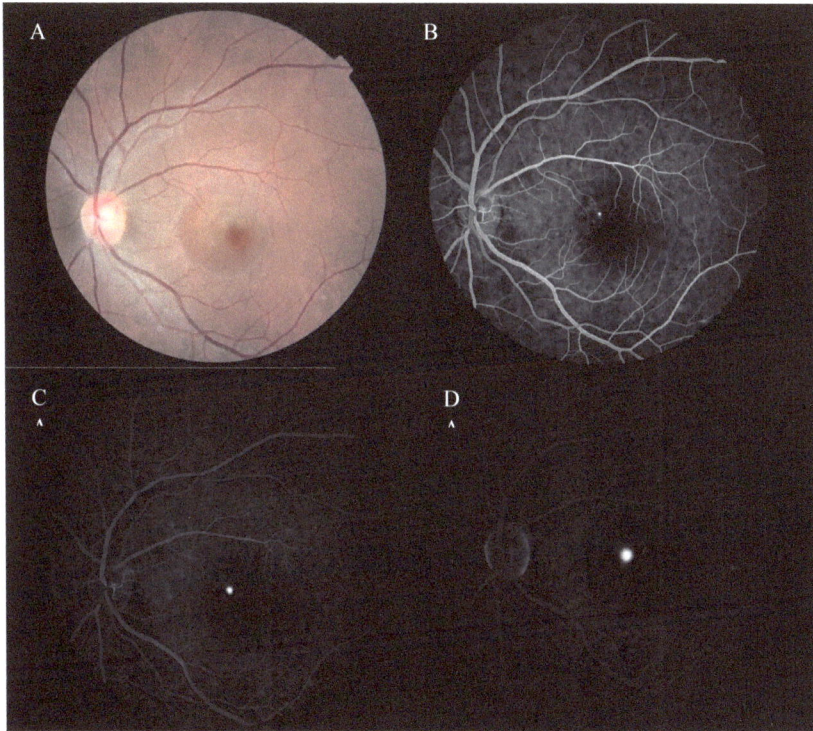

Fig. (7). Central Serous Chorioretinopathy. **A.** Fundus photograph of left eye with serous neurosensory elevation of the central macula. **B-D.** Fluorescein angiography demonstrated focal leakage.

There is evidence of multiples studies that demonstrated intravitreal bevacizumab effectiveness and safety in CSC [45 - 48]; however, large and controlled clinical trials are necessary.

FUTURE THERAPIES

Nowadays, there is an increased interest in the use of anti-PDGF and anti-VEGF combination therapy for the treatment of age-related macular degeneration. This is reasonable since many trials have revealed a poor response of the neovascular structure to anti-VEGF therapy when pericytes create a barrier on proliferating blood vessels.

Ophthotech is conducting three large-scale phase III trials using Fovista anti-PDGF in combination with an anti-VEGF (Ophthotech is neutral about the choice of the anti-VEGF). Although the results are not yet available, previous phase II studies conducted by Ophthotech have proven the effectiveness of anti-VEGF/Fovista combined therapy.

Other companies working on combination therapies for retinal diseases are undertaking controlled trials in humans. Regeneron is studying a combination of Eylea and an anti-PDGF that can be formulated as a single injection. Regeneron is also announcing, along with Bayer, the development of an Angiopoyetina (Ang2) antibody formulated with Eylea in a single injection as a potential therapy for wet AMD. Ang2 is a vascular endothelial growth factor that has been proven to contribute to the development of lymphatic and blood vessels in the eye according to pre-clinical trials.

Allergan is developing a treatment for wet AMD consisting of a combination of an anti-VEGF called DARPin with an anti-PDGF.

Allegro Ophthalmics has designed a peptide integrin called Luminate, whose mechanism of action is meant to stop vascular proliferation in early stages. The company is studying Luminate in the pre-clinical stage in combination with Avastin, and Luminate monotherapy for wet AMD. In previous studies, Luminate has shown a long-lasting response: up to 6 months with a single injection.

Ophthea (Melbourne, Australia) is the novelty regarding combined therapies. Its drug, OPT-302, blocks VEGF-A, VEGF-C and VEGF-D, while not inhibiting VEGF-B, which has a neuroprotective role. Ophthea's drug for the treatment of wet AMD completely inhibits VEGF, especially when used in combination with Lucentis or Eylea. A phase I study on 20 patients has revealed an excellent safety profile, both as monotherapy and in combination with Lucentis. OPT-302 is now being tested in a 30-patient phase IIa trial, which involves the study of its efficacy and durability, as well as the determination of the ideal dosage. This study features two arms: the monotherapy arm and the Lucentis combination therapy arm.

Ohr Pharmaceutical has conducted a phase II trial combining an anti-VEGF aminosterol agent called esqualamina (eye drops) with intravitreal Lucentis. A phase III trial has been scheduled.

The ones described above are the most important and promising initiatives as regards combined therapies. The concept of combined therapies is gaining increased consideration among the scientific community.

More recently, Aerpio Therapeutics has shown promising results in phase II clinical trials using a combined therapy for the treatment of AMD. The company reported successful 3-month results of the AHB-9778 small molecule, which restores proper functioning of the Tie2 receptor by inhibiting a tyrosine phosphatase enzyme, in combination with Lucentis.

The Encapsulated Cell Technology is another innovation that is being studied by Neurotech. It consists of a polymer implant that encompasses one or more microscopic reservoirs, which deliver a drug or a combination of drugs for up to two years, including anti-VEGF, anti-inflammatory drugs and/or a protein with therapeutic potential: Neurotech's ciliary neurotrophic factor (CNTF). Each of the implanted reservoirs can be opened individually at the retina specialist's discretion, which enables a continuous and sustained drug delivery. There have been promising clinical trials conducted in this field [49].

CONSENT FOR PUBLICATION

Not applicable.

CONFLICT OF INTEREST

The editor declares no conflict of interest, financial or otherwise.

ACKNOWLEDGEMENTS

Declared none

REFERENCES

[1]   Dombrow M, Adelman R. Ocular Angiogenesis: The Science Behind the Symptoms. Retinal Physician, January 2011.

[2]   Chan-Ling Tailoi, Gock Bronwyn, Stone Jonathan. The Effect of Oxygen on Vasoformative Cell Division. Ophthalmology and Visual Science, Vol 36 N°7, June 1995.

[3]   Patronas M, Coney J, Singerman LJ. Treating Neovascular Peripheral Retinal Diseases, Retinal Physician, October 2008.

[4]   Adamis AP, Aiello LP, D'Amato RA. Angiogenesis and ophthalmic disease. Angiogenesis 1999; 3(1): 9-14.
[http://dx.doi.org/10.1023/A:1009071601454] [PMID: 14517440]

[5]   Ciardella AP, Donsoff IM, Guyer DR, Adamis A, Yannuzzi LA. Antiangiogenesis agents. Ophthalmol Clin North Am 2002; 15(4): 453-8.
[http://dx.doi.org/10.1016/S0896-1549(02)00042-1] [PMID: 12515077]

[6]   Italiano JE Jr, Richardson JL, Patel-Hett S, *et al.* Angiogenesis is regulated by a novel mechanism: pro- and antiangiogenic proteins are organized into separate platelet α granules and differentially released. Blood 2008; 111(3): 1227-33.
[http://dx.doi.org/10.1182/blood-2007-09-113837] [PMID: 17962514]

[7]   Al-Latayfeh M, Silva PS, Sun JK, Aiello LP. Antiangiogenic therapy for ischemic retinopathies. Cold

Spring Harb Perspect Med 2012; 2(6): a006411.
[http://dx.doi.org/10.1101/cshperspect.a006411] [PMID: 22675660]

[8]   Quiroz-Mercado H, Martinez-Castellanos M, Hernandez-Rojas M. Antiangiogenic therapy with intravitreal Bevacizumab for retinopathy of prematurity, Retina. Journal of Rentinal and Vitreous Diseases 2008; 28(3)

[9]   Stefanini F R, Badaró E, Falabella P. Anti-VEGF for the management of diabetic macular edema. J Immunol Res 2014; ID 632307.

[10]   Torres Soriano ME, Reyna Castelán E, Hernández Rojas M, *et al.* Tractional retinal detachment after intravitreal injection of bevacizumab in proliferative diabetic retinopathy. RETINAL Cases and Brief Reports: Winter 2009 - Volume 3 - Issue 1 - pp 70-73.
[http://dx.doi.org/10.1097/ICB.0b013e3181578dd8]

[11]   Mintz-Hittner H, Kennedy K, Chuang A. Efficacy of intravitreal bevacizumab for stage 3+ retinopathy prematurity. N Engl J Med 2011; 364(7): 603-15.

[12]   Sitohy B, Nagy JA, Dvorak HF. Anti-VEGF/VEGFR therapy for cancer: reassessing the target. Cancer Res 2012; 72(8): 1909-14.
[http://dx.doi.org/10.1158/0008-5472.CAN-11-3406] [PMID: 22508695]

[13]   Hughes S, Yang H, Chan-Ling T. Vascularization of the human fetal retina: roles of vasculogenesis and angiogenesis. Invest Ophthalmol Vis Sci 2000; 41(5): 1217-28.
[PMID: 10752963]

[14]   He X, Cheng R, Benyajati S, Ma JX. PEDF and its roles in physiological and pathological conditions: implication in diabetic and hypoxia-induced angiogenic diseases. Clin Sci 2015; 128(11): 805-23.
[http://dx.doi.org/10.1042/CS20130463] [PMID: 25881671]

[15]   Kumar V, Abbas A, Fausto N. Robins y Cotran. Pathologic Basis of Disease, Elsevier España, séptima edición, 2007.

[16]   Raúl Vélez-Montoya, Jans Fromow-Guerra. Terapia antiangiogénica ocular: experiencia clínica en México. Gac Med Mex 2008; 144(3)

[17]   López-Gálvez MI, García-Campos JM. De la evidencia científica a la práctica clínica: pautas de tratamiento del edema macular diabético. Arch Soc Esp Oftalmol 2012; 87 (Suppl. 1): 38-45.
[http://dx.doi.org/10.1016/S0365-6691(12)70050-3]

[18]   Wecker T, Ehlken C, Bühler A, *et al.* Five-year visual acuity outcomes and injection patterns in patients with pro-re-nata treatments for AMD, DME, RVO and myopic CNV. Br J Ophthalmol 2016; 0: 1-7.
[PMID: 27215744]

[19]   Rosenfeld PJ, Brown DM, Heier JS, *et al.* Ranibizumab for neovascular age-related macular degeneration. N Engl J Med 2006; 355(14): 1419-31.
[http://dx.doi.org/10.1056/NEJMoa054481] [PMID: 17021318]

[20]   Brown DM, Kaiser PK, Michels M, *et al.* Ranibizumab versus verteporfin for neovascular age-related macular degeneration. N Engl J Med 2006; 355(14): 1432-44.
[http://dx.doi.org/10.1056/NEJMoa062655] [PMID: 17021319]

[21]   Regillo CD, Brown DM, Abraham P, *et al.* Randomized, double-masked, sham-controlled trial of ranibizumab for neovascular age-related macular degeneration: PIER Study year 1. Am J Ophthalmol 2008; 145(2): 239-48.
[http://dx.doi.org/10.1016/j.ajo.2007.10.004] [PMID: 18222192]

[22]   Monés J. Safety and tolerability of two dosing regimens of ranibizumab in patients with subfoveal choroidal neovascularization secondary to age-related macular degeneration: outcomes of the EXCITE study. XXVIth Meeting of the Club Jules Gonin.

[23]   Fung AE, Lalwani GA, Rosenfeld PJ, *et al.* An optical coherence tomography-guided, variable dosing

regimen with intravitreal ranibizumab (Lucentis) for neovascular age-related macular degeneration. Am J Ophthalmol 2007; 143(4): 566-83.
[http://dx.doi.org/10.1016/j.ajo.2007.01.028] [PMID: 17386270]

[24]   Holz FG, Meyer C, Eter N. Safety and efficacy of ranibizumab treatment in patients with neovascular age-related macular degeneration: 12-month results of the SUSTAIN study. 2009.

[25]   Boyer DS, Heier JS, Brown DM, Francom SF, Ianchulev T, Rubio RG. A Phase IIIb study to evaluate the safety of ranibizumab in subjects with neovascular age-related macular degeneration. Ophthalmology 2009; 116(9): 1731-9.
[http://dx.doi.org/10.1016/j.ophtha.2009.05.024] [PMID: 19643495]

[26]   Spaide R. Ranibizumab according to need: a treatment for age-related macular degeneration. Am J Ophthalmol 2007; 143(4): 679-80.
[http://dx.doi.org/10.1016/j.ajo.2007.02.024] [PMID: 17386275]

[27]   Berg K, Pedersen TR, Sandvik L, Bragadóttir R. Comparison of ranibizumab and bevacizumab for neovascular age-related macular degeneration according to LUCAS treat-and-extend protocol. Ophthalmology 2015; 122(1): 146-52.
[http://dx.doi.org/10.1016/j.ophtha.2014.07.041] [PMID: 25227499]

[28]   Singer MA, Awh CC, Sadda S, *et al.* HORIZON: an open-label extension trial of ranibizumab for choroidal neovascularization secondary to age-related macular degeneration. Ophthalmology 2012; 119(6): 1175-83.
[http://dx.doi.org/10.1016/j.ophtha.2011.12.016] [PMID: 22306121]

[29]   Sadda SR. HORIZON extension trial of ranibizumab [LUCENTIS] for neovascular age-related macular degeneration [AMD]: first-year safety and efficacy results. Retina Society Annual Meeting. Scottsdale, AZ, USA. 2008.

[30]   Martin DF, Maguire MG, Ying GS, Grunwald JE, Fine SL, Jaffe GJ. Ranibizumab and bevacizumab for neovascular age-related macular degeneration. N Engl J Med 2011; 364(20): 1897-908.
[http://dx.doi.org/10.1056/NEJMoa1102673] [PMID: 21526923]

[31]   Wykoff C. Monthly vs treat and extend for neovascular AMD: TREX-AMD 24-month outcomes. American Academy of Ophthalmology annual meeting. Oct. 14-18, 2016; Chicago.

[32]   Schmidt-Erfurth U, Kaiser PK, Korobelnik JF, *et al.* Intravitreal aflibercept injection for neovascular age-related macular degeneration: ninety-six-week results of the VIEW studies. Ophthalmology 2014; 121(1): 193-201.
[http://dx.doi.org/10.1016/j.ophtha.2013.08.011] [PMID: 24084500]

[33]   Elman MJ, *et al.* Diabetic Retinopathy Clinical Research Network. Expanded 2-year follow-up of ranibizumab plus prompt or deferred laser or triamcinolone plus prompt laser for diabetic macular edema. Ophthalmology 2011; 118: 609-14.

[34]   Wells JA, *et al.* DRCR.net Protocol T: At 2 years, Eylea, Avastin, Lucentis all reduce need for injections, improve visual acuity. Ophthalmology 2016.
[http://dx.doi.org/10.1016/j.ophtha.2016.02.022]

[35]   Ron A. Adelman, Aaron J. Parnes, Silvia Bopp, Ihab Saad Othman, and Didier Ducournau, "Strategy for the Management of Macular Edema in Retinal Vein Occlusion: The European VitreoRetinal Society Macular Edema Study," BioMed Research International, vol. 2015, Article ID 870987, 8 pages, 2015. doi:10.1155/2015/870987

[36]   Shchuko AG, Zlobin IV, Lureva TN, *et al.* Intraocular cytokines in retinal vein occlusion and its relation to the efficiency of anti-vascular endothelial growth factor therapy, Indian J Ophthalmol. 2015 Dec; 63(12): 905–911. doi: 10.4103/0301-4738.176031

[37]   Thach AB, Yau L, Hoang C, Tuomi L. Time to clinically significant visual acuity gains after ranibizumab treatment for retinal vein occlusion: BRAVO and CRUISE trials. Ophthalmology 2014; 121(5): 1059-66.

[http://dx.doi.org/10.1016/j.ophtha.2013.11.022] [PMID: 24424249]

[38]   Heier JS, Campochiaro PA, Yau L, *et al.* Ranibizumab for macular edema due to retinal vein occlusions: long-term follow-up in the HORIZON trial. Ophthalmology 2012; 119(4): 802-9.
[http://dx.doi.org/10.1016/j.ophtha.2011.12.005] [PMID: 22301066]

[39]   Campochiaro PA, Sophie R, Pearlman J, *et al.* RETAIN Study Group. Long-term outcomes in patients with retinal vein occlusion treated with ranibizumab: the RETAIN study. Ophthalmology 2014; 121(1): 209-19.
[http://dx.doi.org/10.1016/j.ophtha.2013.08.038] [PMID: 24112944]

[40]   Rajagopal R, Shah GK, Blinder KJ, *et al.* Bevacizumab Versus Ranibizumab in the Treatment of Macular Edema Due to Retinal Vein Occlusion: 6-Month Results of the CRAVE Study. Ophthalmic Surg Lasers Imaging Retina 2015; 46(8): 844-50.
[http://dx.doi.org/10.3928/23258160-20150909-09] [PMID: 26431300]

[41]   Scott IU, VanVeldhuisen PC, Ip MS, *et al.* SCORE2 Report 3: Effect of bevacizumab versus aflibercept on visual acuity among patients with macular edema due to central retinal vein occlusion 2017.

[42]   Ji L, Lv W, Xiao Y, Xu Z, Zhang X, Zhang W. Therapeutic effect of intravitreal injections of ranibizumab for the treatment of macular choroidal neovascularization caused by pathological myopia. Exp Ther Med 2015; 10(3): 1121-6.
[PMID: 26622450]

[43]   Gross JG, Glassman AR, Jampol LM, *et al.* Writing Committee for the Diabetic Retinopathy Clinical Research Network. Panretinal photocoagulation vs intravitreous ranibizumab for proliferative diabetic retinopathy: A randomized clinical trial. JAMA 2015; 314(20): 2137-46.
[http://dx.doi.org/10.1001/jama.2015.15217] [PMID: 26565927]

[44]   https://www.gene.com/media/press-releases/14661/2017-04-17/fda-approves-genentechs-lu-entis-ranibiz

[45]   Iijima H, Iida T, Murayama K, Imai M, Gohdo T. Plasminogen activator inhibitor 1 in central serous chorioretinopathy. Am J Ophthalmol 1999; 127(4): 477-8.
[http://dx.doi.org/10.1016/S0002-9394(98)00378-X] [PMID: 10218712]

[46]   Torres-Soriano ME, García-Aguirre G, Kon-Jara V, *et al.* A pilot study of intravitreal bevacizumab for the treatment of central serous chorioretinopathy (case reports). Graefes Arch Clin Exp Ophthalmol 2008; 246(9): 1235-9.
[http://dx.doi.org/10.1007/s00417-008-0856-x] [PMID: 18523796]

[47]   Torres Soriano ME, García Aguirre G, Gordon Angelozzi M, *et al.* Intravitreal Bevacizumab for the Treatment of Chronic or Recurrent Central Serous Chorioretinopathy. Open J Ophthalmol 2014; 4: 57-64.
[http://dx.doi.org/10.4236/ojoph.2014.43010]

[48]   Lim JW, Kim MU, Shin MC. Aqueous humor and plasma levels of vascular endothelial growth factor and interleukin-8 in patients with central serous chorioretinopathy. Retina 2010; 30(9): 1465-71.
[http://dx.doi.org/10.1097/IAE.0b013e3181d8e7fe] [PMID: 20526231]

[49]   Helzner J. Coming Advances in Retinal Disease Therapies (2016). Retinal Physician, Volume: 13, Issue: New Retinal Physician July / Aug 2016, page(s): 6-9.

CHAPTER 6

Molecular Targets of Angiogenesis and Future Potential of Anti-angiogensis Therapy in Multiple Sclerosis

Manisha J. Oza[1,2]**, Sachin V. Suryavanshi**[1]**, Mayuresh S. Garud**[1]**, Sandip T. Auti**[1]**, Ankit P. Laddha**[1] **and Yogesh A. Kulkarni**[1,*]

[1] *Shobhaben Pratapbhai Patel School of Pharmacy & Technology Management, SVKM's NMIMS, V.L. Mehta Road, Vile Parle (W), Mumbai-400056, India*

[2] *SVKM's Dr. Bhanuben Nanavati College of Pharmacy, V.L. Mehta Road, Vile Parle (W), Mumbai-400056, India*

Abstract: Multiple sclerosis (MS) is a chronic, inflammatory, gray and white matter demyelinating disease of the central nervous system characterized by axon degeneration, oligodendrocytes damage and astrogliosis. As per epidemiological data obtained from national multiple sclerosis society, 2.3 million people are suffering from MS worldwide. In America and Europe, it is a leading cause of mortality in young adults. The MS international federation reports showed that the prevalence of MS has been increased up to 33/10000 in 2013 from 30/10000 in 2008. Along with degenerative processes, such as axon damage and myelin sheaths destruction, inflammatory components, such as lymphocytes and macrophages also play pivotal role in the pathogenesis of MS. There is an infiltration of immune cells, macrophages and microglia, increased expression of cytokines and chemokines. The structural and functional changes in Blood Brain Barrier occur very commonly in MS.

Angiogenesis is a process of development of new blood vessels from the existing blood vessels. It is commonly involved in various CNS disorders, such as stroke, epilepsy and tumors, indicating that it might have a role in the progression of MS lesions. The inflammatory components involved in pathogenesis of MS have been observed to play significant role to support angiogenesis. Inter cellular cell adhesion molecule-1 (ICAM-1), vascular endothelial growth factor (VEGF), vascular cell adhesion molecule (VCAM) -1, matrix metalloproteinase -1, -2, -3, -7 and 9 (MMP-1,-2,-3,-7,-9), TNF-α /-β, Interferon – γ (IFN– γ) and many other components are involved in angiogenesis processes of MS. Moreover, MMPs and VEGF play significant role in vascular basement membrane degradation and breakdown of BBB in MS. This indicates that there is a firm link between angiogenesis and chronic inflammation for neovascularization in the progression of MS. Since the inflammation and angiogenic processes are very complex and involve multiple biochemical processes, there are

* **Corresponding author Yogesh A. Kulkarni:** Associate Professor, Shobhaben Pratapbhai Patel School of Pharmacy & Technology Management, SVKM's NMIMS,, V.L. Mehta Road, Vile Parle (W), Mumbai- 400056, India; Tel: +91 9930030548; Email: yogeshkulkarni101@yahoo.com

Atta-ur-Rahman & Mohammad Iqbal Choudhary (Eds.)

several molecular targets associated with angiogenesis for therapeutic intervention in MS.

Thus, the aim of the present chapter will be to show the link between angiogenesis and inflammatory processes in the progression of multiple sclerosis. Furthermore, the chapter is also focused on the role of molecular targets of angiogenesis process in MS along with their inhibitors or activators from various sources.

Keywords: Angiogenesis, Blood brain barrier, Demyelination, Experimental autoimmune encephalomyelitis, Hypoxia, Immune cells, Integrins, Interferon, Matrix metalloproteinase, Minocycline, Multiple sclerosis, Quercetin, Vascular endothelial growth factor.

INTRODUCTION

Multiple sclerosis (MS) is an inflammatory neurological disorder characterized by demyelination of neurons and neurodegeneration [1 - 3]. It is known as autoimmune disease that involves both T cells and B cells, causing destruction of oligodendrocytes and CNS myelin which leads to axonal loss [4]. In the pathogenesis of MS, both environmental and genetic factors play major role [5]. The number of people suffering from MS is higher as many people remain undiagnosed throughout the world; approximately 2.3 million people are suffering from MS worldwide. The rate of occurrence of MS in women is double as compared to men which shows the role of hormones in pathogenesis of disease. The rate of prevalence is highest in North America and Europe, while it is unheard in New Zealand and Australia [6].

MS is an immune-mediated disease, a bacterium, virus or other toxin can trigger the immune response against myelin antigens like proteolipid protein, myelin/oligodendrocytes glycoprotein, myelin basic protein, myelin-associated glycoprotein, phosphodiesterases, αB-crystallin, and gangliosides [7, 8]. The plaque formation first starts in the optic nerve, brainstem, spinal cord white matter tracts and cerebral periventricular white matter. Infiltration of inflammatory cells and production of inflammatory cytokines, proteases, generation of free radicals collectively damage myelin and oligodendrocytes and lead to demyelination and result into slow conduction or conduction block [9]. Long-lasting demyelination causes axonal loss which is responsible for chronic, progressive and non-remitting symptoms of MS [7]. Acute MS lesions show the presence of T cells, intense myelin-laden macrophages, B cells, perivascular inflammatory cell infiltrates and plasma cells. Inflammation in active lesion of MS is also responsible for axonal damage [10].

Angiogenesis is a complex, vital and highly regulated process of new blood vessels formation from pre-existing blood vessels not just under physiological conditions but also in various diseases, such as diabetic retinopathy, rheumatoid arthritis, cancer, stroke, epilepsy and other neurological disorders like MS [11 - 13]. Neurons and glial cells are the important cellular components of the central nervous system which requires continuous blood supply to function properly. Blood vessels supplying blood to the brain have specialized protective feature *i.e.* blood brain barrier which restricts the permeability of unwanted molecules from blood to the neuronal structures [14]. Angiogenesis process in the CNS is associated with a series of programmed changes in the endothelial cells to form a tight barrier to maintain CNS homeostasis [15]. It is evident that angiogenesis plays a vital role in MS. Alteration in permeability of blood brain barrier (BBB) and transmigration of mediators and lymphocytes into the CNS is an initial event in the pathogenesis of MS [15]. Alteration of pericytes, vascular basement membrane and modification in the expression of endothelial tight junction proteins have been reported in acute and progressive form of MS [16 - 19]. The preferred location of inflammatory lesions in multiple sclerosis is the sub ventricular zone of the brain, specifically in neurovascular niches and the temporary vascular niches, where angiogenesis is fostering along with neurogenesis [16].

ANGIOGENESIS IN MULTIPLE SCLEROSIS

Angiogenesis is a multifaceted and stepwise process which results into formation of new blood vessels by endothelial cells stimulation, proliferation and migration [20]. Endothelial cells remain dormant throughout their life, however, these cells are able to divide and migrate themselves in some physiological or pathological conditions and initiate the process of angiogenesis [21]. Angiogenesis process activates by angiogenic stimulus, such as hypoxia or injury which leads to activation of degradation processes [22]. The process of angiogenesis can be illustrated into three major steps *i.e.* basement membrane breakdown by substances called proteolytic enzymes, than angiogenic factors causes migration and proliferation of endothelial cells and finally adhesion molecules perform the function of cell matrix and cell-cell interactions [23].

The endothelial cells of the existing blood vessels degrade the basement membrane and enter into the stroma of adjusting tissue. Plasminogen activator system (PAs)(*i.e.* tPA and uPA) and MMPs (Matrix metalloproteinases -group of enzymes which remodel the ECM) play vital role in these processes [24]. First inactive uPAs are activated by cathepsin B, Plasmin or Factor XIIa after binding of uPA with their receptor uPAR on different cells, and lead to signal transduction for cell migration and invasion through uPAR [25]. Additionally, PAs also convert plasminogen into plasmin which activates MMPs. MMP-9 releases VEGF from proteoglycan matrix. MMPs are associated with various functions, such as endothelial cell invasions, migration and capillary tube formation in the angiogenesis cascade. The functions of MMPs in angiogenesis depend on the organ or tissue from which the endothelial cells are obtained [11]. The endothelial cells start migration and proliferation after extracellular matrix degradation and these processes are stimulated by various growth factors, such as VEGF, angiopoietins, cytokines, chemokines, FGF-2, TNF-α, TNF-β, PGDF released from degraded extracellular matrix [26, 27]. Along with these growth factors, cell adhesion molecules, like selectin, cadherin, intercellular adhesion molecule-1(ICAM-1), vascular cell adhesion molecule-1 (VCAM-1) and integrin also play pivotal role in endothelial cell invasion, migration as well as proliferation [28].

The initial event in the pathogenesis of MS is the migration of lymphocytes and other mediators into the CNS because of alteration in the permeability of blood brain barrier. Blood-brain barrier (BBB) is a multifarious structure of pericytes, basal lamina and cerebral endothelial cells and surrounded by perivascular macrophages and astrocytes [29]. In the inflammatory conditions, as observed in the pathogenesis of MS, adherens junctions and tight junctions deregulation leads to loss of BBB permeability [30]. Various study reports showed that angiogenesis is linked with disruption of blood brain barrier [31 - 33]. The important factors responsible for alteration in BBB permeability are angiogenesis mediators, such as VEGF, HIF- α, MMPs, TNF-α, interleukin1 and interferon-γ [34]. Various reports showed that in MS increased angiogenesis leads to increase in the level of angiogenesis mediators, such as VEGF and HIF- α and MMPs which are responsible for degradation of tight junctions, which are associated with maintenance of BBB permeability [31 - 33]. This indicates persistent angiogenesis which is responsible for the deleterious effect on brain tissue mainly because of alteration in the permeability adhesion molecules, like selectin, cadherin, intercellular adhesion of BBB. Proliferation of endothelial cells and increase in vascular network due to angiogenesis have been reported in demyelinating lesions of MS [35]. Angiogenesis further contributes to disease progression by affecting normal appearing white matter and grey matter (NAGM) [36]. In demyelinated axon of MS the energy requirement for impulse conduction is increased along with reduction in axonal ATP production and inducing a virtual hypoxia condition in demyelinated axons which is a stimulator of the angiogenic reaction in normal appearing white matter (NAWM) in MS [37].

MOLECULAR TARGETS OF ANGIOGENESIS IN MS

Hypoxia and Hypoxia-Inducible Factor-1 (HIF-1)

Hypoxia-Inducible Factor-1(HIF-1) is a transcription factor composed of two subunits *i.e.* HIF-1α and HIF-1β proteins. These heterodimeric complexes having helix-loop-helix-per-ARNT-Sim motif, can bind to DNA and causes dimerization of subunits [38]. α-subunit of HIF is rapidly degraded in oxygenated cells because of the presence of oxygen dependent degradation domain present on HIF-1α, where hydroxylation of two proline residues activates ubiquitin ligase proteasomal pathway and degrade HIF-1α [39], whereas, in the hypoxia condition, hydroxylation of the proline residue present on HIF-1α does not occur and this subunit becomes stable. The stabilized form of HIF-1α binds to the HIF-1β and other co-activators like p300/CBP, which ultimately bind to hypoxia responsive element of DNA and starts transcription of the genes involved in angiogenesis [40]. This shows that HIF-1α accumulation is the prerequisite for the activation of HIF-1 and activation of HIF-1 further leads to increased angiogenesis [41, 42]. After activation, HIF-1 translocates to the nucleus and stimulates VEGF transcription and also induces the expression of many other mediators, such as neuropilin-1, VEGFR1, angiopoietins-2, VEGFR2, nitric oxide synthase, PDGF, TGF- β, cyclooxygenase (Fig. **1**) and many more other mediators associated with angiogenesis [43, 44].

Fig. (1). Angiogenesis and multiple sclerosis.

The report shows that in active MS lesion state hypoxia is observed due to a number of changes in the local environment of the lesion. Noticeable increase in the expression of HIF-1α in the MS lesions has been demonstrated by Lassmann and coworkers [45]. Roscoe *et al.* also demonstrated increased expression of HIF-1α in EAE mice, along with other genes associated with cell migration through BBB disruption [46]. In MS lesion, demyelination causes switch of salutatory conduction of impulse to continuous conduction. This leads to increased expression of leaky Na+ channels in the demyelinated axolemma and the energy demand of the tissue increases and depletes the tissue oxygen level which in turn promotes degeneration of axon *via* virtual hypoxia condition [37]. The increased level of NO has been observed in MS lesion due to increased level of inducible nitric oxide synthase, and results into inhibition of mitochondrial respiration. The consequences of these conditions in MS lesions ultimately results into hypoxia and finally increase in angiogenic processes in MS [47, 48]. HIF-1α further degrades extracellular matrix through endothelial cells migration and activation *via* upregulating MMP-2 [49]. The *in-vitro* study data shows that expression of HIF-1α in endothelial cells increases the development of endothelial tubes [50]. The study reports show that in the astrocytes and microglia of the spinal cord of the experimental EAE mice showed increased expression of HIF-1α in the peak level of the disease [51]. Exacerbation of vascular permeability and inflammatory responses is a result of HIF-1α expression in MS [52, 53]. It has been reported that HIF-1 α has desirable or undesirable effect in inflammatory demyelination, depending on its expression in the cell type. Activation and expression of HIF-1 α increases BBB opening and permeability and worsen the pathological condition by infiltration of inflammatory cells. However, HIF-1 α also protects oligodendrocytes, which indicates that future studies are required to find out the effect of HIF-1 α on T-cell subsets and other glial cell types to observe the effect of HIF-1 α in MS [54].

Matrix Metalloproteinases (MMPs)

Matrixins or MMPs are a huge zinc dependent proteolytic enzyme family expressed in response to inflammatory condition and capable to degrade component of extracellular matrix [55]. There are total 23 known MMPs which are classified as gelatinases (MMP-2 & MMP-9), stromelysins (MMP-3, 10 & 11), collagenases (MMP-1, 8,13 & 18), membrane type MMPs (MMP-14 to 17, 24 & 28), matrilysins (MMP-7 & 26) and unnamed type (MMP-11, 12, 19-21, 23, 27 & 28) [56]. MMPs are neutral proteases which mainly affect extracellular matrix components, like elastin, fibronectin, collagen and laminin [57]. MMPs are secreted in inactive form and activated after proteolytic cleavage [58]. The structure of MMPs contains mainly three important binding sites which mainly include predomain, catalytic domain *i.e.* zinc binding site and hemopexin, like domain. Zinc binds to the catalytic site so that the enzyme remains in an inactive zymogen state until the proteolytic cleavage [59]. MMPs are associated with destruction of many tissues thus the expression as well as activity of MMPs must be tightly regulated and this function is done by tissue inhibitors of metalloproteinases (TIMPs) [60].

MMPs are secreted by macrophages, activated T cells and ECs [61]. MMPs are unconditionally essential for angiogenesis. MMPs contribute significantly in pro-angiogenesis and antiangiogenic processes. In physiological angiogenesis, MMPs activity is tightly controlled by MMP inhibitors and balances the process of angiogenesis, while in pathological angiogenesis, this balance is disturbed [62]. MMPs allow the invasion of neighboring stroma into the endothelial cells *via* breaking down vascular basement membrane after pro-angiogenic stimulation [63]. MMPs participate in the migration of endothelial cells and in fibrin barrier invasion. MMP-7 increases proliferation of endothelial cells along with up regulating MMP-1 and MMP-2 expressions which further enhance angiogenesis [64]. MMPs are also involved in the breakdown of cell-cell adhesions by breaking Vascular endothelial-cadherin ectodomain [65, 66].

Several reports showed that MMPs are pathogenic in MS. MMPs are reported to damage basal lamina present in the surrounding blood vessel by degradation of extracellular matrix protein in basal lamina, causing leukocytes to enter into the CNS. In the acute inflammatory stage of Multiple sclerosis MMPs affect myelin sheath [67, 68]. The reported data shows that MMP-7, 9 and 12 levels in the brain of patient suffering from MS are elevated. The increased level of MMP-8 and 9 in the serum of MS patients has been detected by Lee and coworker in their study [69]. MMP-2, 9 and other MMPs also demonstrated BBB disruption *via* damaging junctional complex proteins [70]. MMPs also worsen the disease condition in MS by releasing TNF-α which causes damage to oligodendrocytes. MMPs also increase the production of inflammatory mediators *via* releasing TNF-α and degrading BBB [71]. The increased expression of MMP-9 degrades myelin basic protein which directly disrupts the myelin sheath; additionally, MMP-9 also causes demyelination by releasing the membrane bound TNF-α [59]. It has been reported that interferon-β reduces the symptom of multiple sclerosis by inhibiting the release of MMP-9 by T-cells [72]. This indicates that targeting inhibition of MMP activity by natural inhibitors of specific MMPs, such as interferon-beta or other agents can constitute a novel approach to treat MS.

Vascular Endothelial Growth Factor (VEGF)

Vascular endothelial growth factor (VEGF) is a founder member of growth factor family and has received tremendous attention. It is also named as vascular permeability factor or VEGF-A. The VEGF family is made up of total six members *i.e.* VEGF-A to E and PlGF-1 [73, 74]. It has been recognized as the chief mediator of angiogenesis by increasing vascular permeability as well as inducing endothelial cell proliferation and migration [75, 76]. Gene targeting studies reported that VEGF is a vital regulator in vascular system development [77]. Hypoxia is the substantial regulator of VEGF. The expression of Hypoxia inducible factor (HIF) is increased in hypoxia condition which binds to the VEGF at the promoter region and activates transcription of VEGF mRNA and ultimately increases the expression of VEGF [78]. Other mediators, such as cytokines, transforming growth factor-β, interleukin-1β, epidermal growth factor, and hormones are also responsible for increase in expression of VEGF in numerous cells [79]. The physiological function of VEGF in normal nervous system is to regulate vessel permeability, promote neurogenesis, axon extension, and migrate precursor cells of oligodendrocytes, astrocytes and microglia [80]. VEGF also improves vascular perfusion through angiogenesis. However, the low level of VEGF is necessary to maintain integrity of BBB and endothelial cell survival [81]. High level of VEGF affects CNS homeostasis *via* degrading Blood Brain Barrier [74]. In the animal model of MS, the elevated expression of VEGF in activated Th1 lymphocytes, monocytes and astrocytes was reported to induce BBB breakdown [82]. The dysfunction of BBB through VEGF worsens the neurological diseases condition by various mechanisms, such as increase in inflammatory processes *via* leakage of neurotoxic mediators and generation of ROS, defective waste product disposal, poor nutrient transport, increased level of immune responses due to access of inflammatory cells and formation of leaky vessels [83 - 85]. Breakdown of BBB and vascular leakage are the characteristics of MS. The MRI finding showed that the serum level of VEGF is found to be increased in patients suffering from MS [86]. The increased level of VEGF makes BBB more leaky by increasing vessel permeability factor. Subsequently, the leaky BBB increases invasion of immune cells in the oligodendrocytes and astrocytes and degrade these cells and results into neurodegeneration [87]. VEGF promotes angiogenesis directly by acting as a unique mitogen and chemo attracting endothelia cells, while indirectly VEGF enforces endothelial cells to release other mediators, like MMPs as well as ICAM-1 which are involved in angiogenesis processes [88, 89]. Proescholdt and coworkers have reported that in acute and chronic lesion of MS, the level of VEGF was consistently unregulated. The data also suggest that the increased expression of VEGF also aggravates inflammatory processes by BBB degradation and movement of inflammatory cells in the MS lesions [90]. Kouchaki and coworkers measured the VEGF and its receptor VEGFR1 in the serum of patients suffering from MS. The outcome of the study revealed that the level of both VEGF and VEGFR1 was increased in the MS because of inflammatory and angiogenic processes, which can worsen the symptoms of MS [91].

Integrins

Integrins are the family of structurally related heterodimeric receptors for extracellular matrix proteins. Integrins are membrane glycoproteins having α and β subunits which promote attachment of cell and migration on the extracellular matrix [92]. Endothelial cells can express approximately 10 different integrins as per their location and state of activation [93]. Integrins are the key regulators of migration of endothelial cells during angiogenesis and their activity can be modulated by growth factor or integrin expression which modifies the conformation of integrin [94]. Specific integrins, like α4β1 are able to bind vascular cell adhesion molecule-1 for the promotion of cell-cell adhesion during angiogenesis [95]. In the process of angiogenesis, the growth factors form a pair with specific integrin which activates different signaling cascades to initiate the cell proliferation and cell migration [96].In the inflammatory condition of MS, integrin plays a significant role to increase lymphocyte level in blood, brain and CSF [97].

In the inflammatory conditions, endothelial cell does modification in its cell linings and promotes expression of various cell adhesion molecules, like vascular cell adhesion molecule-1, P and E-selectin, intercellular cell adhesion molecule-1 which help in the adhesion of leukocytes to the endothelium [98]. Subsequently, leukocyte migration across endothelium starts after adhesion of leukocyte to the endothelium in the presence of α4 integrin which is responsible for stable attachment of leukocyte to the endothelial cells of BBB and glial cells. Adhesion of leukocyte to the endothelial cells perpetuates the inflammatory cascade in the presence of fibronectin within the parenchyma of brain and further damage occurs in the brain [99]. This shows that integrin plays a crucial role in inflammation *via* leukocyte activation, differentiation and proliferation in MS brain [100]. It indicates that integrin can be considered as attractive therapeutic target in MS.

Immune Cells

Immune cells indirectly act as supporter of angiogenesis by secreting a number of proangiogenic factors in MS. MMPs and integrins upregulated in MS under inflammatory condition start migration of leukocytes through the CNS and worsen the inflammatory processes in MS [101]. The increased level of neutrophils produces angiogenesis activators, such as VEGF, MMPs, IL-8 and TNF-α [102]. The increased level of eosinophils also supports angiogenesis by producing various cytokines, growth factors and angiogenin. Basophils express mRNA for various isoforms of VEGF which is an important mediator for angiogenesis. Additionally, basophils also release histamine which has been reported to have angiogenic activity [103]. There are two different phenotypes of macrophages observed in MS which include M1-cells (classically activated macrophages) and M2-cell (alternatively activated macrophages). M1-cells increase the severity of MS, while M2-cells decrease the severity of the MS [104]. M1 type of macrophages produces various pro-angiogenic mediators, such as, cytokines, MMPs and growth factors *i.e.* VEGF, PDGF, FGF-2, TNF, TGF-β, IL-8 [105]. The activation of M1 type of macrophages also release iNOs, leading to increased blood flow at the site of inflammation and angiogenesis [106]. Dendritic cells also increases the expression of VEGFR-1, neuropilin and VEGFR-2 directly involved in the angiogenesis processes of MS. Microglia also increases expression of cytokines which ultimately increases the expression of MMP-9, showing indirect association of microglia in the angiogenic processes in MS [107].

ANGIOGENESIS AS THERAPEUTIC TARGET FOR TREATMENT OF MULTIPLE SCLEROSIS

Angiogenesis is a physiological phenomenon which occurs normally during reproduction, development and wound healing. However, the imbalance between pro and anti angiogenic mediators leads to pathological angiogenesis which is generally observed in many inflammatory diseases including MS [108, 109]. Various cytokines and chemokines produced during inflammatory processes in MS are reported to promote angiogenesis [110]. The major problem with anti-angiogenic therapy is impaired healing and thus there is always a controversy for anti-angiogenesis therapy [111]. However, it has been reported that anti-angiogenic treatment using CM101 inhibited angiogenesis in chronic and acute inflammation in CNS along with improved wound healing in the experimental mice suffering from spinal cord injury [112]. Jang and coworkers demonstrated that inhibition of angiogenesis did not affect wound repair processes in their dermal wound healing study using alpha-V integrin blocking antibody [113]. It has been reported that inflammation and angiogenesis possess positive feedback relationship, however, persistent inflammation causes destruction of normal tissue in MS. In fact, induction of anti-angiogenic effect stops the production of endothelial derived soluble factors in the inflamed tissue and provides beneficial effect in MS [114]. Angiogenesis is not a major event in pathogenesis; however, it plays a continuous role in the progression of the disease which makes it as an important therapeutic target for the treatment of MS. Majority of the treatment options currently available for the MS control directly or indirectly are the processes of angiogenesis and its mediators, such as IFN-h which is a multi-function cytokine which has been reported to have anti angiogenic effect in preclinical studies and also used to control tumor growth by suppressing angiogenesis [115]. Immunosuppressive therapy used in patient of RR-MS has been reported to have strong anti-angiogenic effect [116]. Several data reports showed that pro-angiogenic factors, such as hypoxia, HIF-1, VEGF, MMPs, integrins and immune cells are key components for the induction of angiogenic processes in MS [107]. These denote that angiogenesis and its mediators exert their effect directly or indirectly on the pathogenesis of MS.

Desai and coworkers demonstrated that hypoxia is the major factor for the demyelination of the neurons in multiples sclerosis. Their study finding showed that immune mediated hypoxia condition induces hypoxia inducible factor-1α (HIF-1α) which is one of the important mediators of angiogenesis in MS and leads to demyelination. They also reported that oxygen therapy at normobaric pressure at the early stage can protect the neuron from demyelination in MS by reducing hypoxia condition and HIF-1α level which is the root cause of angiogenesis in MS. However, the safety of oxygen therapy, such as reversion of hypoxia due to oxidative stress needs to be investigated [117]. Dimethyl fumarate (DMF) is a newly approved therapy for multiple sclerosis and it is considered as a the first line therapy for MS. Recently, it has been reported that dimethyl fumarate inhibits hypoxia inducible factor-1α and also inhibits vascular endothelial growth factor and interleukin 8 which are considered as its target genes. The study reports showed that DMF causes degradation of HIF-1α by disturbing its maturation and folding [118]. Yu and coworkers revealed that a natural compound 'erianin' suppressed VEGF production through inhibiting activation of HIF-1α and preventing retinal angiogenesis in microglial and endothelial cells [119]. The other natural compounds have also been reported to act on HIF-1α. Epigallocatechin-3-gallate has been reported to suppress HIF-1α induction, and echinomycin inactivate HIF-1α by inhibiting its binding with DNA and digoxin has also been reported to inhibit the synthesis of HIF-1α in autoimmune diseases. However, these compounds have not been evaluated in multiple sclerosis [120 - 122].

MMPs are strongly associated with the process of angiogenesis in MS so they are also considered as a potential target for the therapeutic intervention in MS. Leppert and Stuve in their study reported that interferon-β treatment reduces the progression of disease by inhibiting MMP-9 production in MS [123, 124]. Sternberg and coworkers also demonstrated the effectiveness of quercetin separately and its combination with interferon-beta in reducing immune response partly by inhibiting MMP-9 production in peripheral blood mononuclear cells isolated from patient suffering from MS. The researcher also reported that quercetin shows additive effect on modulating immune response when given as combination therapy in MS. In another study, quercetin showed immunomodulatory effect on the animal model of MS *via* blockade of JAK-STAT pathway. In the same study, the researchers reported that quercetin reduced MMP production *via* inhibiting transcription factor NF-κB activities [125]. Muthian and coworkers also reported that quercetin has the potential effect to reduce demyelination in the animal model of MS. It also reduced the monocyte migration across the endothelial cells of brain and reducing macrophage infiltration [126 - 128]. These reports strongly support the future potential of quercetin as a treatment option in MS as one of the MMP inhibitors. Brundula and coworker studied the effect of a well-known MMP inhibitor minocycline in animal model of MS and reported that there was a minimum inflammation and demyelination in minocycline treated mice. The also reported that minocycline is a direct inhibitor of MMP-9 and MMP-2 and its effect as MMP inhibitor is stronger than interferon- γ. In addition, minocycline also protects myelin sheath by inhibiting MMPs. The reports show that along with MMP inhibition minocycline also reduces inflammatory responses in MS *via* inhibiting T cell proliferation, reduction in the production of interleukin-2, interferon-γ and TNF-α. It also inhibits activation of microglia and provides neuroprotection in MS [129]. Rosenberg and coworkers demonstrated that methylprednisolone may improve capillary function and control the damage to the BBB by inhibiting MMP-9. According to their study, high dose of methylprednisolone reduced MMP-9 level in CSF *via* blocking FOS/JUN dimmer function by inactivating AP-1 site in MMP-9 gene in MS [130]. Foster and coworkers revealed that Fingolimod improves the blood brain barrier damage by inhibiting MMP-9 activity in EAE rats [131]. Mitoxantrone hydrochloride is another drug which has been reported to reduce clinical exacerbation and progression of disability in MS patients partly by inhibiting proteolytic activity of MMP-2 and MMP-9 [132]. Supplementation of Omega-3 fatty acid has been reported to reduce MMP-9 production in patients suffering from relapsing-remitting multiple sclerosis. The study showed that three-month supplementation of omega-3 fatty acid reduced 58% secretion of MMP-9, which showed its potential effect on MMP-9 secretion in MS [133]. A clinical study data showed that dietary supplementation of resveratrol, omega-3 fatty acids, lipoic acid and fish oil along with multivitamin complex for seven months showed 59% reduction in MMP-9 production in primary progressive multiple sclerosis and 51% reduction of MMP-9 production in patients suffering from relapsing-remitting multiple sclerosis. This showed that dietary modification can also help to fight against MS [134]. In animal model of MS, alpha lipoic acid showed significant protective effect against demyelination, inflammation and axonal loss in MS. The researcher also reported that the effect of alpha lipoic acid against MS is mainly by inhibiting production of MMP-9 in the spinal cord [135]. In the clinical study also alpha lipoic acid has proven its effectiveness in patients suffering from MS *via* inhibiting MMP-9 activity as well as by interfering in the migration of T-cell in the CNS [136].

VEGF induces demyelination by migrating inflammatory cells at lesion site and further augment the process of angiogenesis and increases BBB permeability. The study reports showed that treatment to the mice with humanized monoclonal antibody *i.e.* bevacizumab attenuated experimental autoimmune encephalomyelitis after binding with VEGF and suppressing the angiogenesis in the spinal cord [128]. In another *in-vitro* study, it has been shown that treatment of cells with IFN-β stopped angiogenesis *via* suppressing VEGF expression in the inflamed cells [137]. Roscoe and co-workers also reported that in EAE mice acute treatment with semaxinib, a selective inhibitor of VEGFR2 reduced the level of VEGF, demyelination and cell infiltration in the spinal cord of EAE mice [138].

Integrins are other therapeutic targets for the treatment of multiple sclerosis. Natalizumab (humanized monoclonal antibody) is a US FDA approved α4 integrin antagonist used in the treatment of all types of MS by binding with α4β1 and 4β7 integrins present on the activated T lymphocytes, monocytes and other cell types and inhibits the communication with vascular cell-adhesion molecule 1 (VCAM1). It also modulates proliferation of immune cell and disrupts activation of T-cell by hindering the communication of vlA4 with extracellular matrix. The small molecule firategrast has also been reported to treat remitting and relapsing multiple sclerosis and this drug is in clinical trial [139, 140].

The other potential therapeutic interventions indirectly linked with reduction in angiogenesis in MS include treatment based on IL-17 and CD20. IL-17 is a vital immunological player responsible for inflammatory responses in the central nervous system. The cells which produce IL-17 are known to be an important inflammatory mediators in various autoimmune diseases including MS [141]. Recent findings show that IL-17 positive cells promote angiogenesis through upregulating VEGF production *via* activation of STAT-3/GIV pathway [142]. Drug like Secukinumab is an anti-IL-17A monoclonal antibody which binds to human IL-17A and has also been studied clinically in relapsing multiple sclerosis which might inhibit angiogenesis processes in MS [143]. Furthermore, humanized IgG1 monoclonal antibodies, such as ofatumumab which is an antiCD20 antibody, have been reported to have inhibitory potential on angiogenesis *via* Fc gamma receptor I FcγRI [144].

CONCLUSION

Though extensive research has been done, the exact cause of development of multiple sclerosis is still unknown. However, the researchers have added great knowledge which is proving helpful in the discovery of treatment options for MS. It is considered that genetic susceptibility and nongenetic triggers, work together thus finally leading to MS.

No approved treatment options are available for the cure of the MS. The main aim of the currently available treatment is to shorten the duration of acute exacerbations, decrease their frequency, and provide symptomatic relief. The goals of the treatment are to maintain function, reducing disease activity, further progression and improve quality of life.

The infiltrating inflammatory cells, which are the hallmark of MS, are known to secrete many chemical substances which ultimately contribute to accelerate progression of the disease. It promotes and stimulates the process of angiogenesis. Now it is well evident that how angiogenesis plays key role in progression of the MS. Direct or indirect inhibition of process of angiogenesis has great potential to provide clinical benefits to prevent disease progression.

Research is going on finding the new anti-angiogenetic agents. Though the specific mechanism of action for these inhibitors is under investigation, various targets are being studied to inhibit the angiogenesis. Hypoxia-inducible factor-1, matrix metalloproteinases, vascular endothelial growth factor, and integrins are some of the well explored molecular targets intended to inhibit the angiogenesis. There is a wide opportunity to find out new molecular targets as well as new drugs targeting them for inhibiting the angiogenesis. More research is warranted to find out the effective therapy for MS keeping the angiogenesis as significant target.

CONSENT FOR PUBLICATION

Not applicable.

CONFLICT OF INTEREST

The author confirms that he has no conflict of interest to declare for this publication.

ACKNOWLEDGEMENTS

Declared none

ABBREVIATION

BBB   Blood Brain Barrier

CNS   Central Nervous System

CSF   Cerebrospinal Fluid

ECM   Extracellular matrix

EAE   Experimental autoimmune encephalomyelitis

FGF-2 Fibroblast growth factor-2

HIF-1 Hypoxia-Inducible Factor-1

ICAM-1 Inter cellular cell adhesion molecule-1

IFN-γ	Interferon-γ
IL-8	Interleukin-8
MS	Multiple Sclerosis
MMP	Matrix metalloproteinase
NAGM	Normal appearing grey matter
NAWM	Normal appearing white matter
NO	Nitric oxide
PlGF-1	Placental growth factor
PGDF	Platelet-derived growth factor
PAs	Plasminogen activator system
ROS	Reactive oxygen species
TNF-α	Tumor necrosis factor-α
tPA	Tissue plasminogen activator
TGF-β	Transforming growth factor beta 1
uPA	urinary plasminogen activator
uPAR	urinary plasminogen activator receptor
VEGF	Vascular endothelial growth factor
VCAM	Vascular cell adhesion molecule

REFERENCES

[1]   Kulkarni YA, Garud MS, Oza MJ, Gaikwad AB. Biomarkers of Multiple Sclerosis and Their Modulation by Natural Products.Nutrition and lifestyle in neurological autoimmune diseases. USA: Elsevier: Academic Press 2017; pp. 275-84.
[http://dx.doi.org/10.1016/B978-0-12-805298-3.00028-1]

[2]   McFarland HF, Martin R. Multiple sclerosis: a complicated picture of autoimmunity. Nat Immunol 2007; 8(9): 913-9.
[http://dx.doi.org/10.1038/ni1507] [PMID: 17712344]

[3]   Sharief MK, Hentges R. Association between tumor necrosis factor-α and disease progression in patients with multiple sclerosis. N Engl J Med 1991; 325(7): 467-72.
[http://dx.doi.org/10.1056/NEJM199108153250704] [PMID: 1852181]

[4]   Dell'Avvento S, Sotgiu MA, Manca S, Sotgiu G, Sotgiu S. Epidemiology of multiple sclerosis in the pediatric population of Sardinia, Italy. Eur J Pediatr 2016; 175(1): 19-29.
[http://dx.doi.org/10.1007/s00431-015-2588-3] [PMID: 26156052]

[5]   Correale J, Gaitán MI, Ysrraelit MC, Fiol MP. Progressive multiple sclerosis: from pathogenic mechanisms to treatment. Brain 2017; 140(3): 527-46.
[PMID: 27794524]

[6]   Ibiwoye MO, Clement C, Olubadewo JO, *et al.* Blood Vascular Changes Associated with Chronic Active Multiple Sclerosis Plaques: Detection by Anti-Human Brain Vascular Endothelia-Specific Monoclonal Antibodies. J Pharm Sci Pharmacol 2015; 2(1): 26-34.
[http://dx.doi.org/10.1166/jpsp.2015.1039]

[7]   Howard J, Trevick S, Younger DS. Epidemiology of multiple sclerosis. Neurol Clin 2016; 34(4): 919-

39.
[http://dx.doi.org/10.1016/j.ncl.2016.06.016] [PMID: 27720001]

[8]   Tullman MJ. Overview of the epidemiology, diagnosis, and disease progression associated with multiple sclerosis. Am J Manag Care 2013; 19(2) (Suppl.): S15-20.
[PMID: 23544716]

[9]   Waxman SG. Membranes, myelin, and the pathophysiology of multiple sclerosis. N Engl J Med 1982; 306(25): 1529-33.
[http://dx.doi.org/10.1056/NEJM198206243062505] [PMID: 7043271]

[10]   Popescu BF, Lucchinetti CF. Meningeal and cortical grey matter pathology in multiple sclerosis. BMC Neurol 2012; 12: 11.
[http://dx.doi.org/10.1186/1471-2377-12-11] [PMID: 22397318]

[11]   Otrock ZK, Mahfouz RA, Makarem JA, Shamseddine AI. Understanding the biology of angiogenesis: review of the most important molecular mechanisms. Blood Cells Mol Dis 2007; 39(2): 212-20.
[http://dx.doi.org/10.1016/j.bcmd.2007.04.001] [PMID: 17553709]

[12]   Tahergorabi Z, Khazaei M. A review on angiogenesis and its assays. Iran J Basic Med Sci 2012; 15(6): 1110-26.
[PMID: 23653839]

[13]   Yadav L, Puri N, Rastogi V, Satpute P, Sharma V. Tumour angiogenesis and angiogenic inhibitors: A review. J Clin Diagn Res 2015; 9(6): XE01-5.

[14]   Acar G, Tanrıöver G, Demir R. Angiogenesis in neurological disorders: a review. Neurol Res 2012; 34(7): 627-35.
[http://dx.doi.org/10.1179/1743132812Y.0000000068] [PMID: 22889669]

[15]   Lengfeld J, Cutforth T, Agalliu D. The role of angiogenesis in the pathology of multiple sclerosis. Vasc Cell 2014; 6(1): 23.
[http://dx.doi.org/10.1186/s13221-014-0023-6] [PMID: 25473485]

[16]   Girolamo F, Coppola C, Ribatti D, Trojano M. Angiogenesis in multiple sclerosis and experimental autoimmune encephalomyelitis. Acta Neuropathol Commun 2014; 2(1): 84.
[http://dx.doi.org/10.1186/s40478-014-0084-z] [PMID: 25047180]

[17]   Alvarez JI, Cayrol R, Prat A. Disruption of central nervous system barriers in multiple sclerosis. Biochim Biophys Acta 2011; 1812(2): 252-64.
[http://dx.doi.org/10.1016/j.bbadis.2010.06.017] [PMID: 20619340]

[18]   Claudio L, Raine CS, Brosnan CF. Evidence of persistent blood-brain barrier abnormalities in chronic-progressive multiple sclerosis. Acta Neuropathol 1995; 90(3): 228-38.
[http://dx.doi.org/10.1007/BF00296505] [PMID: 8525795]

[19]   Minagar A, Alexander JS. Blood-brain barrier disruption in multiple sclerosis. Mult Scler 2003; 9(6): 540-9.
[http://dx.doi.org/10.1191/1352458503ms965oa] [PMID: 14664465]

[20]   Manetti M, Guiducci S, Ibba-Manneschi L, Matucci-Cerinic M. Mechanisms in the loss of capillaries in systemic sclerosis: angiogenesis versus vasculogenesis. J Cell Mol Med 2010; 14(6A): 1241-54.
[http://dx.doi.org/10.1111/j.1582-4934.2010.01027.x] [PMID: 20132409]

[21]   Blood CH, Zetter BR. Tumor interactions with the vasculature: angiogenesis and tumor metastasis. Biochim Biophys Acta 1990; 1032(1): 89-118.
[PMID: 1694687]

[22]   Gourley M, Williamson JS. Angiogenesis: new targets for the development of anticancer chemotherapies. Curr Pharm Des 2000; 6(4): 417-39.
[http://dx.doi.org/10.2174/1381612003400867] [PMID: 10788590]

[23]   Liekens S, De Clercq E, Neyts J. Angiogenesis: regulators and clinical applications. Biochem

Pharmacol 2001; 61(3): 253-70.
[http://dx.doi.org/10.1016/S0006-2952(00)00529-3] [PMID: 11172729]

[24]   Mignatti P, Rifkin DB. Plasminogen activators and matrix metalloproteinases in angiogenesis. Enzyme Protein 1996; 49(1-3): 117-37.
[http://dx.doi.org/10.1159/000468621] [PMID: 8797002]

[25]   Blasi F. uPA, uPAR, PAI-1: key intersection of proteolytic, adhesive and chemotactic highways? Immunol Today 1997; 18(9): 415-7.
[http://dx.doi.org/10.1016/S0167-5699(97)01121-3] [PMID: 9293155]

[26]   Klagsbrun M, Moses MA. Molecular angiogenesis. Chem Biol 1999; 6(8): R217-24.
[http://dx.doi.org/10.1016/S1074-5521(99)80081-7] [PMID: 10421764]

[27]   Falcone DJ, McCaffrey TA, Haimovitz-Friedman A, Garcia M. Transforming growth factor-beta 1 stimulates macrophage urokinase expression and release of matrix-bound basic fibroblast growth factor. J Cell Physiol 1993; 155(3): 595-605.
[http://dx.doi.org/10.1002/jcp.1041550317] [PMID: 7684044]

[28]   Bischoff J. Cell adhesion and angiogenesis. J Clin Invest 1997; 100(11) (Suppl.): S37-9.
[PMID: 9413399]

[29]   Minagar A, Alexander JS. Blood-brain barrier disruption in multiple sclerosis. Mult Scler 2003; 9(6): 540-9.
[http://dx.doi.org/10.1191/1352458503ms965oa] [PMID: 14664465]

[30]   Alvarez JI, Cayrol R, Prat A. Disruption of central nervous system barriers in multiple sclerosis. Biochim Biophys Acta 2011; 1812(2): 252-64.
[http://dx.doi.org/10.1016/j.bbadis.2010.06.017] [PMID: 20619340]

[31]   Rigau V, Morin M, Rousset MC, *et al.* Angiogenesis is associated with blood-brain barrier permeability in temporal lobe epilepsy. Brain 2007; 130(Pt 7): 1942-56.
[http://dx.doi.org/10.1093/brain/awm118] [PMID: 17533168]

[32]   Biron KE, Dickstein DL, Gopaul R, Jefferies WA. Amyloid triggers extensive cerebral angiogenesis causing blood brain barrier permeability and hypervascularity in Alzheimer's disease. PLoS One 2011; 6(8): e23789.
[http://dx.doi.org/10.1371/journal.pone.0023789] [PMID: 21909359]

[33]   Nag S. The blood-brain barrier and cerebral angiogenesis: lessons from the cold-injury model. Trends Mol Med 2002; 8(1): 38-44.
[http://dx.doi.org/10.1016/S1471-4914(01)02221-3] [PMID: 11796265]

[34]   Mayhan WG. VEGF increases permeability of the blood-brain barrier *via* a nitric oxide synthase/cGMP-dependent pathway. Am J Physiol 1999; 276(5 Pt 1): C1148-53.
[http://dx.doi.org/10.1152/ajpcell.1999.276.5.C1148] [PMID: 10329964]

[35]   Ludwin S. Vascular proliferation and angiogenesis in MS: clinical and pathogenic implications. J Neuropathol Exp Neurol 2001; 60: 505.

[36]   Papadaki EZ, Simos PG, Mastorodemos VC, *et al.* Regional MRI perfusion measures predict motor/executive function in patients with clinically isolated syndrome. Behavioural Neurology 2014; 2014: 252419.
[http://dx.doi.org/10.1155/2014/252419] [PMID: 24825950]

[37]   Trapp BD, Stys PK. Virtual hypoxia and chronic necrosis of demyelinated axons in multiple sclerosis. Lancet Neurol 2009; 8(3): 280-91.
[http://dx.doi.org/10.1016/S1474-4422(09)70043-2] [PMID: 19233038]

[38]   Wang GL, Jiang BH, Rue EA, Semenza GL. Hypoxia-inducible factor 1 is a basic-helix-loop-helix-PAS heterodimer regulated by cellular O2 tension. Proc Natl Acad Sci USA 1995; 92(12): 5510-4.
[http://dx.doi.org/10.1073/pnas.92.12.5510] [PMID: 7539918]

[39]   Huang LE, Gu J, Schau M, Bunn HF. Regulation of hypoxia-inducible factor 1α is mediated by an O2-dependent degradation domain *via* the ubiquitin-proteasome pathway. Proc Natl Acad Sci USA 1998; 95(14): 7987-92.
[http://dx.doi.org/10.1073/pnas.95.14.7987] [PMID: 9653127]

[40]   Ziello JE, Jovin IS, Huang Y. Hypoxia-Inducible Factor (HIF)-1 regulatory pathway and its potential for therapeutic intervention in malignancy and ischemia. Yale J Biol Med 2007; 80(2): 51-60.
[PMID: 18160990]

[41]   Ke Q, Costa M. Hypoxia-inducible factor-1 (HIF-1). Mol Pharmacol 2006; 70(5): 1469-80.
[http://dx.doi.org/10.1124/mol.106.027029] [PMID: 16887934]

[42]   Iyer NV, Kotch LE, Agani F, *et al.* Cellular and developmental control of O_2 homeostasis by hypoxia-inducible factor 1 alpha. Genes Dev 1998; 12(2): 149-62.
[http://dx.doi.org/10.1101/gad.12.2.149] [PMID: 9436976]

[43]   Liu Y, Cox SR, Morita T, Kourembanas S. Hypoxia regulates vascular endothelial growth factor gene expression in endothelial cells. Identification of a 5' enhancer. Circ Res 1995; 77(3): 638-43.
[http://dx.doi.org/10.1161/01.RES.77.3.638] [PMID: 7641334]

[44]   Semenza GL. Hypoxia-inducible factor 1: master regulator of O2 homeostasis. Curr Opin Genet Dev 1998; 8(5): 588-94.
[http://dx.doi.org/10.1016/S0959-437X(98)80016-6] [PMID: 9794818]

[45]   Lassmann H. Hypoxia-like tissue injury as a component of multiple sclerosis lesions. J Neurol Sci 2003; 206(2): 187-91.
[http://dx.doi.org/10.1016/S0022-510X(02)00421-5] [PMID: 12559509]

[46]   Roscoe WA, Welsh ME, Carter DE, Karlik SJ. VEGF and angiogenesis in acute and chronic MOG((35-55)) peptide induced EAE. J Neuroimmunol 2009; 209(1-2): 6-15.
[http://dx.doi.org/10.1016/j.jneuroim.2009.01.009] [PMID: 19233483]

[47]   Bö L, Dawson TM, Wesselingh S, *et al.* Induction of nitric oxide synthase in demyelinating regions of multiple sclerosis brains. Ann Neurol 1994; 36(5): 778-86.
[http://dx.doi.org/10.1002/ana.410360515] [PMID: 7526776]

[48]   Argaw AT, Zhang Y, Snyder BJ, *et al.* IL-1beta regulates blood-brain barrier permeability *via* reactivation of the hypoxia-angiogenesis program. J Immunol 2006; 177(8): 5574-84.
[http://dx.doi.org/10.4049/jimmunol.177.8.5574] [PMID: 17015745]

[49]   Ben-Yosef Y, Miller A, Shapiro S, Lahat N. Hypoxia of endothelial cells leads to MMP-2-dependent survival and death. Am J Physiol Cell Physiol 2005; 289(5): C1321-31.
[http://dx.doi.org/10.1152/ajpcell.00079.2005] [PMID: 16210427]

[50]   Tang N, Wang L, Esko J, *et al.* Loss of HIF-1alpha in endothelial cells disrupts a hypoxia-driven VEGF autocrine loop necessary for tumorigenesis. Cancer Cell 2004; 6(5): 485-95.
[http://dx.doi.org/10.1016/j.ccr.2004.09.026] [PMID: 15542432]

[51]   Le Moan N, Baeten KM, Rafalski VA, *et al.* Hypoxia Inducible Factor-1 in Astrocytes and/or Myeloid Cells Is Not Required for the Development of Autoimmune Demyelinating Disease. eNeuro 2015; 2(2) ENEURO.0050-14.2015.

[52]   Graumann U, Reynolds R, Steck AJ, Schaeren-Wiemers N. Molecular changes in normal appearing white matter in multiple sclerosis are characteristic of neuroprotective mechanisms against hypoxic insult. Brain Pathol 2003; 13(4): 554-73.
[http://dx.doi.org/10.1111/j.1750-3639.2003.tb00485.x] [PMID: 14655760]

[53]   Weidemann A, Kerdiles YM, Knaup KX, *et al.* The glial cell response is an essential component of hypoxia-induced erythropoiesis in mice. J Clin Invest 2009; 119(11): 3373-83.
[PMID: 19809162]

[54]   Guan SY, Leng RX, Tao JH, *et al.* Hypoxia-inducible factor-1α: a promising therapeutic target for

autoimmune diseases. Expert Opin Ther Targets 2017; 21(7): 715-23.
[http://dx.doi.org/10.1080/14728222.2017.1336539] [PMID: 28553732]

[55]   Clements JM, Cossins JA, Wells GM, *et al.* Matrix metalloproteinase expression during experimental autoimmune encephalomyelitis and effects of a combined matrix metalloproteinase and tumour necrosis factor-alpha inhibitor. J Neuroimmunol 1997; 74(1-2): 85-94.
[http://dx.doi.org/10.1016/S0165-5728(96)00210-X] [PMID: 9119983]

[56]   Mirshafiey A, Asghari B, Ghalamfarsa G, Jadidi-Niaragh F, Azizi G. The significance of matrix metalloproteinases in the immunopathogenesis and treatment of multiple sclerosis. Sultan Qaboos Univ Med J 2014; 14(1): e13-25.
[http://dx.doi.org/10.12816/0003332] [PMID: 24516744]

[57]   Nagase H, Woessner JF Jr. Matrix metalloproteinases. J Biol Chem 1999; 274(31): 21491-4. [Review].
[http://dx.doi.org/10.1074/jbc.274.31.21491] [PMID: 10419448]

[58]   Alexander CM, Werb Z. Proteinases and extracellular matrix remodeling. Curr Opin Cell Biol 1989; 1(5): 974-82.
[http://dx.doi.org/10.1016/0955-0674(89)90068-9] [PMID: 2697298]

[59]   Latronico T, Liuzzi GM. Metalloproteinases and their inhibitors as therapeutic targets for multiple sclerosis: current evidence and future perspectives. Metalloproteinases Med 2017; 4: 1-13.
[http://dx.doi.org/10.2147/MNM.S88655]

[60]   Docherty AJ, O'Connell J, Crabbe T, Angal S, Murphy G. The matrix metalloproteinases and their natural inhibitors: prospects for treating degenerative tissue diseases. Trends Biotechnol 1992; 10(6): 200-7.
[http://dx.doi.org/10.1016/0167-7799(92)90214-G] [PMID: 1368394]

[61]   Ferrara N. Vascular endothelial growth factor: basic science and clinical progress. Endocr Rev 2004; 25(4): 581-611.
[http://dx.doi.org/10.1210/er.2003-0027] [PMID: 15294883]

[62]   Vu TH, Shipley JM, Bergers G, *et al.* MMP-9/gelatinase B is a key regulator of growth plate angiogenesis and apoptosis of hypertrophic chondrocytes. Cell 1998; 93(3): 411-22.
[http://dx.doi.org/10.1016/S0092-8674(00)81169-1] [PMID: 9590175]

[63]   Nygårdas PT, Hinkkanen AE. Up-regulation of MMP-8 and MMP-9 activity in the BALB/c mouse spinal cord correlates with the severity of experimental autoimmune encephalomyelitis. Clin Exp Immunol 2002; 128(2): 245-54.
[http://dx.doi.org/10.1046/j.1365-2249.2002.01855.x] [PMID: 11985514]

[64]   Huo N, Ichikawa Y, Kamiyama M, *et al.* MMP-7 (matrilysin) accelerated growth of human umbilical vein endothelial cells. Cancer Lett 2002; 177(1): 95-100.
[http://dx.doi.org/10.1016/S0304-3835(01)00772-8] [PMID: 11809536]

[65]   Herren B, Levkau B, Raines EW, Ross R. Cleavage of β-catenin and plakoglobin and shedding of VE-cadherin during endothelial apoptosis: evidence for a role for caspases and metalloproteinases. Mol Biol Cell 1998; 9(6): 1589-601.
[http://dx.doi.org/10.1091/mbc.9.6.1589] [PMID: 9614196]

[66]   Rundhaug JE. Matrix metalloproteinases and angiogenesis. J Cell Mol Med 2005; 9(2): 267-85.
[http://dx.doi.org/10.1111/j.1582-4934.2005.tb00355.x] [PMID: 15963249]

[67]   Yong VW, Power C, Forsyth P, Edwards DR. Metalloproteinases in biology and pathology of the nervous system. Nat Rev Neurosci 2001; 2(7): 502-11.
[http://dx.doi.org/10.1038/35081571] [PMID: 11433375]

[68]   Rosenberg GA, Yang Y. Vasogenic edema due to tight junction disruption by matrix metalloproteinases in cerebral ischemia. Neurosurg Focus 2007; 22(5): E4.
[http://dx.doi.org/10.3171/foc.2007.22.5.5] [PMID: 17613235]

[69]   Lee MA, Palace J, Stabler G, Ford J, Gearing A, Miller K. Serum gelatinase B, TIMP-1 and TIMP-2

levels in multiple sclerosis. A longitudinal clinical and MRI study. Brain 1999; 122(Pt 2): 191-7.
[http://dx.doi.org/10.1093/brain/122.2.191] [PMID: 10071048]

[70] Liu W, Hendren J, Qin XJ, Shen J, Liu KJ. Normobaric hyperoxia attenuates early blood-brain barrier disruption by inhibiting MMP-9-mediated occludin degradation in focal cerebral ischemia. J Neurochem 2009; 108(3): 811-20.
[http://dx.doi.org/10.1111/j.1471-4159.2008.05821.x] [PMID: 19187098]

[71] Ozenci V, Rinaldi L, Teleshova N, *et al.* Metalloproteinases and their tissue inhibitors in multiple sclerosis. J Autoimmun 1999; 12(4): 297-303.
[http://dx.doi.org/10.1006/jaut.1999.0285] [PMID: 10330301]

[72] Stüve O, Dooley NP, Uhm JH, *et al.* Interferon β-1b decreases the migration of T lymphocytes *in vitro*: effects on matrix metalloproteinase-9. Ann Neurol 1996; 40(6): 853-63.
[http://dx.doi.org/10.1002/ana.410400607] [PMID: 9007090]

[73] Koch S, Tugues S, Li X, Gualandi L, Claesson-Welsh L. Signal transduction by vascular endothelial growth factor receptors. Biochem J 2011; 437(2): 169-83.
[http://dx.doi.org/10.1042/BJ20110301] [PMID: 21711246]

[74] Lange C, Storkebaum E, de Almodóvar CR, Dewerchin M, Carmeliet P. Vascular endothelial growth factor: a neurovascular target in neurological diseases. Nat Rev Neurol 2016; 12(8): 439-54.
[http://dx.doi.org/10.1038/nrneurol.2016.88] [PMID: 27364743]

[75] Ferrara N, Kerbel RS. Angiogenesis as a therapeutic target. Nature 2005; 438(7070): 967-74.
[http://dx.doi.org/10.1038/nature04483] [PMID: 16355214]

[76] Ruiz de Almodovar C, Lambrechts D, Mazzone M, Carmeliet P. Role and therapeutic potential of VEGF in the nervous system. Physiol Rev 2009; 89(2): 607-48.
[http://dx.doi.org/10.1152/physrev.00031.2008] [PMID: 19342615]

[77] Ferrara N, Carver-Moore K, Chen H, *et al.* Heterozygous embryonic lethality induced by targeted inactivation of the VEGF gene. Nature 1996; 380(6573): 439-42.
[http://dx.doi.org/10.1038/380439a0] [PMID: 8602242]

[78] Levy AP, Levy NS, Wegner S, Goldberg MA. Transcriptional regulation of the rat vascular endothelial growth factor gene by hypoxia. J Biol Chem 1995; 270(22): 13333-40.
[http://dx.doi.org/10.1074/jbc.270.22.13333] [PMID: 7768934]

[79] Ferrara N. Molecular and biological properties of vascular endothelial growth factor. J Mol Med (Berl) 1999; 77(7): 527-43.
[http://dx.doi.org/10.1007/s001099900019] [PMID: 10494799]

[80] Licht T, Keshet E. Delineating multiple functions of VEGF-A in the adult brain. Cell Mol Life Sci 2013; 70(10): 1727-37.
[http://dx.doi.org/10.1007/s00018-013-1280-x] [PMID: 23475068]

[81] Carmeliet P, Jain RK. Molecular mechanisms and clinical applications of angiogenesis. Nature 2011; 473(7347): 298-307.
[http://dx.doi.org/10.1038/nature10144] [PMID: 21593862]

[82] Argaw AT, Gurfein BT, Zhang Y, Zameer A, John GR. VEGF-mediated disruption of endothelial CLN-5 promotes blood-brain barrier breakdown. Proc Natl Acad Sci USA 2009; 106(6): 1977-82.
[http://dx.doi.org/10.1073/pnas.0808698106] [PMID: 19174516]

[83] Dvorak HF, Brown LF, Detmar M, Dvorak AM. Vascular permeability factor/vascular endothelial growth factor, microvascular hyperpermeability, and angiogenesis. Am J Pathol 1995; 146(5): 1029-39.
[PMID: 7538264]

[84] Le Guelte A, Dwyer J, Gavard J. Jumping the barrier: VE-cadherin, VEGF and other angiogenic modifiers in cancer. Biol Cell 2011; 103(12): 593-605.
[http://dx.doi.org/10.1042/BC20110069] [PMID: 22054419]

[85]   Zhao Z, Nelson AR, Betsholtz C, Zlokovic BV. Establishment and dysfunction of the blood–brain barrier. Cell 2015; 163(5): 1064-78.
[http://dx.doi.org/10.1016/j.cell.2015.10.067] [PMID: 26590417]

[86]   Su JJ, Osoegawa M, Matsuoka T, *et al.* Upregulation of vascular growth factors in multiple sclerosis: correlation with MRI findings. J Neurol Sci 2006; 243(1-2): 21-30.
[http://dx.doi.org/10.1016/j.jns.2005.11.006] [PMID: 16376944]

[87]   Argaw AT, Asp L, Zhang J, *et al.* Astrocyte-derived VEGF-A drives blood-brain barrier disruption in CNS inflammatory disease. J Clin Invest 2012; 122(7): 2454-68.
[http://dx.doi.org/10.1172/JCI60842] [PMID: 22653056]

[88]   Kolch W, Martiny-Baron G, Kieser A, Marmé D. Regulation of the expression of the VEGF/VPS and its receptors: role in tumor angiogenesis. Breast Cancer Res Treat 1995; 36(2): 139-55.
[http://dx.doi.org/10.1007/BF00666036] [PMID: 8534863]

[89]   Radisavljevic Z, Avraham H, Avraham S. Vascular endothelial growth factor up-regulates ICAM-1 expression *via* the phosphatidylinositol 3 OH-kinase/AKT/Nitric oxide pathway and modulates migration of brain microvascular endothelial cells. J Biol Chem 2000; 275(27): 20770-4.
[http://dx.doi.org/10.1074/jbc.M002448200] [PMID: 10787417]

[90]   Proescholdt MA, Jacobson S, Tresser N, Oldfield EH, Merrill MJ. Vascular endothelial growth factor is expressed in multiple sclerosis plaques and can induce inflammatory lesions in experimental allergic encephalomyelitis rats. J Neuropathol Exp Neurol 2002; 61(10): 914-25.
[http://dx.doi.org/10.1093/jnen/61.10.914] [PMID: 12387457]

[91]   Kouchaki E, Otroshi Shahreza B, Faraji S, Nikoueinejad H, Sehat M. The association between vascular endothelial growth factor-related factors and severity of multiple sclerosis. Iran J Allergy Asthma Immunol 2016; 15(3): 204-11.
[PMID: 27424135]

[92]   Cheresh DA. Structural and biologic properties of integrin-mediated cell adhesion. Clin Lab Med 1992; 12(2): 217-36.
[PMID: 1611819]

[93]   Giancotti FG, Ruoslahti E. Integrin signaling. Science 1999; 285(5430): 1028-32.
[http://dx.doi.org/10.1126/science.285.5430.1028] [PMID: 10446041]

[94]   Avraamides CJ, Garmy-Susini B, Varner JA. Integrins in angiogenesis and lymphangiogenesis. Nat Rev Cancer 2008; 8(8): 604-17.
[http://dx.doi.org/10.1038/nrc2353] [PMID: 18497750]

[95]   Jin H, Varner J. Integrins: roles in cancer development and as treatment targets. Br J Cancer 2004; 90(3): 561-5.
[http://dx.doi.org/10.1038/sj.bjc.6601576] [PMID: 14760364]

[96]   Stupack DG, Cheresh DA. Integrins and angiogenesis. Curr Top Dev Biol 2004; 64: 207-38.
[http://dx.doi.org/10.1016/S0070-2153(04)64009-9] [PMID: 15563949]

[97]   Shimonkevitz R, Colburn C, Burnham JA, Murray RS, Kotzin BL. Clonal expansions of activated gamma/delta T cells in recent-onset multiple sclerosis. Proc Natl Acad Sci USA 1993; 90(3): 923-7.
[http://dx.doi.org/10.1073/pnas.90.3.923] [PMID: 8430106]

[98]   Springer TA. Traffic signals for lymphocyte recirculation and leukocyte emigration: the multistep paradigm. Cell 1994; 76(2): 301-14.
[http://dx.doi.org/10.1016/0092-8674(94)90337-9] [PMID: 7507411]

[99]   Guan JL, Hynes RO. Lymphoid cells recognize an alternatively spliced segment of fibronectin *via* the integrin receptor alpha 4 beta 1. Cell 1990; 60(1): 53-61.
[http://dx.doi.org/10.1016/0092-8674(90)90715-Q] [PMID: 2295088]

[100] Rice GP, Hartung HP, Calabresi PA. Anti-α4 integrin therapy for multiple sclerosis: mechanisms and

rationale. Neurology 2005; 64(8): 1336-42.
[http://dx.doi.org/10.1212/01.WNL.0000158329.30470.D0] [PMID: 15851719]

[101] Yong VW, Krekoski CA, Forsyth PA, Bell R, Edwards DR. Matrix metalloproteinases and diseases of the CNS. Trends Neurosci 1998; 21(2): 75-80.
[http://dx.doi.org/10.1016/S0166-2236(97)01169-7] [PMID: 9498303]

[102] Muhs BE, Plitas G, Delgado Y, *et al.* Temporal expression and activation of matrix metalloproteinases-2, -9, and membrane type 1-matrix metalloproteinase following acute hindlimb ischemia. J Surg Res 2003; 111(1): 8-15.
[http://dx.doi.org/10.1016/S0022-4804(02)00034-3] [PMID: 12842442]

[103] Sörbo J, Jakobsson A, Norrby K. Mast-cell histamine is angiogenic through receptors for histamine1 and histamine2. Int J Exp Pathol 1994; 75(1): 43-50.
[PMID: 7511407]

[104] Cheng Y, Sun L, Xie Z, *et al.* Diversity of immune cell types in multiple sclerosis and its animal model: Pathological and therapeutic implications. J Neurosci Res 2017; 95(10): 1973-83.
[http://dx.doi.org/10.1002/jnr.24023] [PMID: 28084640]

[105] Klimp AH, Hollema H, Kempinga C, van der Zee AGJ, de Vries EGE, Daemen T. Expression of cyclooxygenase-2 and inducible nitric oxide synthase in human ovarian tumors and tumor-associated macrophages. Cancer Res 2001; 61(19): 7305-9.
[PMID: 11585770]

[106] Jenkins DC, Charles IG, Thomsen LL, *et al.* Roles of nitric oxide in tumor growth. Proc Natl Acad Sci USA 1995; 92(10): 4392-6.
[http://dx.doi.org/10.1073/pnas.92.10.4392] [PMID: 7538668]

[107] Hamid KM, Mirshafiey A. Role of proangiogenic factors in immunopathogenesis of multiple sclerosis: a systematic review. Iran J Allergy Asthma Immunol 2016; 15(1): 1-12.
[PMID: 26996106]

[108] Gallin JI, Snyderman R. Inflammation: Basic principles and clinical correlates. 3rd ed. Philadelphia: Lippincott Williams & Wilkins 1999; p. 1335.

[109] Ribatti D, Iaffaldano P, Marinaccio C, Trojano M. First evidence of in vivo pro-angiogenic activity of cerebrospinal fluid samples from multiple sclerosis patients. Clin Exp Med 2016; 16(1): 103-7.
[http://dx.doi.org/10.1007/s10238-014-0334-1] [PMID: 25539984]

[110] Heissig B, Nishida C, Tashiro Y, *et al.* Role of neutrophil-derived matrix metalloproteinase-9 in tissue regeneration. Histol Histopathol 2010; 25(6): 765-70.
[PMID: 20376783]

[111] Paleolog EM. Angiogenesis in rheumatoid arthritis. Arthritis Res 2002; 4 (Suppl. 3): S81-90.
[http://dx.doi.org/10.1186/ar575] [PMID: 12110126]

[112] Wamil AW, Wamil BD, Hellerqvist CG. CM101-mediated recovery of walking ability in adult mice paralyzed by spinal cord injury. Proc Natl Acad Sci USA 1998; 95(22): 13188-93.
[http://dx.doi.org/10.1073/pnas.95.22.13188] [PMID: 9789063]

[113] Jang YC, Arumugam S, Gibran NS, Isik FF. Role of alpha(v) integrins and angiogenesis during wound repair. Wound Repair Regen 1999; 7(5): 375-80.
[http://dx.doi.org/10.1046/j.1524-475X.1999.00375.x] [PMID: 10564566]

[114] Griffioen AW, Molema G. Angiogenesis: potentials for pharmacologic intervention in the treatment of cancer, cardiovascular diseases, and chronic inflammation. Pharmacol Rev 2000; 52(2): 237-68.
[PMID: 10835101]

[115] Lindner DJ, Borden EC. Synergistic antitumor effects of a combination of interferon and tamoxifen on estrogen receptor-positive and receptor-negative human tumor cell lines in vivo and in vitro. J Interferon Cytokine Res 1997; 17(11): 681-93.
[PMID: 9402106]

[116] Billington DC. Angiogenesis and its inhibition: potential new therapies in oncology and non-neoplastic diseases. Drug Des Discov 1991; 8(1): 3-35.
[PMID: 1725722]

[117] Desai RA, Davies AL, Tachrount M, *et al.* Cause and prevention of demyelination in a model multiple sclerosis lesion. Ann Neurol 2016; 79(4): 591-604.
[http://dx.doi.org/10.1002/ana.24607] [PMID: 26814844]

[118] Zhao G, Liu Y, Fang J, Chen Y, Li H, Gao K. Dimethyl fumarate inhibits the expression and function of hypoxia-inducible factor-1α (HIF-1α). Biochem Biophys Res Commun 2014; 448(3): 303-7.
[http://dx.doi.org/10.1016/j.bbrc.2014.02.062] [PMID: 24569076]

[119] Yu Z, Zhang T, Gong C, *et al.* Erianin inhibits high glucose-induced retinal angiogenesis *via* blocking ERK1/2-regulated HIF-1α-VEGF/VEGFR2 signaling pathway. Sci Rep 2016; 6: 34306.
[http://dx.doi.org/10.1038/srep34306] [PMID: 27678303]

[120] Yang EJ, Lee J, Lee SY, *et al.* EGCG attenuates autoimmune arthritis by inhibition of STAT3 and HIF-1α with Th17/Treg control. PLoS One 2014; 9(2): e86062.
[http://dx.doi.org/10.1371/journal.pone.0086062] [PMID: 24558360]

[121] Zhang H, Qian DZ, Tan YS, *et al.* Digoxin and other cardiac glycosides inhibit HIF-1alpha synthesis and block tumor growth. Proc Natl Acad Sci USA 2008; 105(50): 19579-86.
[http://dx.doi.org/10.1073/pnas.0809763105] [PMID: 19020076]

[122] Kong D, Park EJ, Stephen AG, *et al.* Echinomycin, a small-molecule inhibitor of hypoxia-inducible factor-1 DNA-binding activity. Cancer Res 2005; 65(19): 9047-55.
[http://dx.doi.org/10.1158/0008-5472.CAN-05-1235] [PMID: 16204079]

[123] Leppert D, Waubant E, Bürk MR, Oksenberg JR, Hauser SL. Interferon beta-1b inhibits gelatinase secretion and in vitro migration of human T cells: a possible mechanism for treatment efficacy in multiple sclerosis. Ann Neurol 1996; 40(6): 846-52.
[http://dx.doi.org/10.1002/ana.410400606] [PMID: 9007089]

[124] Stüve O, Dooley NP, Uhm JH, *et al.* Interferon β-1b decreases the migration of T lymphocytes in vitro: effects on matrix metalloproteinase-9. Ann Neurol 1996; 40(6): 853-63.
[http://dx.doi.org/10.1002/ana.410400607] [PMID: 9007090]

[125] Moon SK, Cho GO, Jung SY, *et al.* Quercetin exerts multiple inhibitory effects on vascular smooth muscle cells: role of ERK1/2, cell-cycle regulation, and matrix metalloproteinase-9. Biochem Biophys Res Commun 2003; 301(4): 1069-78.
[http://dx.doi.org/10.1016/S0006-291X(03)00091-3] [PMID: 12589822]

[126] Muthian G, Bright JJ. Quercetin, a flavonoid phytoestrogen, ameliorates experimental allergic encephalomyelitis by blocking IL-12 signaling through JAK-STAT pathway in T lymphocyte. J Clin Immunol 2004; 24(5): 542-52.
[http://dx.doi.org/10.1023/B:JOCI.0000040925.55682.a5] [PMID: 15359113]

[127] Hendriks JJ, Alblas J, van der Pol SM, van Tol EA, Dijkstra CD, de Vries HE. Flavonoids influence monocytic GTPase activity and are protective in experimental allergic encephalitis. J Exp Med 2004; 200(12): 1667-72.
[http://dx.doi.org/10.1084/jem.20040819] [PMID: 15611292]

[128] MacMillan CJ, Furlong SJ, Doucette CD, Chen PL, Hoskin DW, Easton AS. Bevacizumab diminishes experimental autoimmune encephalomyelitis by inhibiting spinal cord angiogenesis and reducing peripheral T-cell responses. J Neuropathol Exp Neurol 2012; 71(11): 983-99.
[http://dx.doi.org/10.1097/NEN.0b013e3182724831] [PMID: 23037326]

[129] Brundula V, Rewcastle NB, Metz LM, Bernard CC, Yong VW. Targeting leukocyte MMPs and transmigration: minocycline as a potential therapy for multiple sclerosis. Brain 2002; 125(Pt 6): 1297-308.
[http://dx.doi.org/10.1093/brain/awf133] [PMID: 12023318]

[130]   Rosenberg GA, Dencoff JE, Correa N Jr, Reiners M, Ford CC. Effect of steroids on CSF matrix metalloproteinases in multiple sclerosis: relation to blood-brain barrier injury. Neurology 1996; 46(6): 1626-32.
[http://dx.doi.org/10.1212/WNL.46.6.1626] [PMID: 8649561]

[131]   Foster CA, Mechtcheriakova D, Storch MK, *et al.* FTY720 rescue therapy in the dark agouti rat model of experimental autoimmune encephalomyelitis: expression of central nervous system genes and reversal of blood-brain-barrier damage. Brain Pathol 2009; 19(2): 254-66.
[http://dx.doi.org/10.1111/j.1750-3639.2008.00182.x] [PMID: 18540945]

[132]   Kopadze T, Dehmel T, Hartung HP, Stüve O, Kieseier BC. Inhibition by mitoxantrone of in vitro migration of immunocompetent cells: a possible mechanism for therapeutic efficacy in the treatment of multiple sclerosis. Arch Neurol 2006; 63(11): 1572-8.
[http://dx.doi.org/10.1001/archneur.63.11.1572] [PMID: 17101825]

[133]   Shinto L, Marracci G, Baldauf-Wagner S, *et al.* Omega-3 fatty acid supplementation decreases matrix metalloproteinase-9 production in relapsing-remitting multiple sclerosis. Prostaglandins Leukot Essent Fatty Acids 2009; 80(2-3): 131-6.
[http://dx.doi.org/10.1016/j.plefa.2008.12.001] [PMID: 19171471]

[134]   Riccio P, Rossano R, Larocca M, *et al.* Anti-inflammatory nutritional intervention in patients with relapsing-remitting and primary-progressive multiple sclerosis: A pilot study. Exp Biol Med (Maywood) 2016; 241(6): 620-35.
[http://dx.doi.org/10.1177/1535370215618462] [PMID: 26785711]

[135]   Marracci GH, Jones RE, McKeon GP, Bourdette DN. Alpha lipoic acid inhibits T cell migration into the spinal cord and suppresses and treats experimental autoimmune encephalomyelitis. J Neuroimmunol 2002; 131(1-2): 104-14.
[http://dx.doi.org/10.1016/S0165-5728(02)00269-2] [PMID: 12458042]

[136]   Yadav V, Marracci G, Lovera J, *et al.* Lipoic acid in multiple sclerosis: a pilot study. Mult Scler 2005; 11(2): 159-65.
[http://dx.doi.org/10.1191/1352458505ms1143oa] [PMID: 15794388]

[137]   Taylor KL, Leaman DW, Grane R, Mechti N, Borden EC, Lindner DJ. Identification of interferon-beta-stimulated genes that inhibit angiogenesis in vitro. J Interferon Cytokine Res 2008; 28(12): 733-40.
[http://dx.doi.org/10.1089/jir.2008.0030] [PMID: 18937547]

[138]   Roscoe WA, Welsh ME, Carter DE, Karlik SJ. VEGF and angiogenesis in acute and chronic MOG((35-55)) peptide induced EAE. J Neuroimmunol 2009; 209(1-2): 6-15.
[http://dx.doi.org/10.1016/j.jneuroim.2009.01.009] [PMID: 19233483]

[139]   Sternberg Z, Chadha K, Lieberman A, *et al.* Quercetin and interferon-β modulate immune response(s) in peripheral blood mononuclear cells isolated from multiple sclerosis patients. J Neuroimmunol 2008; 205(1-2): 142-7.
[http://dx.doi.org/10.1016/j.jneuroim.2008.09.008] [PMID: 18926575]

[140]   Millard M, Odde S, Neamati N. Integrin targeted therapeutics. Theranostics 2011; 1: 154-88.
[http://dx.doi.org/10.7150/thno/v01p0154] [PMID: 21547158]

[141]   Gold R, Lühder F. Interleukin-17--extended features of a key player in multiple sclerosis. Am J Pathol 2008; 172(1): 8-10.
[http://dx.doi.org/10.2353/ajpath.2008.070862] [PMID: 18063700]

[142]   Pan B, Shen J, Cao J, *et al.* Interleukin-17 promotes angiogenesis by stimulating VEGF production of cancer cells *via* the STAT3/GIV signaling pathway in non-small-cell lung cancer. Sci Rep 2015; 5: 16053.
[http://dx.doi.org/10.1038/srep16053] [PMID: 26524953]

[143]   Havrdová E, Belova A, Goloborodko A, *et al.* Activity of secukinumab, an anti-IL-17A antibody, on

brain lesions in RRMS: results from a randomized, proof-of-concept study. J Neurol 2016; 263(7): 1287-95.
[http://dx.doi.org/10.1007/s00415-016-8128-x] [PMID: 27142710]

[144] Bogdanovich S, Kim Y, Mizutani T, *et al.* Human IgG1 antibodies suppress angiogenesis in a target-independent manner. Signal Transduct Target Ther 2016; 1: 15001.
[http://dx.doi.org/10.1038/sigtrans.2015.1] [PMID: 26918197]

CHAPTER 7

Angiogenesis and Portal Hypertension: An Update

Dmitry Victorovich Garbuzenko[*], Nikolay Olegovich Arefyev and **Evgeniy Leonidovich Kazachkov**

South Ural State Medical University, Chelyabinsk, Russia

Abstract: Developing medicines for hemodynamic disorders that are characteristic of cirrhosis of the liver is a relevant problem in modern hepatology. The increase in hepatic vascular resistance to portal blood flow and subsequent hyperdynamic circulation underlie portal hypertension (PH) and promote its progression, despite the formation of portosystemic collaterals. Angiogenesis and vascular bed restructurization play an important role in PH pathogenesis as well. In this regard, strategic directions in the therapy for PH in cirrhosis include selectively decreasing hepatic vascular resistance while preserving or increasing portal blood flow, and correcting hyperdynamic circulation and pathological angiogenesis. The aim of this review is to describe the mechanisms of angiogenesis in PH, methods for studying angiogenesis in experimental research, and the perspectives of antiangiogenic therapy. Although most angiogenesis inhibitors were studied only in animal experiments, this selective therapy for abnormally growing newly formed vessels is pathogenetically reasonable to treat PH and associated complications.

Keywords: Angiogenesis, Antiangiogenic Therapy, Liver Cirrhosis, Portal Hypertension, Pathogenesis, Vascular Remodeling.

INTRODUCTION

Developing medicines to treat hemodynamic disorders that are characteristic of liver cirrhosis and promote portal hypertension (PH) and related complications is a relevant problem in modern hepatology. In accordance with the current clinical recommendations, nonselective β-blockers are the drugs of choice [1, 2]. However, their influence on portal pressure is variable. A number of studies showed that they did not lead to a clinically significant decrease in portal pressure, and the weakening of their therapeutic effect was noted in 50–70% of cases in the long-term period. Also, the question of the appropriateness of using nonselective β-adrenergic blockers in patients with decompensated cirrhosis has not been finally resolved [3].

[*] **Corresponding author Dmitry Victorovich Garbuzenko:** South Ural State Medical University, Chelyabinsk, Russia; E-mail: garb@inbox.ru

Atta-ur-Rahman & Mohammad Iqbal Choudhary (Eds.)

Ideally, the pharmacotherapy of PH should lessen the severity of morphofunctional disorders in the liver, contributing to the reduction of the vascular resistance to portal blood flow. Also, it should successfully correct a hyperdynamic circulatory state. As a result, the hepatic venous pressure gradient (HVPG), the most accurate equivalent of portal pressure, should be reduced to values less than 12 mmHg or be 20% lower than an original value. In addition, it is necessary to avoid arterial hypotension and at the same time reduce the influx of splanchnic blood into the portal vein, keeping unchanged the portal blood flow, which participates in liver perfusion [4].

Angiogenesis plays an important role in the pathogenesis of many chronic liver diseases, including fibrosis, cirrhosis, and hepatocellular carcinoma [5]. It can also accompany PH, underlying its development and causing related complications. Indeed, the newly formed blood vessels, which bypass sinusoids in response to the gross morphofunctional rearrangement of the liver in cirrhosis, fail to provide oxygen and nutrients to the tissues, which worsens the course of the disease and increases hepatic vascular resistance to portal blood flow [6]. Further progression of PH is a consequence of complex processes including angiogenesis, vascular remodeling, and endothelial dysfunction, which contribute to splanchnic congestion, portosystemic shunt formation, and a hyperdynamic circulatory state [7] (Fig. **1**). From this, it can be inferred that antiangiogenic therapy, which is selectively aimed at suppressing newly formed vessels' formation and growth, is a pathogenetically grounded method of treating PH and associated complications [8].

MORPHOFUNCTIONAL REARRANGEMENT OF THE HEPATIC MICROVASCULAR BED IN CIRRHOSIS-ASSOCIATED PORTAL HYPERTENSION PATHOGENESIS

It is generally accepted that pathologically modified sinusoids are the main sites of resistance to portal blood flow in cirrhosis. Endothelial cells lining sinusoids (SEC) become dysfunctional and among other features acquire a vasoconstrictor phenotype. In this situation, SEC sensitivity to endogenous vasoconstrictors (such as endothelin, norepinephrine, angiotensin II, vasopressin, leukotrienes, thromboxane A2) is elevated. At the same time, SEC produce less nitric oxide (NO), the most studied vasodilator that takes part in the regulation of hepatic vascular tone [9]. This may be due to the lower activity of endothelial nitric oxide synthase (eNOS) caused by increased interaction of eNOS with caveolin-1. Moreover, endotelin-1 stimulates G-protein-coupled receptor kinase-2, which directly interacts with and decreases protein kinase B (Akt) phosphorylation and NO production.

Fig. (1). Potential mechanisms of portal hypertension pathogenesis in cirrhosis. The newly formed blood vessels, which bypass sinusoids in response to the gross morphofunctional rearrangement of the liver in cirrhosis, fail to provide oxygen and nutrients to the tissues. This process is accompanied by endothelial dysfunction and impaired paracrine interaction between hepatocytes, sinusoidal endothelial cells, Kupffer cells, and activated hepatic stellate cells, and leads to an increase in hepatic vascular resistance to portal blood flow. Further progression of portal hypertension is a consequence of complex processes including angiogenesis, vascular remodeling, and endothelial dysfunction, which contribute to splanchnic congestion, systemic vasodilation, and portosystemic shunt formation. The subsequent hyperdynamic circulatory state worsens the course of the disease [7].

Intrahepatic oxidative stress is one of the main factors of sinusoidal endothelial dysfunction in cirrhosis. Oxidative stress is associated with a decrease in NO bioavailability and eNOS expression. For example, cyclooxygenase attenuates Akt-eNOS signalization by activating Rho-kinase and thromboxane A2 that inhibits Akt phosphorylation in endothelial cells. Asymmetric dimethylarginine, an endogenous inhibitor of NOS, causes uncoupling of NOS, which leads to a higher production of reactive nitrogen species such as peroxynitrite. Down-regulated tetrahydrobiopterin expression increases eNOS inability to generate NO but to produce O^2 instead, leading to a further decrease in NO production. Additionally, a probable reason for the insufficient bioavailability of NO may be a reduction of superoxide dismutase («an enzyme that saves NO») and an increase in homocysteine serum level caused by a reduced expression of cystathionine-β - synthase and cystathionine-γ-lyase [10].

Activated hepatic stellate cells (HSC) and its paracrine interaction with SEC significantly affect the sinusoidal microcirculation in cirrhosis. In pathological conditions, structural and functional damage to HSC includes a loss of retinoids reserve and HSC transformation into myofibroblasts. Activated HSC start functioning as pericytes. This transformation is confirmed by the expression of phenotypic markers of pericytes, such as α-smooth muscle actin (α-SMA), desmin, NG2, glial fibrillary acidic protein, and emergence or increase in the amount of receptors for growth factors, endothelin and cytokines, as well as a number of cell adhesion molecules on HSC surface [11].

HSC, located in the subendothelial Disse spaces between the SEC and hepatocytes, contact with nerve endings by means of the long branching cytoplasmic processes. The nerve endings contain various neurotransmitters such as substance P, vasoactive intestinal peptide, somatostatin, cholecystokinin, neurotensin, NO, calcitonin gene-related peptide, and neuropeptide Y. Some vasoactive substances are capable of regulating HSC tone. Some substances, such as endothelin-1, substance P, angiotensin II, prostaglandin F2, norepinephrine, thromboxane A2, platelet activating factor (PAF), and thrombin trigger HSC contractility. On the contrary, acetylcholine, prostaglandin E2, NO, vasoactive intestinal peptide, carbon monoxide, hydrogen sulfide, and adrenomedullin are known for the ability to cause HSC relaxation [12].

HSC contraction involves myosin II and is mediated by Ca^{2+}-dependent and Ca^{2+}-independent pathways. In a Ca^{2+}-dependent pathway, an increase in intracellular Ca^{2+} concentration ($[Ca^{2+}]i$) and subsequent formation of the Ca^{2+}/calmodulin complex induce activation of myosin light chain kinase that phosphorylates myosin light chains. In a Ca^{2+}-independent pathway, Rho kinase and protein kinase C inhibit the activity of myosin light chain phosphatase, an enzyme that dephosphorylates phosphorylated myosin light chains and induces relaxation [13].

Endothelins (ET) are potent endogenous vasoconstrictors that may change HSC tone. ET have three kinds of isoforms: ET-1, 2, and 3. The isoforms are synthesized from their precursor "large endothelin" by endothelin-converting enzymes. ET interact with conjugated protein G receptors type A and B, which are well expressed on the HSC. Endothelin-1 is the most studied. The main site of its synthesis in cirrhosis is activated HSC. Stimulation of endothelin A receptors leads to their proliferation [14]. Angiotensin II has a similar effect. In cirrhosis, HSC positively affect angiotensin II synthesis, which is due to the increased expression of angiotensin-converting enzyme [15]. HSC constriction may also be mediated by decreased NO production and/or bioavailability in cirrhotic liver. In contrast, Kupffer cells overproduce carbon monoxide, causing the dilation of sinusoids, and hence decrease hepatic vascular resistance because of paracrine impact on HSC and SEC [16].

Mobility and migration of HSC are necessary to promote enhanced coverage of HSC around sinusoids, which is important for sinusoidal remodeling in liver cirrhosis [17]. Cellular locomotion requires dynamic but regulated actin remodeling to form membrane structures that promote cell extension. These membrane structures include lamellipodia, which are membrane protrusions that form the leading edge toward directed cell migration, and filopodia, which are thin, actin filament-structured spikes emanating from the plasma membrane. Small guanosine triphosphatases from the Rho family, including RhoA (Rho), Rac1 (Rac), and Cdc42, coordinate the formation of actin-based structures. While Rac contributes to filopodia formation and migration of HSC, Rho creates the resistance to the inhibitory action of NO and restores the chemotactic response to platelet-derived growth factor (PDGF) in the absence of a functional Rac [18].

PDGF is a key factor responsible for proliferation, migration, mobility, and recruitment of HSC, which is secreted by endothelial cells. PDGF binds to its receptor (PDGFR-β) on pericytes, which is mediated by an ephrin-B2/EphB4 signaling pathway [19]. Moreover, activated PDGFR-β stimulates Raf-1 kinase, MEK kinase, and extracellular-signal regulated kinase (ERK), leading to HSC proliferation. Phosphatidylinositol 3-kinase (PI 3-K) activation is also required for both PDGF-induced mitogenesis and chemotaxis [20]. In addition, the axonal guidance molecule neuropilin-1 takes part in the chemotactic response to PDGF as well [21].

Activated HSC are a rich source of polypeptides, eicosanoids, and various other molecules with paracrine, juxtacrine, autocrine signalization, or chemoattractant activity, which include:

- polypeptides that increase cell proliferation in an autocrine and paracrine manner: vascular endothelial growth factor (VEGF), hepatocyte growth factor (HGF), transforming growth factor (TGF)-α, endothelin-1, epidermal growth factor (EGF), insulin-like growth factor (IGF), and acidic fibroblast growth factor (aFGF);
- members of the TGF-β family;
- neurotrophins; and
- hematopoietic growth factors such as erythropoietin [22].

When the liver is damaged, activated HSC proliferate and migrate to areas of inflammation and necrosis of hepatocytes, producing high amounts of extracellular matrix components. TGF-β1, PDGF, connective tissue growth factor (CTGF), and FGF regulate this process [23].

Three general sources of fibrogenic cells in the liver include:

- endogenous (resident) fibroblast or myofibroblast-like cells, mainly represented by HSC, but also by portal fibroblasts, vascular smooth muscle cells, and pericytes;
- the epithelial–mesenchymal transition that may occur in the liver as well as in other organs and lead to transdifferentiation of parenchymal cells; and
- recruitment of fibrocytes from the bone marrow [24].

Intrahepatic Angiogenesis in Cirrhosis

In 1983, Rappaport *et al* [25] were among the first to report the collateral microcirculation in the cirrhotic liver. Nowadays, pathological angiogenesis is well studied in experimental liver fibrosis [26] and in patients with chronic viral and autoimmune liver diseases and nonalcoholic steatohepatitis [27, 28].

Angiogenesis is a complicated physiological process through which new blood vessels form from pre-existing vessels. It includes endothelial cell activation, protease expression, extracellular matrix destruction, proliferation, migration, and the formation of highly permeable primary vascular structures by endothelial cells. These structures become stabilized and "mature" because of pericyte and smooth muscle cell involvement and transform into a three-dimensional vascular network [29].

Molecular Insights into the Angiogenic Process

The primary inducer of angiogenesis in physiological and pathological conditions is hypoxia. Cells respond to hypoxic stress through multiple mechanisms, including the stabilization of hypoxia-inducible factors (HIF), which directly regulate the expression of angiogenic growth factors. The family of HIF includes three α-subunits, which are associated with a common β-subunit (HIF-1β). HIF-1α appears to be ubiquitously expressed, whereas HIF-2α is detected in a more restricted set of cell types, including vascular endothelial cells, hepatocytes, type II pneumocytes, and macrophages. A third mammalian HIF-α subunit, HIF-3α, has also been described, although its role in hypoxic responses is less well understood [30].

NADPH oxidase is an important mediator of angiogenic signaling pathways. It was noted that the increased NADPH oxidase expression increases the reactive oxygen species (ROS) levels because of NADPH oxidase subunit p47phox phosphorylation, contributing to HIF-1α induction, VEGF-receptor (VEGFR) activation, and EGF-receptor transactivation [31].

Recently, an important role of miRNA has been shown in the regulation of cellular response to hypoxia. In particular, Let-7 and miR-103/107 favor the

VEGF induction by targeting argonaute 1 protein [32].

The most studied angiogenic growth factors are VEGF family consisting of five homologs: VEGF-A, -B, -C, -D, and placental growth factor (PlGF). VEGF stimulate both physiological and pathological angiogenesis. All members of this family are connected to different homologous receptors: VEGFR-1 (Flt-1), VEGFR-2 (KDR/Flk-1), VEGFR-3 (Flt-4), of which only the first and second are responsible for angiogenic signal transmitting. Besides that, the binding of VEGF-A to VEGFR-2 and increasing vascular permeability through NO are the mechanisms that start angiogenesis and vasculogenesis.

PlGF, a homolog of VEGF binding VEGFR-1, enhances angiogenesis only in pathological conditions. PlGF directly and indirectly affects multiple cell types, including endothelial cells. Also, PlGF possibly breaks the binding of VEGF with VEGFR-1, making the binding of VEGF with VEGFR-2 more probable. Mass spectrometry studies showed that PlGF and VEGF each induce the phosphorylation of distinct tyrosine residues in VEGFR-1, further indicating that PlGF and VEGF transmit distinct angiogenic signals through VEGFR-1.

Different mechanisms are the basis of synergism between PlGF and VEGF. By activating VEGFR-1, PlGF induces an intermolecular cross talk between VEGFR-1 and VEGFR-2, which thereby is more responsive to VEGF. PlGF, as a subunit of PlGF/VEGF heterodimer, induces the formation of VEGFR-1/2 heterodimers, which transphosphorylate each other in an intramolecular reaction. By producing PlGF, endothelial cells are able to improve their own responsiveness to VEGF but adjacent stromal or inflammatory cells may also release PlGF.

PlGF directly affects smooth muscle cells and fibroblasts, which express VEGFR-1, but may also indirectly influence its proliferation and migration through cytokine release from activated endothelial cells. In this way, PlGF recruits smooth muscle cells around nascent vessels, thereby stabilizing them into mature, durable, and non-leaky vessels.

PlGF also mobilizes VEGFR-1 positive hematopoietic progenitor cells from the bone marrow and recruits (indirectly, via upregulation of VEGF expression) VEGFR-2-positive endothelial progenitor cells to the ischemic tissue. PlGF is also chemoattractive for monocytes and macrophages, which express VEGFR-1 [33].

FGF family members are also able to induce angiogenesis. Cellular response to FGF occurs through specific binding with FGF-receptors (FGFR), which have internal tyrosine kinase activity. FGFR dimerization is a prerequisite for phosphorylation and activation of signaling molecules with the participation of heparin-binding proteins. This causes migration, proliferation, cell differentiation, and destruction of extracellular matrix. It should be noted that while VEGF family members are involved mainly in the formation of the capillaries, FGF is primarily involved in arteriogenesis [34].

Although the angiogenic effect of PDGF is not as expressed as that of VEGF, PlGF, and FGF, studies *in vivo* have shown that it may induce the formation of blood vessels and regulate their tone [35].

Tie-2 (Tek), an endothelial-specific receptor tyrosine kinase, and its ligands, the angiopoietins, have been identified as critical mediators of vascular development. Angiopoetin-1 induces migration, inhibits apoptosis, and stimulates the formation of endothelial cells, promoting stabilization of vessels. At the same time, NADPH oxidase is involved in the ang-1-mediated activation of Akt and mitogen-activated protein kinase (p42/p44 MAPK or ERK2 and ERK1) and the subsequent modulation of endothelial cell migration and angiogenesis [36]. In contrast, angiopoietin-2 causes vascular destabilization by shifting endothelial cells from stable to proliferative phenotype. However, it may also stimulate angiogenesis in the presence of VEGF [37].

Integrins $\alpha V\beta 3$ and $\alpha V\beta 5$ are adhesion receptors stimulating angiogenesis by mediating endothelial cell migration, proliferation, and the formation of new blood vessels [38].

Endothelial-specific adhesion molecule vascular endothelial VE-cadherin contributes to cell-cell junctions during neovascularization and controls the passage of molecules through the endothelial lining [39].

Thrombospondin-1, one of the five known thrombospondins, is an adhesive protein that controls the interaction of cells with each other and with the extracellular matrix. The increased expression of thrombospondin-1 strongly correlates with the severity of fibrosis and angiogenesis during the progression of cirrhosis. However, the precise role of thrombospondin-1 in this process is not determined. It may serve as a promoter or inhibitor of angiogenesis, which may depend on its concentration, the type of domain being activated, and the type of receptors on endothelial cells [40].

Angiostatin, a fragment of plasminogen, and endostatin, a fragment of the C-terminal part of the collagen XVIII $\alpha 1$-chain, inhibit the migration of human endothelial cells stimulated with FGF and VEGF and do not have an impact on intracellular signaling pathways stimulated by FGF and VEGF [41].

Toll-like receptor 4 (TLR4), which recognizes bacterial lipopolysaccharide, is expressed by SEC involved in fibrosis-associated angiogenesis in cirrhotic liver. It acts through the cytosolic adapter protein MyD88 involved in the production of extracellular protease regulating the invasive ability of SEC [42].

Hepatic apelin system (apelin/APJ-receptor) is a connecting link between chronic inflammation and subsequent fibrogenic and angiogenic processes in cirrhosis. On the one hand, hypoxia and inflammation initiate the expression of APJ. On the other hand, the profibrogenic activation of APJ mediates the induction of profibrogenic genes, HSC proliferation, and secretion of pro-angiogenic factors [43].

Aquaporin-1 is an integral membrane channel protein, overexpressed in cirrhosis, that promotes angiogenesis by enhancing endothelial invasion [44].

It is known that chemokines from CXC family are involved in angiogenesis. ELR-positive chemokines stimulate this process, and ELR-negative suppress it [45].

Neuropilin-1 and neuropilin-2 are transmembrane glycoproteins with large extracellular domains that interact with both class 3 semaphorins, VEGF, and the classical receptors for VEGF, VEGF-R1, and -R2, mediating signal transduction. Neuropilin-1 is mainly expressed by arterial endothelium, whereas neuropilin-2 is only expressed by venous and lymphatic endothelium. Both neuropilins are commonly over-expressed in the regions of physiological and pathological angiogenesis, but the definitive role of neuropilins in angiogenic processes is not fully studied [46].

Mechanisms of Intrahepatic Angiogenesis in Cirrhosis

Hepatic angiogenesis may substantially differ from homologous processes in other organs or tissues on the basis of: (a) the rather unique phenotypic profile and functional role of activated HSC and of other liver myofibroblasts; (b) the presence of two different microvascular structures described (*i.e.*, sinusoids lined by fenestrated endothelium versus large vessels lined by a continuous one); and (c) the existence of ANGPTL3, a liver-specific angiogenic factor.

There are two main ways of angiogenesis in cirrhosis [47] (Fig. **2**).

One of them is associated with the increased expression of pro-angiogenic growth factors, cytokines, and matrix metalloproteinases on the background of chronic inflammation. Proinflammatory mediators produced by Kupffer cells, mast cells, and leukocytes may cause angiogenic response because of the induction and increased transcriptional activity of HIF-1α [48].

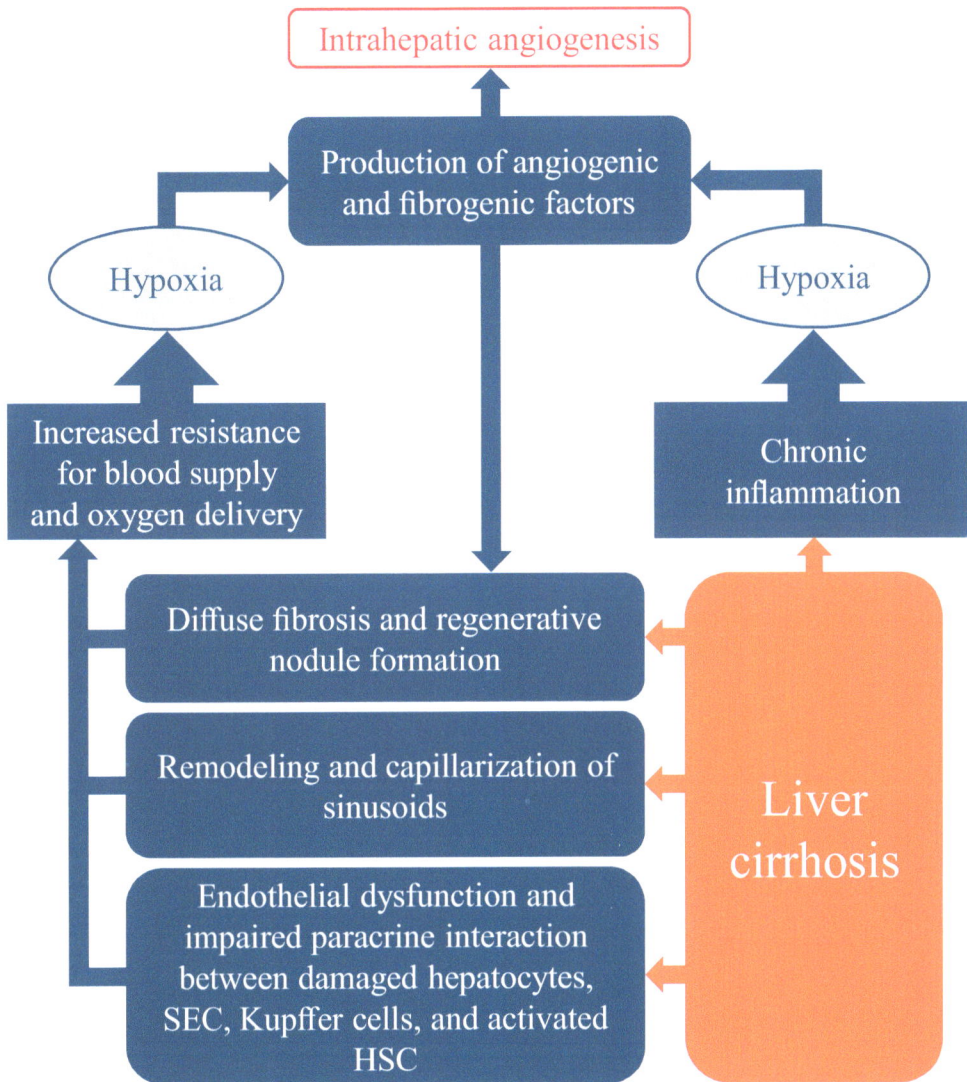

Fig. (2). Two main pathways of intrahepatic angiogenesis in liver cirrhosis [6].

It is believed that macrophages, when in the normal state, are not directly involved in angiogenesis. In contrast, activated Kupffer cells contribute to the formation of new blood vessels through the production of cytokines, ROS, and PAF in cirrhosis [49]. Kupffer cells also release tumor necrosis factor-α (TNF-α), which promotes the migration of cells and coordinates apoptosis and angiogenesis [50]. The increase of ROS in the liver induces angiogenesis via the enhanced expression of TNF-α, NO, HIF-1, and VEGF [51]. PAF promote the development of VEGF by activating nuclear transcription factor kappa-light-chain-enhancer of activated B cells (NF-κB) [52]. Mast cells take part in angiogenesis by producing heparin, histamine, tryptase, cytokines (TGF-β1, TNF-α, interleukins), and VEGF. They are also able to increase the number of SEC *in vitro* [53]. Soluble mediators, in particular, pro-inflammatory cytokines, growth factors, proteases, and products of oxidative stress regulate the increased expression of chemokines in chronic inflammation of the liver. Due to this process, leukocytes can penetrate into the liver tissue, where they produce angiogenic factors, such as VEGF, PIGF, PDGF, FGF, TGF-β1, EGF, ang-2, and different interleukins [54].

On the one hand, hypoxia, that is caused by HIF-1α stimulation, activates HSC and leads to the production of various angiogenic and fibrogenic factors (PIGF, VEGF, NO, HGF, PDGF) [55], promoting angiogenesis and progression of hepatic fibrosis [56]. On the other hand, diffuse fibrosis, regenerative nodules formation, and sinusoidal capillarization cause an increase in hepatic vascular resistance and impair the oxygen supply to the liver cells [57]. Accumulation of HIF, in particular, HIF-1α, increases the VEGF, angiopoietin-1, and their receptors expression on activated HSC. This leads to the involvement and stimulation of SEC, stabilizing the newly formed vessels and providing them with strength [5]. In turn, SEC generate PDGF and TGF-β, attracting HSC. This process includes ROS-mediated activation of ERK and c-Jun-NH2-terminal kinase (JNK) followed by a delayed- and HIF-1α-dependent up-regulation and release of VEGF [58].

Respectively, there are two different phases of an angiogenic process occurring in cirrhosis. Initially, the formation of blood vessels occurs in developing incomplete septa, in which concomitant expression of VEGF, Flk-1, and Tie-2 is restricted by HSC. In a later phase, angiogenesis occurs in large bridging septa, and the expression of this proangiogenic panel is limited to endothelial cells and aims to stabilize the newly formed blood vessels [59]. Some of them are located mainly around and inside of the fibrous septa and probably needed for compensation of the insufficient intrahepatic blood flow. Others form intrahepatic shunts bypassing sinusoids and draining blood from the portal to the central venules. Although they decompress the portal system, this may lead to liver dysfunction because of declining oxygen delivery and nutrients to the liver tissues and limiting the free exchange between hepatocytes and sinusoids [60].

During last years it has been found that endothelial progenitor cells produced by stem cells of the bone marrow are capable of causing *in situ* neovascularization in both physiological and pathological conditions (postnatal vasculogenesis). In particular, they may stimulate angiogenesis in patients with cirrhosis by activating

SEC through the secretion of paracrine factors, such as PDGF and VEGF [61]. However, their angiogenic ability is significantly reduced in patients of this category, and especially in those with severe hepatic dysfunction. This may be due to chronic inflammation stimulating the release of angiogenic factors by resident HSC and SEC and inhibiting the endothelial progenitor cells mobilization into the bloodstream [62].

Thus, in addition to structural changes associated with diffuse fibrosis and regenerative nodule formation in cirrhosis, there are endothelial dysfunction, impaired paracrine interaction between activated HSC and SEC, and sinusoidal remodeling and capillarization, which play an important role in increasing the hepatic vascular resistance to portal blood flow. The development of intrahepatic angiogenesis may be considered as a compensatory mechanism aimed at portal system decompression. However, the newly formed vessels bypass sinusoids. Therefore, they are unable to provide oxygen and nutrients to the liver tissue, which worsens its morphofunctional state and leads to an increase in portal pressure.

ADAPTATION OF THE VASCULAR BED TO HEMODYNAMIC DISTURBANCES IN PORTAL HYPERTENSION

At the early stages of portal hypertension, a moderate increase in portal pressure leads to blood flow redistribution towards the muscle layer of the small intestine. The appearance of mucosal hypoxia causes a significant increase in NAD(P)H oxidase activity, the main source of reactive oxygen species (ROS) in the mucous membrane, and also leads to the increased production of VEGF and NO by arterioles, contributing to splanchnic vasodilation [63]. In addition, multiple signaling pathways are stimulated, such as mitogen-activated protein kinases, tyrosine kinases, and transcription factors that are involved in VEGF-induced neovascularization [64]. It was shown that overexpression of Kruppel-like factor 2 in duodenal tissue, with the assistance of microRNA, causes hemodynamic stimuli integration and VEGF-driven angiogenesis in patients with cirrhosis [65]. Besides the small intestinal wall [66], the elevated levels of VEGF, VEGFR-2, and CD31 (PECAM-1) are observed in the mesentery [47].

After PH induction, vascular stem/progenitor cells (VSPC) of the mesentery become activated and produce daughter cells (*i.e.*, proliferative progenitors or transit-amplifying cells), which divide and differentiate into endothelial cells or smooth muscle cells lineages and readily incorporate into newly formed mesenteric blood vessels, making a physical and functional contribution to neovascularization *in vivo* in PH. The differentiation potential of VSPC may be regulated by various factors including VEGF, PDGF, and their receptors, which are increased within the precise tissue microenvironment of neovascularisation sites during PH, creating a suitable setting to promote VSPC differentiation towards either endothelial cells or smooth muscle cells [67].

Mechanism of the Formation of Portal-Systemic Collaterals

These pathophysiological disturbances may be an initial step in the development of portosystemic collateral circulation in portal hypertension [68]. Monocytes adhere to the surface of activated endothelial cells and produce growth factors and proteases, such as urokinase plasminogen activator and MMP, promoting the division and migration of smooth muscle cells. Proinflammatory cytokines (macrophage chemotactic protein-1, granulocyte-macrophage colony-stimulating factor, transforming growth factor $\beta1$ (TGF-$\beta1$), TNF-alpha) also promote the growth of blood vessels. PlGF stimulates the growth of endothelial and smooth muscle cells. FGF upregulates PDGF and VEGF-receptor expression via Ang-1. At the same time, anti-inflammatory cytokines (*e.g.*, interleukin-10) inhibit this process [33].

It was shown in animal models of prehepatic portal hypertension induced by partial portal vein ligation, that the blockade of VEGFR-2 with anti-VEGFR-2 monoclonal antibodys for 5-7 days and inhibition of VEGF/VEGFR-2 signalization using autophosphorylation inhibitor VEGFR-2 for 5 days after the operation resulted in a 50% reduction of portosystemic collateral vessel formation [69, 70]. Blockade of NAD(P)H also contributed to this owing to the reduced splanchnic expression of VEGF, VEGFR-2, and CD31 [71]. In addition, fourfold sequential intravenous administration of siRNA KDR-lipoplexes reduced the portosystemic collateralization by 73%, violated the angiogenic potential of endothelial cells and reduced pathological neovascularization in the mesenteric vascular bed [72].

It should be noted that the emerging shunts are very dynamic vascular structures because of the expression of various receptor types on the surface of the endothelial lining, for example, α and β-adrenoreceptors and 5-HT2 receptors. Furthermore, vasoactive substances such as NO, ET-1, and prostaglandins may affect vessel tonus [73]. In particular, the excessive shunting of blood through portosystemic collaterals at the time of postprandial splanchnic hyperemia promotes their dilation due to shear stress activating the overproduction of NO by endothelial cells [74].

Although natural portosystemic anastomoses are found in all patients with portal hypertension, they acquire the highest clinical significance in the development of gastroesophageal varices, because their rupture leads to life-threatening bleeding. The determining factor of their formation is the hepatofugal blood flow, and a gastroesophageal drainage path is the most important in this situation. The left gastric vein plays the main role in this path. It drains blood from both surfaces of the stomach, ascends from right to left along the lesser curvature into the lesser omentum, to the esophageal opening of the diaphragm, where it receives esophageal veins. It then turns backward and passes from left to right behind the omental bursa and drains into the portal vein. Anastomoses between the left and right gastric veins and the left and short gastric veins, respectively indicated by the terms "coronary vein" and "posterior gastric vein", have clinical significance only in portal hypertension, because they are involved in the formation of esophageal and paraesophageal varices [75].

Immunohistochemical studies, which were conducted in patients with portal hypertension, revealed the existence of the pronounced expression of PDGF, basic fibroblast growth factors (FGF-2), EGF, and transforming growth factor-α (TGF-α) in the wall of the coronary vein of the stomach. This fact shows that the increase in pressure in this vein activates smooth muscle cells and induces the release of growth factors that stimulate their proliferation, differentiation, and migration, as well as contribute to the disruption of the metabolism of collagen and elastin fibers. Phenotypic changes of smooth muscle cells are a response to chronic mechanical stimuli. They lead to venous wall thickening and elasticity reduction [76].

Vascular Structure of the Lower Esophagus in Clinical Portal Hypertension

The venous system of the distal portion of the esophagus includes intraepithelial, subepithelial superficial, deep submucosal, and adventitial veins. The largest varices are generally localized 2-3 cm above and 2 cm below the cardia, mainly in the lamina propria of the mucous membrane. They have two types of vascular structure: palisading type and bar type. The palisading type has dilated intraepithelial channels and numerous small superficial collateral veins. The bar type has triply dilated subepithelial superficial veins and deep submucosal veins which erode the epithelium [77].

Structural changes in the veins of the distal portion of the esophagus in portal hypertension are characterized by thickening of the medial layer because of hyperplasia of elastic and collagen fibers. Elastic fibers become fragmented and sharply tortuous directly in the varicose veins of the esophagus in the background of increasing sclerosis of the vascular wall [78].

Four distinct intramural vascular zones of the gastroesophageal junction were defined as follows: gastric zone, palisade zone, perforating zone, and truncal zone. Portacaval shunts in this area are formed because of increased pressure in the portal venous system [79].

Gastric Zone

The longitudinal veins of the gastric area are located in the submucosa and the lamina propria of the proximal portion of the stomach. They are more abundant near the esophagus, have a small diameter, and form a group of several longitudinal vessels. The veins merge in the submucosa of the distal part of the gastric zone and form large tortuous trunks draining blood into the portal vein system.

Palisade Zone

The palisade zone is an extension of the gastric zone. It begins in the projection of the gastroesophageal junction and ends 2-3 cm above it. Veins in that zone are located randomly, close to each other, and are arranged longitudinally and in parallel as a palisade.

Numerous anastomoses are identified between vessels of both gastric and palisade zones. They are localized in the submucosa of the gastroesophageal junction, penetrate the muscularis mucosa, and pass into the lamina propria mainly in a longitudinal direction.

The veins of a proximal portion of the palisade zone simultaneously converge at one point and, perforating the muscularis mucosa, pass into the submucosa again as four or five big trunks. There are arched transverse anastomoses between them. Veins perforating the muscular layer of the esophagus were not detected in this zone.

Perforating Zone

Veins of the perforating zone, which is located 3-5 cm above the gastroesophageal junction, are not so homogeneous and constant. Vessels form five polygonal networks in the lamina propria of the esophageal mucosa (as a continuation of the veins of the palisade zone) and perforate the muscular layer, communicating with adventitial veins located on the outer esophageal surface. They were referred to as «treble clef» veins because of their similarity with music symbols.

The perforating zone is the "critical area" for variceal rupture in portal hypertension. This is due to increased resistance to blood flow in this anatomical area, as well as increased fragility and superficial location of perforating veins [80].

Truncal Zone

The truncal zone is a region from 8 to 10 cm in length with the bottom edge 5 cm above the gastroesophageal junction. Large longitudinal venous trunks, discovered here in the lamina propria, constitute a continuation of the polygon vascular networks of the perforating zone. They have a small diameter in the proximal portion. Between them, there are several transversely oriented anastomoses. Perforating veins, locating randomly along the zone, pass from the submucosa of the esophagus to its outer surface and communicate with adventitial veins.

In physiological terms, palisade zone is the most important part of the vascular structure of the gastroesophageal junction. Veins are located there mainly in the lamina propria. Their superficial location decreases venous blood flow resistance to a minimum, which would otherwise arise in the high-pressure zone in the area of the lower esophageal sphincter.

Small longitudinal vessels in the palisade zone are perfectly adapted to the physiological pressure variations that lead to a bi-directional flow during breathing. When the venous outflow is caudal, the gastric zone collects and drains the blood into the portal vein system.

Deep submucosal veins are enlarged because of the blood outflow in the cranial direction in portal hypertension. They drain the blood into the enlarged adventitial veins (periesophageal collateral veins) through the numerous veins perforating the esophageal smooth muscle layer in the perforating zone. Adventitial veins, in turn, communicate with paraesophageal collateral veins, which are located in the posterior mediastinum. The blood flows from them usually into the azygos vein [81], which structural changes in response to increased blood flow are characterized by focal destruction, hyperplasia, and chaotic arrangement of elastic fibers [78].

The Systemic and Splanchnic Adaptive Response of Vascular Bed to Hemodynamic Disturbances in Portal Hypertension

The development of portosystemic collateral circulation is a compensatory mechanism aimed at decreasing portal pressure. However, this does not happen. Conversely, there is a hyperdynamic circulatory state accompanied by increased cardiac output, decreased peripheral vascular resistance, and the opening of arteriovenous communications, which exacerbate portal hypertension. The cause of these disorders may be the flow of vasodilator substances (*e.g.*, glucagon, endocannabinoid, atrial natriuretic peptide, bacterial endotoxin) through the network of portosystemic shunts, as well as the increased production of topical vasodilators by endothelium, such as NO, carbon monoxide, PGI2, endothelium-derived hyperpolarizing factor, adrenomedullin, and hydrogen sulfide. Furthermore, in spite of increased circulating levels of endogenous vasoconstrictors (noradrenaline, ET-1, angiotensin II), vascular sensitivity to them is significantly reduced [82].

Abdominal Aorta

In the conditions of the hyperdynamic circulation, adaptive response of the abdominal aorta to shear stress induced by the blood flow may be associated with oxidative stress. The production of ROS, such as superoxide and hydrogen peroxide, which are cell toxic metabolic products, leads to non-specific damage of nucleic acids, proteins, lipids, and other cellular components. ROS regulate vascular tone, endothelial cells sensitivity to oxygen, their growth, proliferation, and apoptosis. Furthermore, they promote the expression of inducible genes *via* transcription factors, such as NF-kB. These genes contribute to the synthesis of proinflammatory cytokines, chemokines, chemokine receptors, and adhesion molecules, inducing an inflammatory response. Potential sources of ROS are various enzyme systems: NAD(P)H oxidase, xanthine oxidase, enzymes of arachidonic acid metabolism (cyclooxygenase and lipoxygenase), and the mitochondrial respiratory chain [83].

Increased levels of TNF-α, IL-1β, and IL-6 in the aorta, as a result of oxidative stress, play an important role in the induction of immune-mediated systemic vascular process in portal hypertension. The subsequent increase in expression of connective tissue growth factor (CTGF) may enhance the synthesis of extracellular matrix proteins, particularly, collagen I type, whereas the decrease of the level of MMP-2 / TIMP-2 complex (tissue inhibitor of metalloproteinase-2) contributes to reducing the degradation of extracellular matrix proteins. These processes lead to significant histological changes in the aorta. Its wall thickness decreases, as well as the ratio of medial layer thickness to lumen diameter. Elastic fibers lose their ordered arrangement, and well-marked collagen fibers become more narrow and separated because of the increase in the extracellular matrix in the media interstitium with a significant decrease in the number of smooth muscle cells [84, 85].

The left gastric artery is the first branch of the celiac artery. It is assumed that the hemodynamics in the left gastric artery in portal hypertension may act as the initiator of variceal formation, showing close linkage with variceal recurrence [86].

Mesenteric Resistance Arteries

Similar infringements also occur in mesenteric resistance arteries. The mechanical stimuli, generated by shear stress, activate endothelial cells and induce hyperproduction of NO and prostaglandins, causing vasodilation [87]. The significantly reduced isometric stiffness of blood vessels and their increased elongation may cause structural changes in the internal elastic membrane and increase fenestrations in it [88]. This contributes to excessive NO-mediated vascular permeability and angiogenic processes in the mesentery of the small intestine because of the high VEGF and eNOS expression in microvessels located there [89].

Portal Vein and Hepatic Artery

Splanchnic congestion leads to increased portal inflow. At the same time, portal blood flow decreases as a result of the development of collateral circulation [90]. The portal vein becomes dilated, and shear stress simultaneously decreases [91]. Intima and media of the portal vein are thickened due to the high amount of collagen fibers, hypertrophy, and hyperplasia of smooth muscle cells, which significantly reduce the vascular wall elasticity [92]. *In vitro* studies have revealed that transmembrane protein 16A can be associated with the proliferation of portal vein smooth muscle cells and portal vein remodeling in PH. Upregulation of transmembrane protein 16A promotes the proliferation of portal vein smooth muscle cells, whereas inhibition reduces it [93].

In this situation, so-called hepatic arterial buffer response maintains hepatic perfusion constancy. This phenomenon, first described by Lautt in 1981 [94], was identified in physiological and in various pathological conditions, including cirrhosis. It maintains oxygen delivery to the liver, protecting its structure and function [95]. However, increased blood flow through the hepatic artery causes its remodeling and decreases its elasticity with time [96].

Splenic Artery and Vein

Significant histopathological changes also occur in the blood vessels of the spleen. Damaged splenic artery intima becomes thicker, and smooth muscle cells grow into it. The internal elastic lamina is stratified, that is accompanied by the destruction of both included in its structure and localized in media elastic fibers. Smooth muscle cells, randomly located in the media, have a different size and morphology, and the content of separating them collagen fibers, as well as the extracellular matrix, increases significantly, causing the "collagenization" of the vascular wall, thickening, and rigidity [97]. The splenic vein expanding and its intima and media thickening is due to high content of collagen fibers, hypertrophy, and hyperplasia of smooth muscle cells [98]. These pathologic changes in the blood vessels of the spleen lead to a significant reduction of their elasticity.

Thus, in addition to pathophysiological disorders related to endothelial dysfunction in cirrhosis, there is the restructuring of the splanchnic and systemic vasculature, which includes vascular remodeling and angiogenesis. In spite of the fact that these changes are the compensatory-adaptive response to the deteriorating conditions of blood circulation, taken together, they contribute to the development and progression of portal hypertension and cause severe complications, one of which is bleeding from esophageal varices.

MODERN METHODS FOR STUDYING PORTAL HYPERTENSION-ASSOCIATED ANGIOGENESIS IN EXPERIMENTAL RESEARCH

Various experimental models and methods, both *in vitro* and *in vivo*, of qualitative and quantitative evaluation are used to study angiogenesis [99].

Intrahepatic Angiogenesis Assays

Appearing simultaneously with fibrosis, intrahepatic angiogenesis causes abnormal angioarchitecture formation characteristic of cirrhosis, which is the endpoint of the disease. Therefore, evaluation of intrahepatic angiogenesis is necessary to assess disease progression and search for therapeutic targets (Table **1**).

Scanning Electron Microscopy

Scanning electron microscopy is the traditional method for studying the three-dimensional (3D) structure of microcirculation. It is visualized by an electron beam after intravascular injection of colored gelatin, latex, or plastic casting material followed by tissue clearing or corrosion. Unlike tissue sections, this approach makes it possible to not only quantify vessel dimensions, intervascular distances, branching order, and luminal surface features, but also to mathematically calculate the wall shear stress [100].

Table 1. Intrahepatic angiogenesis assays.

Assay	Advantages	Disadvantages
Scanning electron microscopy	Quantification of vessel dimensions, intervascular distances, branching order and luminal surface features, as well as the wall shear stress.	Perfusion difficulties of casting materials, especially for microvascular perfusion. Biloma formation after bile duct ligation causes holes in the cast.

(Table 1) cont.....

Assay	Advantages	Disadvantages
Intravital fluorescence microscopy	Evaluation of microcirculatory structural changes *in vivo*. HSC visualization. Possibility to estimate the number of rolling and adherent leukocytes, relative vascular density, the diameter and perfusion of sinusoids, and flow and volume velocity of blood.	Visualization of only superficial structures; not capable of estimating the diameter of portal venules. Hard to perform if intraperitoneal injections of CCl_4 or bile duct ligation are used.
Three-dimensional microcomputed tomography *in vivo*	May be re repeatedly conducted, thereby allowing gradual monitoring. 3D images of vasculature.	Resolution is relatively low, therefore it is not possible to evaluate microcirculation. Perfusion difficulties of casting materials.
Three-dimensional microcomputed tomography *ex vivo*	Higher resolution, if compared to *in vivo* microCT. Analysis of the microcirculation, as well as large vessels. 3D images of vasculature.	Perfusion difficulties of casting materials.
Immunohistochemical methods	Evaluation of newly formed vessels without a lumen. Evaluation of proangiogenic factors expression.	Analysis of microcirculation only.
Confocal laser scanning microscopy after immunohistochemical staining	3D images of vasculature. High resolution. Provides volumetric data on microcirculation.	Tissue shrinkage and deformation hampers confocal microscopy. Limited diffusion of (primary) antibody penetration.

Using scanning electron microscopy in rats with cirrhosis caused by subcutaneous injections of carbon tetrachloride (CCl_4) (0.3 mL 50% CCl_4 diluted with oil per 100 g of body weight twice a week for 3 months), it was determined that the number of sinusoidal endothelial fenestrae decreased and the sinusoids within the regenerative nodules surrounded by fibrous septa were narrow [14]. In mice with biliary cirrhosis, this technique allowed for the identification of numerous blindly terminating and chaotically located sinusoids, as well as large portosystemic collaterals bypassing them and shunting blood towards the hepatic veins. The disadvantage of bile duct ligation is biloma formation, causing irregular saccular deformation of sinusoids, which presents as holes in the cast. Moreover, limitations of the casting technique include perfusion difficulties, especially for microvascular perfusion, and bloating of the sinusoids due to the injection pressure. This makes it difficult to perform a more thorough morphometric analysis of the hepatic microvasculature [101].

Intravital Fluorescence Microscopy

Intravital fluorescence microscopy is necessary for the intravital evaluation of structural changes at the microcirculatory level in experimental cirrhosis. For this purpose, different models of cirrhosis may be used, such as bile duct ligation and subcutaneous or intraperitoneal administration of CCl_4. Although subcutaneous CCl_4 administration can induce necrosis at the site of injection and should be carried out for 16 weeks, this route of administration is preferable for intravital fluorescence microscopy. In contrast to intraperitoneal injections or bile duct ligation, subcutaneous CCl_4 administration does not cause adhesions between the liver and the neighboring organs that can later limit the possibility of carrying out *in vivo* studies in the abdominal cavity [102].

After performing midline and subcostal incisions, the hepatic ligaments are dissected, and the left liver lobe is placed on a fixed plate to minimize respiratory movements. A fluorescent dye was injected into the jugular or tail vein, and, while tissue contrast is increased, liver microcirculation was analyzed with a fluorescent microscope.

Intravital fluorescence microscopy makes it possible to visualize HSC due to autofluorescence of vitamin A; estimate the number of rolling and adherent leukocytes; and measure relative vascular density, the diameter and perfusion of sinusoids, and flow and volume velocity of blood [103].

The maximal number and diameters of portosystemic shunts were observed 3 weeks after bile duct ligation and 12 weeks after the first administration of CCl_4 (0.1 mL 50% oil solution per 100 g of body weight subcutaneously twice a week for 4 months; 5% alcohol was added to drinking water). Fibrosis and the activated HSC were located in periportal areas in biliary cirrhosis and in pericentral areas in CCl_4-induced cirrhosis. The sinusoids in these regions became narrow, whereas the distance between them increased.

The major drawback of intravital fluorescence microscopy is that it can only visualize superficial structures; therefore, it does not give an opportunity to estimate the diameter of portal venules. This may be due to the displacement of portal tracts deeper into the tissue as a result of pericentral fibrosis.

Three-Dimensional Microcomputed Tomography

Microcomputed tomography (microCT) provides high-resolution 3D images that are composed of two-dimensional (2D) trans-axial projections, or 'slices', of a target object. For live animal imaging, the slices are obtained by rotating the emitter and detector. To evaluate microcirculation, *ex vivo* microCT requires vascular casting with contrast agents, such as microfil MV-122 and BaSO4/gelatin, whereas *in vivo* microCT can be performed with iodinated monomer-based bolus or lipid emulsion-based blood-pool contrast agents [104].

Intravital microCT is performed with a dual-energy flat-panel microCT scanner before and immediately after intravenous injection of 100 μl of specially optimised iodine-based contrast agent eXIA™160XL (Binitio Biomedical Inc., Ottawa, Canada). A Feldkamp-type algorithm is used to reconstruct 2D images into 3D with a voxel size of 35x35x35 μm. The relative blood volume value determination is based on the mean brightness of the liver tissue after a contrast agent injection. The value correlates with the number of angiogenic vessels. In this way, a statistically significant increase in the relative blood volume was observed in the murine cirrhotic liver 6 weeks after the first intraperitoneal administration of CCl_4 (0.06 mL 50% oil solution per 100 g of body weight twice a week for 6 weeks) and 2 weeks after bile duct ligation. The advantage of the technique is that it can be conducted repeatedly, thereby allowing gradual monitoring of the process.

The merit of *ex vivo* microCT is the higher resolution image obtained [105, 106]. It was used in different models of cirrhosis in mice and rats. In its classical version, the inferior vena cava is crossed above the diaphragm, and the radiopaque lead oxide diluted in a liquid silicone polymer (microfil) is injected into the portal vein at the rate of 8–10 mL/min and at a pressure of 10–12 mmHg; or alternatively, injection into the heart at a pressure not higher than that of the artery, this is carried out using an automatic pump. The specimens are kept at 4°C for 12 hours. Subsequently, the liver is taken, cut into lobes, fixed in formalin, and then dehydrated in increasing concentrations of a glycerol aqueous solution at 24-hour intervals. Using a microCT scanner and the special computer processing algorithm, 3D images of the intrahepatic microvasculature are obtained and then analyzed using software [107].

MicroCT *ex vivo* makes it possible to estimate the ratio of vascular volume to total liver volume and enables precise analysis of the branching of medium and large hepatic vessels. They are detected in the liver, particularly at the periphery, 6 weeks after the first intraperitoneal injection of CCl_4 (0.06 mL 50% oil solution per 100 g of body weight twice a week for 6 weeks) and 21 days after bile duct ligation. By Week 4 of biliary cirrhosis development, the vascular volume increased one and a half times and the number of branches doubled [108], which reflected the severity of angiogenesis [109].

The limitations of the technique include perfusion difficulties, especially for microcirculatory perfusion, and the reactivity of casting resins with other chemical compounds and surrounding tissue. Moreover, dual casting, which is necessary for contrast-based differentiation between venous and arterial systems, is not possible. This is due to the presence of shunts between the hepatic arterioles and portal venules, functioning as a one-way valve that allows blood to flow only from the arterial to venous system [110].

To overcome this shortcoming, Peeters *et al* [111] sequentially injected yellow or blue contrast agents, PU4ii, into the abdominal aorta or portal vein, respectively, after clamping the thoracic aorta and renal arteries. In order to prevent damage to the microvessels by the pumped substance, a polyethylene drainage tube was installed into the inferior vena cava through the right atrium. The thoracic section of the inferior vena cava, the abdominal aorta, and the portal vein were clamped to eliminate leakage of the substance during polymerization. After 72 hours, the casted liver was macerated using a 25% potassium hydroxide bath for 5 days. The vascular replica was then flushed with distilled water and laid to dry under a vented hood for a further 5 days. MicroCT with 3D reconstruction was performed with a resolution of 1.89 μm for microcirculation and 40 μm for larger vessels. To morphologically analyze microcirculation, a sample with the dimensions 350x350x200 μm was virtually dissected in between portal triads. The average radius of the sinusoidal vessels, branch length, tortuosity, and porosity (the total sinusoidal volume divided by the volume of its envelope) of the vascular network was assessed with the in-house developed software. Using this technique in animals with macronodular cirrhosis induced by thioacetamide (first, 0.03% thioacetamide was added to drinking water, and then the concentration was adapted every week for 18 weeks to keep body weight within a 250–300 g range), these authors have identified the compression of the hepatic venules and an increase in the diameter of the hepatic artery [112].

Immunohistochemical Methods

Intravascular injection of contrast agents only revealed the structure of functioning vessels. Immunohistochemical staining of tissue sections is used for a more accurate evaluation of the newly formed vessels, including the nascent capillaries without a lumen. The most common specific markers are VEGF and membrane proteins CD31 and CD34 for endothelial cell detection. In particular, VEGF and angiopoietin-1 expression shows an increase in intrahepatic vascular density in rats with biliary cirrhosis [109]. Immunofluorescence is a variant of immunohistochemical staining. It requires the use of secondary antibodies such as streptavidin conjugated with carbocyanine CY2 [113].

Confocal laser scanning microscopy after immunohistochemical staining makes it possible to study 3D structures with a resolution of up to 0.2 μm. This technique is based on improved protocols for the chemical purification of samples allowing a dye and photons to penetrate deeper into tissue before and after immunohistochemistry [114, 115]. Subsequent confocal laser scanning provides detailed volumetric data on microcirculation at a voxel size of 0.63x0.63x1.40 μm. The data are processed by a specially developed software (DeLiver). In a study involving rats with thioacetamide-induced cirrhosis, a decrease in mean radius and porosity as well as an increase in tortuosity and length of sinusoids were determined using this technique [112].

Extrahepatic Angiogenesis Assays

The advantages and disadvantages of different extrahepatic assays are listed below (Table **2**).

Intravital Microscopy of the Small Bowel Mesentery

Intravital microscopy enables imaging of structural changes in microvasculature, vascular permeability, and mesenteric vascular density, that characterizes splanchnic angiogenesis. After performing a midline laparotomy, a small intestinal

Table 2. Extrahepatic angiogenesis and portosystemic shunting assays.

Assay	Advantages	Disadvantages
Intravital microscopy of the small bowel mesentery	Enables imaging of structural changes of microvasculature, vascular permeability, adhesion and rolling of leukocytes, and mesenteric vascular density.	The need for surgical intervention, which limits repeated procedures because of adhesions formation. Rapid increase in the number of leukocyte rolling.
Teflon rings implantation	Corresponds to an *in vivo* situation with an intact circulation. Evaluation of newly formed vessels without a lumen. Evaluation of proangiogenic factors expression.	The need for surgical intervention.
Immunohistochemical methods	Evaluation of newly formed vessels without a lumen. Evaluation of proangiogenic factors expression.	Analysis of microcirculation only.
Scanning electron microscopy	Quantification of vessel dimensions, intervascular distances, branching order and luminal surface features, as well as the wall shear stress.	Perfusion difficulties of casting materials, especially for microvascular perfusion.

(Table 2) cont.....

Assay	Advantages	Disadvantages
Microsphere technique	Evaluation of total shunting degree, as well as spleno-renal shunting.	The need to sacrifice laboratory animals.
3D micro-single-photon emission computed tomography	Serial measurements of portosystemic shunting. 3D imaging *in vivo*. Pre-interventional measurement of portosystemic shunting that is important for selection of animals with similar baseline characteristics in studies evaluating anti-angiogenic therapy.	Requires the use of radioactive material.

loop should be exteriorized, placed on a heated Plexiglas plate, and continuously superfused with an Earle's balanced salt solution to prevent dehydration. Observations are carried out with the Axiotech Vario 100HD microscope (Carl Zeiss AG, Oberkochen, Germany) equipped with water immersion objectives (x10 and x40). The obtained image is recorded for the subsequent computer analysis. This enables study of all the types of mesenteric microvessels and calculation of their density, which is defined as the ratio of a vessel's length to the area it occupies [116].

Epifluorescence microscopy is used to measure vascular permeability. After the selection of a venular segment with a diameter of 20–40 mm and an unbranched length of about 150 mm, fluorescent isothiocyanate-bovine serum albumin was injected intravenously. As the intraluminal grey scale value fell, the perivascular grey scale value rose when the fluorescent isothiocyanate-bovine serum albumin molecule leaked through the vascular wall, quantified using black and white image and taking black for 0 and white for 255. Intravital microscopy revealed an increased vascular density and gross disturbance of the mesenteric microcirculation in rats with PH induced by partial portal vein ligation (PPVL) and in rats with biliary cirrhosis. Moreover, the changes in the latter were more significant, which may be due to the time required for cirrhosis development. In addition, vascular permeability was significantly increased in these animals, in contrast to permeability in animals with extrahepatic PH. This is explained by the higher levels of eNOS and VEGF [102].

In addition to the aforementioned uses, intravital microscopy is used to quantify adhesion and rolling of leukocytes, a well-known hallmark of inflammation, which in turn leads to angiogenesis. In particular, in rats with cirrhosis induced by CCl_4 (0.04 mL administered intragastrically and increased weekly in increments of 0.04 mL to a maximum dose of 0.4 mL; 35 mg/100 mL phenobarbital was added to drinking water once 2 weeks before the first administration of CCl_4), the index of leukocyte-endothelial interaction was increased in the microcirculation of the liver and small bowel mesentery [117]. The disadvantage of this method is the need for surgical intervention and extraction of the mesentery from the abdominal cavity. This causes a rapid and pronounced increase in the number of leukocyte rolling in response to partial degranulation of perivascular mast cells and endothelium expression of P-selectin in a matter of minutes [118].

The Requirements for the Analysis of Microcirculation Images Obtained with Intravital Microscopy

Intravital microscopy requires video recording for the analysis of microvasculature. It is recommended that the following requirements are met [119]:

- At least three, or preferably five, arbitrary regions of microcirculation should be included in the analysis.
- Optical magnification should be x10 for microcirculation imaging in small laboratory animals.
- It is necessary to avoid pressure artifacts occurring when a microscope objective contacts the region of interest; excess pressure applied to the area may collapse the microcirculation and stop venous blood flow.
- Video images should be stored in full size without compression to the form of DV-AVI files in order to provide the possibility of computer frame-by-frame analysis. The optimal video recording time is 20 seconds.

A report on the analysis of images obtained with intravital microscopy must include the following parameters calculated for all vessels and capillaries separately:

- Total vascular density and perfused vessel density, which are calculated as the ratio of total vessel length to image area.
- Proportion of perfused vessels expressed as a percentage.
- Microvascular flow index.
- Heterogeneity index, which is calculated as the ratio of the difference between the maximum and minimum blood flow velocity to its average velocity in the five selected areas of an image.

Calculations can be made directly by the researcher using semiquantitative scales for visual evaluation [120, 121]. For a more accurate analysis of the required parameters, the CapImage software is used. It was specially developed for intravital microscopy [122].

In Vivo Evaluation of Angiogenesis in the Small Bowel Mesentery by Implantation of Teflon Rings

Implantation of Teflon rings is another technique for intravital evaluation of angiogenesis of the small bowel mesentery in PH. The rings have a diameter of 7 mm, a height of 3 mm, and an internal diameter of 5 mm. The rings are placed into polyester mesh bags and filled with a mixture of bovine Type I collagen and bovine serum albumin. After performing a midline incision and PPVL, the rings are implanted between the two mesenteric membranes and fixed with single sutures in rats. After 16 days, the rats are euthanized, the implant is removed, fixed in a 4% formalin, and paraffinized. Then, 3-μm-thick tissue sections are prepared. The tissue is stained for further video morphometry and vascular density calculation. This technique makes it possible to determine the number of vessels and the mechanisms of their formation [123].

Immunofluorescence Assay

Vascular network imaging can be carried out by immunological reaction of fluorescent antibodies with membrane proteins of endothelial cells. Anti-CD31 and anti-VEGF antibodies are most often used for these purposes [124]. The small intestinal wall or its mesentery is washed in sodium phosphate buffer, dried on gelatin-coated slides, and fixed in 100% methanol at -20°C for 30 minutes. The sections are then incubated with the corresponding primary murine anti-rat antibodies at 4°C for 12 hours. Streptavidin conjugated with carbocyanine CY2 is used as a secondary antibody. It is applied at room temperature and held for 1 hour. The image obtained after fluorescence microscopy may be analyzed using ImageJ software [125].

An alternative technique consists of the fixation of frozen sections in acetone at -20°C for 10 minutes. After which, the tissue is blocked with 5% bovine serum albumin solution for 45 minutes [38]. Besides CD31, endothelial cell identification is possible with the use of BSI-lectin. Perivascular cell markers include Neural/glial antigen 2, desmin, α-SMA, PDGFR-β, and class III β-tubulin [126].

Immunohistochemical Staining

Immunohistochemical staining is performed to study not only intrahepatic but also extrahepatic angiogenesis, including angiogenesis in the small bowel mesentery and the gastric wall. The presence of angiogenesis in the small bowel mesentery was confirmed by numerous experimental studies in laboratory animals with different PH models [127].

Tissue oxidative stress, which occurs in PH, aggravates the pathophysiological changes that occur in the gastric wall. The oxidative stress is detected by the reaction of antibodies with metabolites that arise during free radical oxidation, such as nitrotirosine. In particular, an increased expression of eNOS, VEGF, and nitrotyrosine was found in the gastric wall of rats with prehepatic PH induced by PPVL, indicating the presence of stimuli for further development of collateral circulation [128].

Aperio [129] or the CAIMAN algorithm [130] may be used to calculate the number of vessels on images of immunohistochemically stained samples. The program called AngioPath can quantify microvessels and determine the size and shape of all vessels as well as each vessel individually. As such, it is an important tool for characterizing angiogenesis [131].

Scanning Electron Microscopy

Scanning electron microscopy of vascular casts is helpful for imaging of the splanchnic vascular network's 3D structure with its subsequent quantitative analysis. The technique was used in animals with PPVL and biliary cirrhosis and revealed the presence of newly formed tortuous vessels serving as shunts between the branches of the inferior vena cava and the portal vein. In addition, holes were found in the walls of some capillaries, serving as a sign of intussusceptive angiogenesis, which is one of the two known types of microvessel growth [101].

Assessment of Portosystemic Shunting

Portosystemic Shunting Assay Using Microspheres

In 1981, Chojkier and Groszmann [132] proposed to use ^{51}Cr-labelled microspheres to assess the degree of portosystemic shunting. The modification of Chojkier and Groszmann's technique through the use of color polystyrene fluorescent microspheres has become widespread at the present time, because this technique excludes any contact with the dangerous radioactive material and maintains accuracy [133].

Approximately 30,000 yellow microspheres (15 μm in diameter) are slowly injected into the spleen. An injection of microspheres of a different colour into the ileocolic vein should be completed for a more detailed haemodynamic assessment of total shunting from the splanchnic area. The liver and lungs of the animal models are removed and placed in centrifuge tubes. Approximately 3,000 blue microspheres are added as an internal control. The tissue is digested in unilocular potassium hydroxide at 60°C for 12 hours and then sonicated. After centrifugation, the supernatant is removed and the pellets are washed once in 10%

Triton X-100 solution and twice in acidified ethanol.

The precipitate containing microspheres was dried for 12 hours, diluted in acidified Cellosolve™ acetate (The Dow Chemical Company, Midland, Michigan, USA), and the number of microspheres was counted using a spectrophotometer. A hemocytometer and an epifluorescent microscope are also adequate for this procedure [134]. The degree of portosystemic shunting is calculated as the ratio of the number of pulmonary microspheres to their sum in the lungs and liver [135].

The microsphere technique confirmed that portosystemic collaterals had started forming in rats with PH 2 days after PPVL and became fully developed on Day 7 post PPVL [69]. At the same time, portosystemic collaterals developed later in rats with biliary cirrhosis. Therefore, it is expedient to evaluate them 1 month after bile duct ligation [136].

Three-Dimensional Micro-Single-Photon Emission Computed Tomography

Since a significant disadvantage of the microsphere method is the need to use laboratory animals, micro-single-photon emission computed tomography (3D micro-SPECT) with technetium (^{99m}Tc) macro aggregated albumin was developed as an alternative. It provides a possibility of conducting serial measurements of portosystemic shunting at different time points after the creation of a model. ^{99m}Tc macro aggregated albumin particles are injected into the splenic pulp; accumulation of the particles in the liver and lungs is determined by using colour scales and computer processing.

3D micro-SPECT was used in mice with PPVL and biliary cirrhosis. The results correlated with the results obtained by using ^{51}Cr-labelled microspheres, and there were no lethality or changes in animals' behaviour after its reusing on the 8th, 12th, and 15th day after the model creation [137].

The application of modern techniques for studying angiogenesis in experimental research made it possible to establish the important role of new vessel formation in cirrhosis-associated PH pathogenesis and has created the prerequisites for the development of antiangiogenic therapy aimed at threating PH-associated hemodynamic disorders.

PERSPECTIVES OF ANTIANGIOGENIC THERAPY FOR PORTAL HYPERTENSION IN LIVER CIRRHOSIS

The efforts to develop angiogenesis inhibitors began in the 1970s at Harvard University under the guidance of Judah Folkman. The drugs were actively introduced into clinical practice a decade after the first were developed [29].

Inhibitors of Intrahepatic Angiogenesis

Tyrosine Kinase Inhibitors

The introduction of antiangiogenic therapy into hepatological practice began with the treatment of hepatocellular carcinoma, a well-vascularized tumor that needs intense angiogenic activity for its development [138]. The most studied drug used for this purpose is sorafenib, a multi-targeted inhibitor of receptor and nonreceptor tyrosine kinases, which are responsible for transmitting various signals to cells, including proliferative stimuli. The antitumor and antiangiogenic effect of sorafenib is achieved mainly through the suppression of the Raf/MEK/ERK signaling pathway and blockade of signaling from the receptors of VEGF (VEGFR), PDGF (PDGFR), and c-kit (SCFR) [139].

Experimental studies have shown the antiangiogenic effect of sorafenib during the early stage of hepatic fibrosis [140]. In animals with various models of cirrhosis, it had positive effects on some pathogenetic pathways of fibrogenesis and angiogenesis in the liver by blocking the receptor tyrosine kinases located on the surface of HSC, the expression of which, especially VEGFR and PDGFR, was increased [141] (Fig. **3**):

- the suppression of activated HSC proliferation and the activation of apoptosis;
- the inhibition of cyclin D1 and cyclin-dependent kinase 4 (Cdk-4) with a simultaneous increase in the expression of Fas, Fas-L, and Caspase-3, and a decrease in the ratio of Bcl-2 to Bax;
- an increase in the ratio of matrix metalloproteinases to the tissue inhibitor of matrix metalloproteinases, and also a decrease in the synthesis of collagen by HSC;
- the inhibition of phosphorylation of ERK, Akt, and ribosomal protein kinase S6 with a molecular mass of 70 kDa (p70S6K) [143]; and
- the disturbance of the Kruppel-like factor 6–Ang1–fibronectin molecular triad functioning [108].

Sorafenib decreased the severity of inflammation, fibrogenesis, and angiogenesis in rats with biliary cirrhosis, which led to a reduction in hepatic vascular resistance to portal blood flow [144].

Another multi-targeted tyrosine kinase inhibitor sunitinib is less studied but known to block VEGFR1/2/3, PDGFR-α/β, fibroblast growth factor receptor (FGFR), and c-kit signaling [145]. In addition, an *in vitro* study by Majumder *et al* [146] showed that sunitinib can slow HSC collagen synthesis by 47%, reduce

HSC contractility by 65%, and decrease cellular migration by 28%, as well as inhibit the angiogenic capacity of SEC.

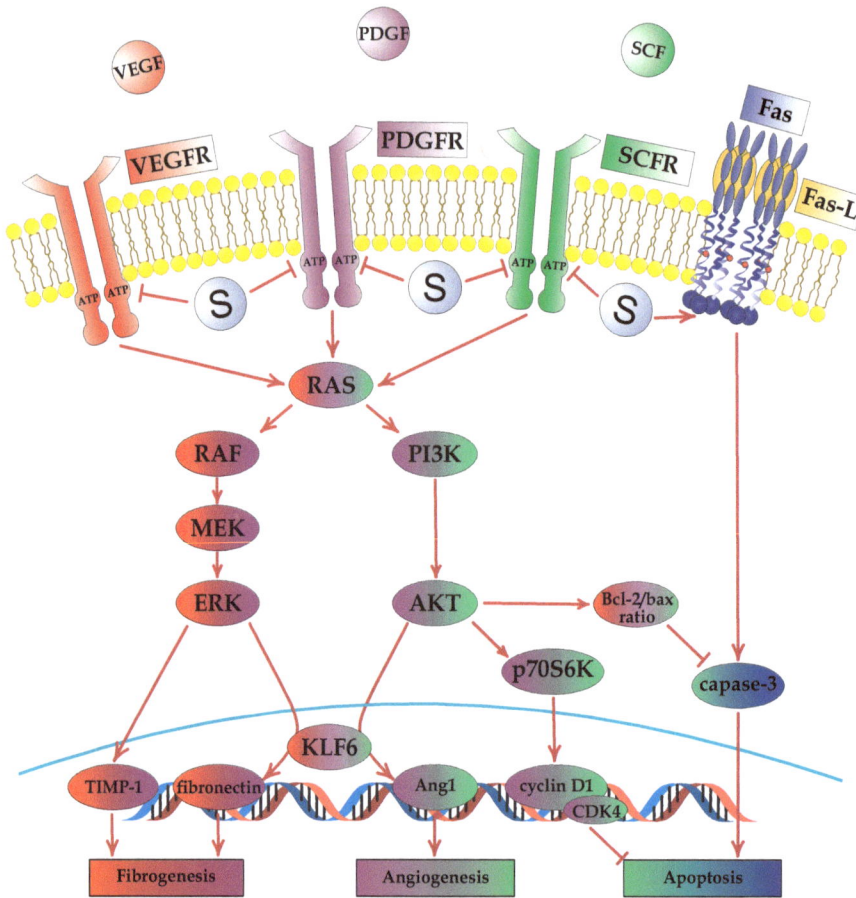

Fig. (3). Positive effects of sorafenib on some pathogenetic pathways of fibrogenesis and angiogenesis in the liver. Sorafenib (S) blocks the ATP-binding site of the vascular endothelial growth factor receptor (VEGFR), platelet-derived growth factor receptor (PDGFR), and stem cell growth factor receptor (SCFR) tyrosine kinases located on the surface of HSC, inhibiting the two main cellular pathways of the RAS protein. At the same time, sorafenib increases the expression of Fas and its ligand. This decreases the severity of fibrogenesis and angiogenesis and increases apoptosis, leading to a reduction in hepatic vascular resistance to portal blood flow [142].

Branivib is a double inhibitor of VEGFR and FGFR signaling. It significantly suppressed intrahepatic angiogenesis and reduced PH in rats with biliary cirrhosis [109]. Additionally, it improved blood circulation in the liver and hindered the formation of ascites in rats with liver cirrhosis caused by nonalcoholic steatohepatitis [147].

Statins

The positive effect of statins on hepatic fibro- and angiogenesis in cirrhosis is associated with the induction of Krüppel-like factor 2 (KLF2) in SEC [148]. KLF2 is a member of a family of widely expressed transcription factors that regulate cell and tissue growth. KLF2 is well represented in the vascular endothelium and is necessary for the normal development of vessels; in addition, it is a well-known antiangiogenic factor that modulates the severity of many endothelial vasoprotective genes [149]. KLF2 can effectively inhibit HIF-1α, reducing the expression of such proangiogenic factors as VEGF and Ang2 [150].

The mechanical stimuli generated by shear stress are the main physiological impulse for triggering and maintaining endothelial KLF2 expression [151]. In the cirrhotic liver, KLF2 expression was elevated in both SEC [152] and activated HSC [153]. This serves as a compensatory mechanism aimed at eliminating vascular dysfunction and preventing angiogenesis by suppressing the proliferation and migration of SEC, as well as downregulating the ERK1/2 signaling pathway to inhibit the formation of tubular structures [154].

In an *in vitro* study conducted by Miao *et al* [155], simvastatin eliminated the pro-angiogenic environment for TGF-β-activated HSC as a result of the following processes:

- the reduction of cell migration and proliferation;
- the inhibition of the α-SMA expression, and the elevation of mRNA and KLF2 levels in HSC;
- an increase in the production of eNOS and suppression of the various proangiogenic proteins expression in HSC, such as VEGF, HIF-1α, and pro-inflammatory NF-κB; and
- the reduction of the hyperactivity of interferon γ, which participates in angiogenesis.

In rats with CCL4-induced liver cirrhosis, it was noted that statins (atorvastatin, mevastatin, simvastatin, and lovastatin) enhanced the effect of KLF2. By doing this, they deactivated SEC and reduced the severity of fibrosis and associated angiogenesis, thereby exerting a positive effect on PH [156].

Rifaximin

Endotoxemia, which is due to the translocation of gram-negative bacteria from the intestine, plays an important role in the pathogenesis of both cirrhosis and associated complications [157]. During the development of cirrhosis, bacterial lipopolysaccharide influences Kupffer cells and HSC. Nevertheless, SEC are affected first. TLR4, which are located on their surface and capable of binding bacterial lipopolysaccharide, are involved in fibrosis-associated angiogenesis. These receptors manifest such properties through the related cytosolic adapter protein MyD88, which is involved in the production of extracellular protease regulating the invasive ability of SEC [42].

In mice with biliary cirrhosis, it was shown that rifaximin, a nonabsorbable antibiotic with broad antimicrobial activity against aerobic and anaerobic gram-negative bacteria, reduced the severity of fibrosis and angiogenesis in the liver by inhibiting bacterial lipopolysaccharide binding to TLR4. As a consequence, it reduced PH [158]. This drug is already used to treat hepatic encephalopathy. It has an acceptable safety profile when applied in patients with chronic liver diseases and is approved by the US Food and Drug Administration [159]. This experimental study may be a basis for evaluation of rifaximin in other complications of cirrhosis.

Largazole

The histone deacetylase inhibitor largazole is a natural compound derived from marine cyanobacteria Symploca sp. With a strong antiproliferative and cytotoxic effect, it has a wide spectrum but differential activity against several different lines of cancer cells [160]. In addition, in experimental studies *in vitro* and *in vivo*, largazole attenuated the severity of liver fibrosis and associated angiogenesis through numerous independent mechanisms:

- the reduction of VEGF production by HSC;
- the inhibition of VEGF-stimulated HSC proliferation;
- the downregulation of TGF-β1- and VEGF-induced Akt phosphorylation in activated HSC, as well as the downregulation of VEGFR2-dependent p38MAPK phosphorylation in SEC; and
- the suppression of CD34, VEGF, and VEGFR2 expression [161].

The ability of largazole to affect the main fibrogenic and angiogenic pathways in the cirrhotic liver can be used to test its effectiveness in PH.

Ribavirin

In addition to antiviral activity against certain DNA- and RNA-containing viruses, ribavirin may have a positive effect on the morphological changes underlying the development of cirrhosis [162]. In addition, at therapeutic concentrations, it is able to inhibit angiogenesis both *in vitro* and *in vivo*, which is due to the inhibition of inosine-5'-monophosphate dehydrogenase 1 activity and a decrease in tetrahydrobiopterin, NO, and cyclic guanosine monophosphate (cGMP) levels in

SEC [163].

Inhibitors of Extrahepatic Angiogenesis

It was traditionally thought that portosystemic shunts are formed when increased portal pressure "opens" pre-existing vessels in the areas of embryonic connection between the portal and systemic circulation. This paradigm was challenged by Fernandez *et al*, who first reported that portosystemic collaterals in PH are formed due to active angiogenesis. It should be noted that VEGF is of the greatest importance only at the initial stages of angiogenesis, when it activates endothelial cell proliferation and the subsequent formation of endothelial tubules. Vascular maturation is modulated mainly by PDGF, which regulates the introduction of endothelial tubules into the population of intramural cells and pericytes, thus stabilizing the newly formed vasculature [47]. The simultaneous suppression of the signaling caused by both VEGF and PDGF appears more promising than suppressing them individually.

Tyrosine Kinase Inhibitors

Fernandez *et al* [164] studied the combined effect of rapamycin (mTOR inhibitor) and glivec (tyrosine protein kinase inhibitor) on VEGF and PDGF signaling, respectively, in rats with extrahepatic PH caused by partial portal vein ligation and with well-developed portosystemic collateral circulation. It was noted that rapamycin and glivec in combination markedly reduced the splanchnic neovascularization and pericyte coverage of new vessels through the decreased expression of VEGF, VEGFR2, CD31, PDGF, PDGFR-β, and α-SMA. In addition, there was a reduction of portal pressure and blood flow along the superior mesenteric artery by 40% and 30% from the baseline level, respectively.

Similar results were obtained by Mejias *et al* [144], who found that multi-kinase inhibitor sorafenib triggered blockade of VEGF and PDGF signaling transduction and the Raf/MEK/ERK signaling pathways. Sorafenib significantly reduced intraorgan and systemic blood flow, and increased splanchnic neovascularization by 80% and portosystemic shunting by 18%. This led to a reduction in hepatic vascular resistance and decrease in portal pressure by 25% from the baseline. It was also noted that the positive effect of sorafenib on PH was more significant when it was combined with propranolol [165].

Somatostatin and its Synthetic Analogs

Somatostatin is a cyclic 14-amino acid peptide, which is secreted by nerve, endocrine, and enteroendocrine cells in the hypothalamus and digestive system (in the stomach, intestine, and pancreatic δ-cells). Somatostatin and its synthetic analogs (octreotide, vapreotide, and others) are used in patients with cirrhosis to treat bleeding from esophageal varices by affecting both intra- and extrahepatic mechanisms of PH [166].

The ability of octreotide to inhibit cell proliferation and neovascularization through the high-affinity somatostatin subtype receptor 2 (SSTR2) was an impetus for studying its antiangiogenic properties in various diseases [167]. In studies involving rats with extrahepatic PH caused by partial portal vein ligation, octreotide significantly weakened the expression of VEGF and CD31 in the internal organs, reduced the development of splanchnic neovascularization by 64%, and lessened the severity of a portosystemic collateral circulation by 16%. At the same time, its angioinhibitory effect manifested only in the first four days of the experiment and completely disappeared after a week, as PH progressed. This is possibly due to a decrease in SSTR2 expression in mucosa, intestinal vessels, and portosystemic collaterals [168].

Spironolactone

Pathophysiological disturbances inherent to PH underlie the occurrence of ascites in cirrhosis. Systemic arterial vasodilation and the activation of various neurohormonal pathways, including the renin-angiotensin-aldosterone system, cause renal dysfunction. This decreases Na+ and water excretion and reduces the glomerular filtration rate. The drug of choice for treatment is spironolactone, an antagonist of aldosterone, a mineralocorticoid, that mediates the reabsorption of Na+ and water in the distal part of the nephron [169]. In addition to the important role in maintaining water–salt metabolism, aldosterone has angiogenic properties. In particular, it enhances ischemia-induced neovascularization [170], stimulates pathological angiogenesis in the retina [171], and promotes the proliferation of endothelial cells of the heart [172] by activating angiotensin II signaling. At the same time, its antagonist spironolactone inhibits these processes both *in vitro* and *in vivo* [173]. In rats with biliary cirrhosis, spironolactone significantly reduced the degree of mesenteric angiogenesis and portosystemic shunting by suppressing the VEGF signal transduction pathway [174].

N-acetylcysteine

Because hypoxia serves as the main inducer of angiogenesis both under physiological and pathological conditions, angiogenesis inhibitors may be drugs with antioxidant properties. One of them is N-acetylcysteine, which is a derivative of amino acid cysteine, the thiol groups of which directly interact with electrophilic groups of free radicals. N-acetylcysteine can also enhance the activity of glutathione-S-transferase, glutathione peroxidase, glutathione reductase, and a number of other enzymes involved in maintaining the oxidant/antioxidant balance [175].

Long-term application of N-acetylcysteine in rats with biliary cirrhosis lessened oxidative stress in the mesentery of the small intestine, reduced the level of circulating inflammatory cytokines, and inhibited mesenteric angiogenesis by decreasing angiogenic marker expression (VEGF, VEGFR2, Ang1, and CD31). This eventually improved splanchnic and systemic hemodynamics.

In addition, N-acetylcysteine inhibited VEGF-induced endothelial tubule formation and endothelial cell migration by suppressing TNF-α and Akt/eNOS/NO angiogenic signaling cascade *in vitro*. It also reduced the number of reactive oxygen species (including reactive compounds of thiobarbituric acid and malondialdehyde) and inflammatory cytokines in the human umbilical vein endothelial cell supernatant [136].

Endothelin Receptor Blockers

ET-1 is one of the mediators whose synthesis is enhanced in conditions of tissue hypoxia. It is directly involved in intra- and extrahepatic mechanisms of PH pathogenesis, and its circulating level is increased in cirrhosis because of "large endothelin" hyperproduction and increased expression of endothelin-converting enzyme [176]. Experimental studies have shown that ET-1 induces angiogenic responses in cultured endothelial cells through endothelial ETB-type receptors and, in combination with VEGF, stimulates neovascularization *in vivo* [177]. The nonselective endothelin receptor blocker bosentan and the selective ETA receptor blocker ambrisentan reduced the degree of mesenteric angiogenesis and portosystemic shunting in rats with biliary cirrhosis by suppressing inducible nitric oxide synthase (iNOS), cyclooxygenase 2, VEGF and VEGFR2, and Akt signaling [178].

Pioglitazone

Pioglitazone, a potent selective agonist of peroxisome proliferator-activated receptors-γ (PPAR-γ), is able to reduce the level of systemic inflammation in patients with a high cardiovascular disease risk. It blocks the activity of pro-inflammatory genes by post-transcriptional modification of their products (by attaching small SUMO proteins to them) and suppresses NF-κB expression by transrepression. All PPAR isomers (PPAR-α, PPAR-β/-δ, and PPAR-γ) are anti-inflammatory nuclear transcription factors and NF-κB antagonists. Dominant negative mutation of PPAR-γ leads to systemic inflammation and rapid development of related diseases: arterial hypertension, atherosclerosis, type 2 diabetes, nonalcoholic steatohepatitis, psoriasis, and premature aging [179].

In addition to systemic inflammation reduction, PPAR-γ agonists are also capable of inhibiting oxidative stress and angiogenesis [180]. In rats with models of biliary cirrhosis and extrahepatic PH caused by partial portal vein ligation, pioglitazone reduced the degree of portosystemic shunting by 22–30% by suppressing angiogenic and pro-inflammatory cytokines, chemokines, and growth factors (VEGF, PDGF, and PIGF) [181].

Thalidomide

Thalidomide, a glutamic acid derivative with antiangiogenic, anti-inflammatory, and immunomodulatory properties, is able to hinder TNF-α/interleukin-1β production for which activated immune cells are responsible [182]. It was also shown in rats with biliary cirrhosis that thalidomide blocked the TNFα-VEG--NOS-NO pathway by downregulating elevated inflammasome expression in the intestinal and mesenteric tissues, which weakened mesenteric angiogenesis and portosystemic shunting [183].

Polyphenols

The possibility of influencing the pathogenetic mechanisms of extrahepatic angiogenesis was found in polyphenols, the chemicals of plant origin with a strong antioxidant effect.

The tea catechins extracted from the dried leaves of Camellia sinensis reduced the severity of mesenteric angiogenesis and portosystemic shunting in rats with biliary cirrhosis by reducing HIF-1α expression, Akt signaling, and VEGF synthesis [135].

2'-hydroxyflavonoid, which is contained in citruses, prevented the formation of new splanchnic vessels and portosystemic collaterals in rats with thioacetamide-induced liver cirrhosis by downregulating apoptosis [184].

The long-term use of curcumin, a polyphenol extracted from turmeric roots, improved the course of PH in liver cirrhosis by positively affecting liver fibrosis and reducing portal influx. These effects were achieved through inhibiting mesenteric angiogenesis and restoring mesenteric vessel contractility, as well as decreasing the degree of portosystemic collateral circulation and hyperdynamic circulatory state. Moreover, its favorable effects on the splanchnic and systemic blood flow included the suppression of VEGF, cyclooxygenase 2, and eNOS [113].

Clinical Experience of Antiangiogenic Therapy for Portal Hypertension

The effect of the drugs described above was studied only in experiments involving animals (Tables **3**, **4**), and only tyrosine kinase inhibitors were tested as an antiangiogenic therapy in patients with cirrhosis and PH.

Coriat *et al* [185] were the first to assess the effect of sorafenib on the portal and systemic hemodynamics, in seven patients with cirrhosis and hepatocellular carcinoma. Five of them had Child–Turcotte–Pugh (CTP) class A, and two had CTP class B. Sorafenib was administered for one month at 400 mg twice a day. In one patient, this was first reduced to 400 mg once a day and then to 400 mg every two days because side effects appeared. A decrease in portal blood flow by at least 36% was noted, while no changes in blood flow were found in the azygos vein and abdominal aorta.

In a pilot study, Pinter *et al* [186] investigated the effects of sorafenib on HVPG and systemic hemodynamics, as well as the expression of mRNA genes involved in fibrogenesis, angiogenesis, and inflammation in the liver in 13 patients suffering from cirrhosis and hepatocellular carcinoma (10 patients had CTP class A and three patients had CTP class B). The drug was administered at 400 mg twice a day for two weeks. Four of the 11 patients with PH (eight of whom had clinically significant PH) had a reduction in HVPG by more than 20% from the baseline values and, in addition, a decrease in the levels of mRNA, VEGF, PDGF, PIGF, RhoA kinase, and TNF-α.

However, the results were not as optimistic in a randomized double-blind placebo-controlled study that assessed the effects of sorafenib administered at 400 mg twice a day on HVPG in nine patients with cirrhosis and hepatocellular carcinoma [187].

The main drawback of tyrosine kinase inhibitors is hepatotoxicity. A study of possibilities of their selective delivery to target cells, in particular, HSC, seems to be a promising direction in solving this problem.

Achievements in understanding the pathogenesis of PH in cirrhosis stimulated the development of new pharmacotherapeutic methods. Currently, the drugs of choice

Table 3. Drugs that can inhibit intrahepatic angiogenesis in portal hypertension.

Ref.	Drugs	Experimental models	Effects
Liu *et al* [133], Qu *et al* [134], Wang *et al* [135], Thabut *et al* [101], Mejias *et al* [136]	Sorafenib	Biliary cirrhosis, non-alcoholic steatohepatitis, thioacetamide-, diethylnitrosamine-, dimethylnitrosamine-, and CCl$_4$-induced cirrhosis.	Suppresses the Raf/MEK/ERK signaling pathway and blocks the signaling from the VEGFR, PDGFR, and SCFR; therefore, increases apoptosis and decreases inflammation, fibrogenesis, angiogenesis, and hepatic vascular resistance.

(Table 3) cont.....

Ref.	Drugs	Experimental models	Effects
Tugues *et al* [137], Majumder *et al* [138]	Sunitinib	CCl_4-induced cirrhosis and cell cultures (immortalized human activated HSC cell line, human HSC, and isolated primary human liver sinusoidal endothelial cells).	Blocks VEGFR1/2/3, PDGFR-α/β, FGFR, and SCFR; reduces HSC collagen synthesis, contractility, cellular migration, and SEC angiogenic capacity.
Lin *et al* [102], Yang *et al* [139]	Brivanib	Biliary cirrhosis, non-alcoholic steatohepatitis.	Inhibits VEGFR and FGFR; therefore, suppresses intrahepatic angiogenesis and portal hypertension, improves blood circulation, and hinders ascites formation.
Miao *et al* [147], Marrone *et al* [148]	Simvastatin	CCl_4-induced cirrhosis and LX-2 cell line.	Enhances KLF2, through which deactivates SEC and reduces the severity of fibrosis and associated angiogenesis.
Zhu *et al* [150]	Rifaximin	Biliary cirrhosis.	Downregulates bacterial lipopolysaccharide binding to TLR4; therefore, reduces the severity of fibrosis and associated angiogenesis.
Liu *et al* [152], Liu *et al* [153]	Largazole	Human colorectal carcinoma cells (HCT116, HT29, and HCT15), human HSC, and CCl_4-induced cirrhosis.	Suppresses the effects of CD34, VEGF, TGF-β1, and VEGFR2, blocking the main fibrogenic and angiogenic pathways.
Michaelis *et al* [155]	Ribavirin	Human umbilical vein endothelial cells.	Hinders angiogenesis by inhibiting inosine-5'-monophosphate dehydrogenase 1, tetrahydrobiopterin, NO, and cGMP.

Table 4. Drugs that can inhibit extrahepatic angiogenesis in portal hypertension.

Ref.	Drugs	Experimental models	Effects
Fernandez *et al* [156]	Rapamycin and glivec	Partial portal vein ligation	Downregulates VEGF, VEGFR2, CD31, PDGF, PDGFR-β, and α-SMA.
Mejias *et al* [136]	Sorafenib	Partial portal vein ligation and CCl_4-induced cirrhosis	Blocks VEGF, PDGF, and Raf/MEK/ERK signaling pathway; therefore, reduces intraorgan and systemic blood flow, splanchnic neovascularization, portosystemic shunting, hepatic vascular resistance, and portal pressure.
Woltering *et al* [159], Mejias *et al* [160]	Somatostatin and its synthetic analogs	Partial portal vein ligation	Reduces VEGF and CD31 expression, splanchnic neovascularization, and portosystemic collateral circulation by blocking SSTR2.

(Table 4) cont.....

Ref.	Drugs	Experimental models	Effects
Miternique-Grosse *et al* [165]	Spironolactone	Biliary cirrhosis	Suppresses the effects of aldosterone and the VEGF signal transduction pathway
Lee *et al* [129]	N-acetylcysteine	Biliary cirrhosis	Reduces oxidative stress, inflammatory cytokine levels, TNF-α, VEGF, VEGFR2, Ang1, CD31 expression, and suppresses Akt/eNOS/NO pathway.
Hsu *et al* [170]	Bosentan and ambrisentan	Biliary cirrhosis	Block endothelin receptors and suppress iNOS, cyclooxygenase 2, VEGF, VEGFR2, and Akt signaling.
Schwabl *et al* [173]	Pioglitazone	Biliary cirrhosis	Downregulates inflammatory genes and NF-κB expression, suppresses angiogenic and pro-inflammatory cytokines, chemokines, and growth factors (VEGF, PDGF, and PIGF).
Li *et al* [175]	Thalidomide	Biliary cirrhosis	Hinders TNF-α/interleukin-1β production and blocks the TNFα-VEGF-NOS-NO pathway.
Hsu *et al* [128]	Catechins of *Camellia sinensis*	Biliary cirrhosis	Reduce HIF-1α expression, Akt signaling, and VEGF synthesis.
Hsin *et al* [176]	2'-hydroxyflavonoid	Thioacetamide-induced liver cirrhosis	Downregulates apoptosis.
Hsu *et al* [106]	Curcumin	Biliary cirrhosis	Suppresses VEGF, cyclooxygenase 2, and eNOS.

are nonselective β-blockers. However, nonselective β-blockers are not recommended during the subclinical stage of the disease, when the most justified treatment is etiotropic and pathogenetic. Such treatment may be aimed at, for example, affecting fibro- and angiogenesis in the liver, as well as angiogenesis underlying the formation of portosystemic shunts. Etiopathogenic approach, as part of a complex correction of pathophysiological disorders that contribute to the development of PH, may be the key to success in preventing related complications.

CONCLUSION

When choosing the therapy for PH, one should take into account a clinical stage of cirrhosis, which largely determines the prognosis of the disease [188].

• Stage 1. An absence of esophageal varices in patients with compensated cirrhosis. In this case, they may have both subclinical (HVPG is within 6-10 mmHg) and clinically significant PH (HVPG is more than 10 mmHg).

- Stage 2. The presence of esophageal varices in patients with compensated cirrhosis.
- Stage 3. Bleeding from esophageal varices in patients with cirrhosis in the absence of such signs of decompensation as ascites, jaundice, or encephalopathy.
- Stage 4. Patients with cirrhosis have one of the following signs of decompensation: ascites, jaundice, or encephalopathy, regardless of esophageal varices.
- Stage 5. Patients with cirrhosis have more than one of the following signs of decompensation: ascites, jaundice, or encephalopathy, regardless of esophageal varices.

Patients with the first and second stages should be divided on those who have subclinical PH and need pre-primary prophylaxis, which prevents the formation of esophageal varices, and those who have clinically significant PH and need measures aimed at variceal bleeding prevention [189] (Fig. **4**). HVPG values >10 mmHg measured using the balloon wedge method are the "gold standard" for clinically significant PH diagnosis. Alternatively, liver stiffness could be measured using transient elastography (TE). The liver stiffness values ≥20-25 kPa indicate clinically significant PH in patients with cirrhosis of viral etiology [1].

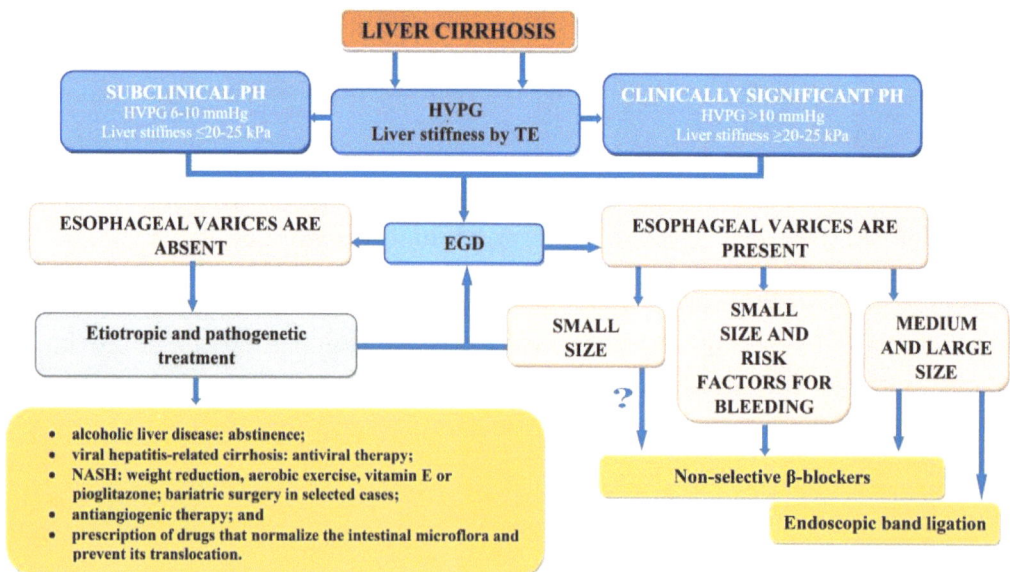

Fig. (4). The therapeutic and diagnostic algorithm in patients with cirrhosis who have not had bleeding from esophageal varices.

The ability of nonselective β-blockers to positively affect portal pressure by reducing cardiac output (blockade of β1-adrenergic receptors) and splanchnic vasodilation (blockade of β2-adrenergic receptors) allowed them to be considered the drugs of choice for primary prevention of bleeding from esophageal varices. However, the absence of a hyperdynamic circulatory status makes it inappropriate to use them in patients with subclinical PH [190]. At this stage, treatment of PH should be etiological and pathogenetic [191].

Certainly, abstinence is the most substantial and fundamental etiological treatment for alcoholic liver disease. In patients with alcoholic cirrhosis, abstinence may lead to regression of liver fibrosis, improve liver function, and help reduce portal pressure [192]. In the past decade, with the progress of antiviral therapy, viral hepatitis-related cirrhosis has undergone a radical change in its natural course following antiviral therapy. At the same time, a sustained virologic response has a positive effect on the histological structure of the liver and significantly reduces HVPG [193, 194]. Angiogenesis plays an important role in the pathogenesis of cirrhosis, underlies the development of associated PH, and is the cause of PH-related complications. Experimental studies made it possible to study the mechanism of action of drugs inhibiting angiogenesis and their effect on PH. However, only tyrosine kinase inhibitors have been tested in patients with cirrhosis as an anti-angiogenic therapy for PH [142]. Although these studies look promising, the complete blockade of the angiogenic pathways can be detrimental, since angiogenesis is also necessary to repair liver tissue and resolve fibrosis. In our opinion, the future of anti-angiogenic therapy lies in its selective effect on target cells in patients with compensated cirrhosis and subclinical PH.

Nonselective β-blockers *should be* prescribed to patients with clinically significant PH, who have small esophageal varices and risk factors for bleeding (severe liver dysfunction (CTP class B or C), alcoholic etiology of the disease, and the presence of so-called red signs on varicose veins during initial esophagogastroduodenoscopy (EGD)). The use of nonselective β-blockers is *possible* in the absence of these risk factors. The use of nonselective β-blockers is also a first-line therapy for the primary prevention of bleeding from esophageal varices of medium and large size. Endoscopic band ligation is indicated for patients who are tolerant or have contraindications to nonselective β-blockers [1].

CONFLICT OF INTEREST

Dr. Arefyev reports a grant from RFBR (Russian Foundation for Basic Research), during the writing of the manuscript. The information included in this manuscript is not related to the interests of RFBR. Prof. Garbuzenko and Prof. Kazachkov have nothing to disclose.

ACKNOWLEDGEMENT

This work is supported by RFBR according to the research project N° 18-315-00434.

ABBREVIATION LIST

Akt	protein kinase B
Ang	angiopoietin
α-SMA	alpha smooth muscle actin
CTGF	connective tissue growth factor
cGMP	cyclic guanosine monophosphate
CTP	Child-Turcotte-Pugh
CCl$_4$	carbon tetrachloride
ET	endothelin-1
eNOS	endothelial nitric oxide synthase
EGF	epidermal growth factor
FGF	fibroblast growth factor
EGD	esophagogastroduodenoscopy
FGFR	fibroblast growth factor receptor
HVPG	hepatic venous portal gradient
HSC	hepatic stellate cells
HGF	hepatocyte growth factor
HIF	hypoxia-inducible factor
iNOS	inducible nitric oxide synthase
IGF	insulin-like growth factor
IL	interleukin
KLF	Krupple-like factor
KLF2	Krüppel-like factor 2
NF-κB	factor kappa-light-chain-enhancer of activated B cells
NO	nitric oxide
PAF	platelet activation factor
PDGF	platelet-derived growth factor
PDGFR	platelet-derived growth factor receptor-β
PlGF	placental growth factor
PPAR	peroxisome proliferator-activated receptor
PH	portal hypertension

ROS	reactive oxygen species
SEC	sinusoidal endothelial cells
SCFR	stem cell growth factor receptor
SSTR2	somatostatin receptor type 2
TGF	transforming growth factor
TNF	tumor necrosis factor
TE	transient elastography
VEGF	vascular endothelial growth factor
VEGFR	vascular endothelial growth factor receptor
VSPC	vascular stem/progenitor cells

REFERENCES

[1]   de Franchis R, Baveno VI. Expanding consensus in portal hypertension: Report of the Baveno VI Consensus Workshop: Stratifying risk and individualizing care for portal hypertension. J Hepatol 2015; 63(3): 743-52.
[http://dx.doi.org/10.1016/j.jhep.2015.05.022] [PMID: 26047908]

[2]   EASL Clinical Practice Guidelines for the management of patients with decompensated cirrhosis. J Hepatol 2019; 69(2): 406-60.
[http://dx.doi.org/10.1016/j.jhep.2018.03.024] [PMID: 29653741]

[3]   Garbuzenko DV. Contemporary concepts of the medical therapy of portal hypertension under liver cirrhosis. World J Gastroenterol 2015; 21(20): 6117-26.
[http://dx.doi.org/10.3748/wjg.v21.i20.6117] [PMID: 26034348]

[4]   Berzigotti A, Bosch J. Pharmacologic management of portal hypertension. Clin Liver Dis 2014; 18(2): 303-17.
[http://dx.doi.org/10.1016/j.cld.2013.12.003] [PMID: 24679496]

[5]   Coulon S, Heindryckx F, Geerts A, Van Steenkiste C, Colle I, Van Vlierberghe H. Angiogenesis in chronic liver disease and its complications. Liver Int 2011; 31(2): 146-62.
[http://dx.doi.org/10.1111/j.1478-3231.2010.02369.x] [PMID: 21073649]

[6]   Garbuzenko DV, Arefyev NO, Belov DV. Mechanisms of adaptation of the hepatic vasculature to the deteriorating conditions of blood circulation in liver cirrhosis. World J Hepatol 2016; 8(16): 665-72.
[http://dx.doi.org/10.4254/wjh.v8.i16.665] [PMID: 27326313]

[7]   Garbuzenko DV, Arefyev NO, Belov DV. Restructuring of the vascular bed in response to hemodynamic disturbances in portal hypertension. World J Hepatol 2016; 8(36): 1602-9.
[http://dx.doi.org/10.4254/wjh.v8.i36.1602] [PMID: 28083082]

[8]   Rosmorduc O. Antiangiogenic therapies in portal hypertension: a breakthrough in hepatology. Gastroenterol Clin Biol 2010; 34(8-9): 446-9.
[http://dx.doi.org/10.1016/j.gcb.2010.05.007] [PMID: 20630674]

[9]   García-Pagán JC, Gracia-Sancho J, Bosch J. Functional aspects on the pathophysiology of portal hypertension in cirrhosis. J Hepatol 2012; 57(2): 458-61.
[http://dx.doi.org/10.1016/j.jhep.2012.03.007] [PMID: 22504334]

[10]   Hu LS, George J, Wang JH. Current concepts on the role of nitric oxide in portal hypertension. World J Gastroenterol 2013; 19(11): 1707-17.
[http://dx.doi.org/10.3748/wjg.v19.i11.1707] [PMID: 23555159]

[11]   Hellerbrand C. Hepatic stellate cells--the pericytes in the liver. Pflugers Arch 2013; 465(6): 775-8.
[http://dx.doi.org/10.1007/s00424-012-1209-5] [PMID: 23292551]

[12]   Ueno T, Bioulac-Sage P, Balabaud C, Rosenbaum J. Innervation of the sinusoidal wall: regulation of the sinusoidal diameter. Anat Rec A Discov Mol Cell Evol Biol 2004; 280(1): 868-73.
[http://dx.doi.org/10.1002/ar.a.20092] [PMID: 15382014]

[13]   Iizuka M, Murata T, Hori M, Ozaki H. Increased contractility of hepatic stellate cells in cirrhosis is mediated by enhanced Ca2+-dependent and Ca2+-sensitization pathways. Am J Physiol Gastrointest Liver Physiol 2011; 300(6): G1010-21.
[http://dx.doi.org/10.1152/ajpgi.00350.2010] [PMID: 21393429]

[14]   Takashimizu S, Kojima S, Nishizaki Y, *et al.* Effect of endothelin A receptor antagonist on hepatic hemodynamics in cirrhotic rats. Implications for endothelin-1 in portal hypertension. Tokai J Exp Clin Med 2011; 36(2): 37-43.
[PMID: 21769771]

[15]   Lugo-Baruqui A, Muñoz-Valle JF, Arévalo-Gallegos S, Armendáriz-Borunda J. Role of angiotensin II in liver fibrosis-induced portal hypertension and therapeutic implications. Hepatol Res 2010; 40(1): 95-104.
[http://dx.doi.org/10.1111/j.1872-034X.2009.00581.x] [PMID: 19737316]

[16]   Reynaert H, Urbain D, Geerts A. Regulation of sinusoidal perfusion in portal hypertension. Anat Rec (Hoboken) 2008; 291(6): 693-8.
[http://dx.doi.org/10.1002/ar.20669] [PMID: 18484616]

[17]   Lee JS, Semela D, Iredale J, Shah VH. Sinusoidal remodeling and angiogenesis: a new function for the liver-specific pericyte? Hepatology 2007; 45(3): 817-25.
[http://dx.doi.org/10.1002/hep.21564] [PMID: 17326208]

[18]   Lee JS, Kang Decker N, Chatterjee S, Yao J, Friedman S, Shah V. Mechanisms of nitric oxide interplay with Rho GTPase family members in modulation of actin membrane dynamics in pericytes and fibroblasts. Am J Pathol 2005; 166(6): 1861-70.
[http://dx.doi.org/10.1016/S0002-9440(10)62495-9] [PMID: 15920170]

[19]   Semela D, Das A, Langer D, Kang N, Leof E, Shah V. Platelet-derived growth factor signaling through ephrin-b2 regulates hepatic vascular structure and function. Gastroenterology 2008; 135(2): 671-9.
[http://dx.doi.org/10.1053/j.gastro.2008.04.010] [PMID: 18570897]

[20]   Pinzani M. PDGF and signal transduction in hepatic stellate cells. Front Biosci 2002; 7: d1720-6.
[http://dx.doi.org/10.2741/A875] [PMID: 12133817]

[21]   Cao S, Yaqoob U, Das A, *et al.* Neuropilin-1 promotes cirrhosis of the rodent and human liver by enhancing PDGF/TGF-beta signaling in hepatic stellate cells. J Clin Invest 2010; 120(7): 2379-94.
[http://dx.doi.org/10.1172/JCI41203] [PMID: 20577048]

[22]   Friedman SL. Hepatic stellate cells: protean, multifunctional, and enigmatic cells of the liver. Physiol Rev 2008; 88(1): 125-72.
[http://dx.doi.org/10.1152/physrev.00013.2007] [PMID: 18195085]

[23]   Seki E, Brenner DA. Recent advancement of molecular mechanisms of liver fibrosis. J Hepatobiliary Pancreat Sci 2015; 22(7): 512-8.
[http://dx.doi.org/10.1002/jhbp.245] [PMID: 25869468]

[24]   Svegliati-Baroni G, De Minicis S, Marzioni M. Hepatic fibrogenesis in response to chronic liver injury: novel insights on the role of cell-to-cell interaction and transition. Liver Int 2008; 28(8): 1052-64.
[http://dx.doi.org/10.1111/j.1478-3231.2008.01825.x] [PMID: 18783548]

[25]   Rappaport AM, MacPhee PJ, Fisher MM, Phillips MJ. The scarring of the liver acini (Cirrhosis). Tridimensional and microcirculatory considerations. Virchows Arch A Pathol Anat Histopathol 1983;

402(2): 107-37.
[http://dx.doi.org/10.1007/BF00695054] [PMID: 6420982]

[26] Lemos QT, Andrade ZA. Angiogenesis and experimental hepatic fibrosis. Mem Inst Oswaldo Cruz 2010; 105(5): 611-4.
[http://dx.doi.org/10.1590/S0074-02762010000500002] [PMID: 20835605]

[27] Elpek GÖ. Angiogenesis and liver fibrosis. World J Hepatol 2015; 7(3): 377-91.
[http://dx.doi.org/10.4254/wjh.v7.i3.377] [PMID: 25848465]

[28] Guido M, Sarcognato S, Russo FP, *et al.* Focus on histological abnormalities of intrahepatic vasculature in chronic viral hepatitis. Liver Int 2019; 38(10): 1770-6.
[http://dx.doi.org/10.1111/liv.13718] [PMID: 29427537]

[29] Folkman J. Angiogenesis: an organizing principle for drug discovery? Nat Rev Drug Discov 2007; 6(4): 273-86.
[http://dx.doi.org/10.1038/nrd2115] [PMID: 17396134]

[30] Skuli N, Majmundar AJ, Krock BL, *et al.* Endothelial HIF-2α regulates murine pathological angiogenesis and revascularization processes. J Clin Invest 2012; 122(4): 1427-43.
[http://dx.doi.org/10.1172/JCI57322] [PMID: 22426208]

[31] Brandes RP, Miller FJ, Beer S, *et al.* The vascular NADPH oxidase subunit p47phox is involved in redox-mediated gene expression. Free Radic Biol Med 2002; 32(11): 1116-22.
[http://dx.doi.org/10.1016/S0891-5849(02)00789-X] [PMID: 12031896]

[32] Chen Z, Lai TC, Jan YH, *et al.* Hypoxia-responsive miRNAs target argonaute 1 to promote angiogenesis. J Clin Invest 2013; 123(3): 1057-67.
[http://dx.doi.org/10.1172/JCI65344] [PMID: 23426184]

[33] Carmeliet P. Manipulating angiogenesis in medicine. J Intern Med 2004; 255(5): 538-61.
[http://dx.doi.org/10.1111/j.1365-2796.2003.01297.x] [PMID: 15078497]

[34] Klein S, Roghani M, Rifkin DB. Fibroblast growth factors as angiogenesis factors: new insights into their mechanism of action. EXS 1997; 79: 159-92.
[http://dx.doi.org/10.1007/978-3-0348-9006-9_7] [PMID: 9002232]

[35] Hellberg C, Ostman A, Heldin CH. PDGF and vessel maturation. Recent Results Cancer Res 2010; 180: 103-14.
[http://dx.doi.org/10.1007/978-3-540-78281-0_7] [PMID: 20033380]

[36] Chen JX, Zeng H, Lawrence ML, Blackwell TS, Meyrick B. Angiopoietin-1-induced angiogenesis is modulated by endothelial NADPH oxidase. Am J Physiol Heart Circ Physiol 2006; 291(4): H1563-72.
[http://dx.doi.org/10.1152/ajpheart.01081.2005] [PMID: 16679392]

[37] Pauta M, Ribera J, Melgar-Lesmes P, *et al.* Overexpression of angiopoietin-2 in rats and patients with liver fibrosis. Therapeutic consequences of its inhibition. Liver Int 2015; 35(4): 1383-92.
[http://dx.doi.org/10.1111/liv.12505] [PMID: 24612347]

[38] Patsenker E, Popov Y, Stickel F, *et al.* Pharmacological inhibition of integrin alphavbeta3 aggravates experimental liver fibrosis and suppresses hepatic angiogenesis. Hepatology 2009; 50(5): 1501-11.
[http://dx.doi.org/10.1002/hep.23144] [PMID: 19725105]

[39] Kevil CG, Payne DK, Mire E, Alexander JS. Vascular permeability factor/vascular endothelial cell growth factor-mediated permeability occurs through disorganization of endothelial junctional proteins. J Biol Chem 1998; 273(24): 15099-103.
[http://dx.doi.org/10.1074/jbc.273.24.15099] [PMID: 9614120]

[40] Elpek GO, Gokhan GA, Bozova S. Thrombospondin-1 expression correlates with angiogenesis in experimental cirrhosis. World J Gastroenterol 2008; 14(14): 2213-7.
[http://dx.doi.org/10.3748/wjg.14.2213] [PMID: 18407596]

[41] Eriksson K, Magnusson P, Dixelius J, Claesson-Welsh L, Cross MJ. Angiostatin and endostatin inhibit

endothelial cell migration in response to FGF and VEGF without interfering with specific intracellular signal transduction pathways. FEBS Lett 2003; 536(1-3): 19-24.
[http://dx.doi.org/10.1016/S0014-5793(03)00003-6] [PMID: 12586331]

[42]   Jagavelu K, Routray C, Shergill U, O'Hara SP, Faubion W, Shah VH. Endothelial cell toll-like receptor 4 regulates fibrosis-associated angiogenesis in the liver. Hepatology 2010; 52(2): 590-601.
[http://dx.doi.org/10.1002/hep.23739] [PMID: 20564354]

[43]   Melgar-Lesmes P, Pauta M, Reichenbach V, *et al.* Hypoxia and proinflammatory factors upregulate apelin receptor expression in human stellate cells and hepatocytes. Gut 2011; 60(10): 1404-11.
[http://dx.doi.org/10.1136/gut.2010.234690] [PMID: 21450694]

[44]   Huebert RC, Jagavelu K, Hendrickson HI, *et al.* Aquaporin-1 promotes angiogenesis, fibrosis, and portal hypertension through mechanisms dependent on osmotically sensitive microRNAs. Am J Pathol 2011; 179(4): 1851-60.
[http://dx.doi.org/10.1016/j.ajpath.2011.06.045] [PMID: 21854740]

[45]   Sahin H, Borkham-Kamphorst E, Kuppe C, *et al.* Chemokine Cxcl9 attenuates liver fibrosis-associated angiogenesis in mice. Hepatology 2012; 55(5): 1610-9.
[http://dx.doi.org/10.1002/hep.25545] [PMID: 22237831]

[46]   Staton CA, Kumar I, Reed MW, Brown NJ. Neuropilins in physiological and pathological angiogenesis. J Pathol 2007; 212(3): 237-48.
[http://dx.doi.org/10.1002/path.2182] [PMID: 17503412]

[47]   Fernández M, Semela D, Bruix J, Colle I, Pinzani M, Bosch J. Angiogenesis in liver disease. J Hepatol 2009; 50(3): 604-20.
[http://dx.doi.org/10.1016/j.jhep.2008.12.011] [PMID: 19157625]

[48]   Chaparro M, Sanz-Cameno P, Trapero-Marugan M, Garcia-Buey L, Moreno-Otero R. Mechanisms of angiogenesis in chronic inflammatory liver disease. Ann Hepatol 2007; 6(4): 208-13.
[PMID: 18007549]

[49]   Steib CJ. Kupffer cell activation and portal hypertension. Gut 2011; 60(10): 1307-8.
[http://dx.doi.org/10.1136/gut.2011.242560] [PMID: 21708827]

[50]   Lochhead PA, Gilley R, Cook SJ. ERK5 and its role in tumour development. Biochem Soc Trans 2012; 40(1): 251-6.
[http://dx.doi.org/10.1042/BST20110663] [PMID: 22260700]

[51]   Dewhirst MW, Cao Y, Moeller B. Cycling hypoxia and free radicals regulate angiogenesis and radiotherapy response. Nat Rev Cancer 2008; 8(6): 425-37.
[http://dx.doi.org/10.1038/nrc2397] [PMID: 18500244]

[52]   Ko HM, Seo KH, Han SJ, *et al.* Nuclear factor kappaB dependency of platelet-activating factor-induced angiogenesis. Cancer Res 2002; 62(6): 1809-14.
[PMID: 11912159]

[53]   Franceschini B, Ceva-Grimaldi G, Russo C, Dioguardi N, Grizzi F. The complex functions of mast cells in chronic human liver diseases. Dig Dis Sci 2006; 51(12): 2248-56.
[http://dx.doi.org/10.1007/s10620-006-9082-8] [PMID: 17103041]

[54]   Marra F. Chemokines in liver inflammation and fibrosis. Front Biosci 2002; 7(7): d1899-914.
[http://dx.doi.org/10.2741/A887] [PMID: 12161342]

[55]   Copple BL, Bai S, Burgoon LD, Moon JO. Hypoxia-inducible factor-1α regulates the expression of genes in hypoxic hepatic stellate cells important for collagen deposition and angiogenesis. Liver Int 2011; 31(2): 230-44.
[http://dx.doi.org/10.1111/j.1478-3231.2010.02347.x] [PMID: 20880076]

[56]   Lemoinne S, Cadoret A, El Mourabit H, Thabut D, Housset C. Origins and functions of liver myofibroblasts. Biochim Biophys Acta 2013; 1832(7): 948-54.
[http://dx.doi.org/10.1016/j.bbadis.2013.02.019] [PMID: 23470555]

[57]   Yokomori H, Oda M, Yoshimura K, Hibi T. Enhanced expressions of apelin on proliferative hepatic arterial capillaries in human cirrhotic liver. Hepatol Res 2012; 42(5): 508-14.
[http://dx.doi.org/10.1111/j.1872-034X.2011.00945.x] [PMID: 22502744]

[58]   Novo E, Povero D, Busletta C, *et al.* The biphasic nature of hypoxia-induced directional migration of activated human hepatic stellate cells. J Pathol 2012; 226(4): 588-97.
[http://dx.doi.org/10.1002/path.3005] [PMID: 21959987]

[59]   Novo E, Cannito S, Zamara E, *et al.* Proangiogenic cytokines as hypoxia-dependent factors stimulating migration of human hepatic stellate cells. Am J Pathol 2007; 170(6): 1942-53.
[http://dx.doi.org/10.2353/ajpath.2007.060887] [PMID: 17525262]

[60]   Vanheule E, Geerts AM, Van Huysse J, *et al.* An intravital microscopic study of the hepatic microcirculation in cirrhotic mice models: relationship between fibrosis and angiogenesis. Int J Exp Pathol 2008; 89(6): 419-32.
[http://dx.doi.org/10.1111/j.1365-2613.2008.00608.x] [PMID: 19134051]

[61]   Kaur S, Tripathi D, Dongre K, *et al.* Increased number and function of endothelial progenitor cells stimulate angiogenesis by resident liver sinusoidal endothelial cells (SECs) in cirrhosis through paracrine factors. J Hepatol 2012; 57(6): 1193-8.
[http://dx.doi.org/10.1016/j.jhep.2012.07.016] [PMID: 22824816]

[62]   Chen CH, Chang LT, Tung WC, *et al.* Levels and values of circulating endothelial progenitor cells, soluble angiogenic factors, and mononuclear cell apoptosis in liver cirrhosis patients. J Biomed Sci 2012; 19: 66.
[http://dx.doi.org/10.1186/1423-0127-19-66] [PMID: 22809449]

[63]   Abraldes JG, Iwakiri Y, Loureiro-Silva M, Haq O, Sessa WC, Groszmann RJ. Mild increases in portal pressure upregulate vascular endothelial growth factor and endothelial nitric oxide synthase in the intestinal microcirculatory bed, leading to a hyperdynamic state. Am J Physiol Gastrointest Liver Physiol 2006; 290(5): G980-7.
[http://dx.doi.org/10.1152/ajpgi.00336.2005] [PMID: 16603731]

[64]   Angermayr B, Mejias M, Gracia-Sancho J, Garcia-Pagan JC, Bosch J, Fernandez M. Heme oxygenase attenuates oxidative stress and inflammation, and increases VEGF expression in portal hypertensive rats. J Hepatol 2006; 44(6): 1033-9.
[http://dx.doi.org/10.1016/j.jhep.2005.09.021] [PMID: 16458992]

[65]   Kobus K, Kopycinska J, Kozlowska-Wiechowska A, *et al.* Angiogenesis within the duodenum of patients with cirrhosis is modulated by mechanosensitive Kruppel-like factor 2 and microRNA-126. Liver Int 2012; 32(8): 1222-32.
[http://dx.doi.org/10.1111/j.1478-3231.2012.02791.x] [PMID: 22574900]

[66]   Huang HC, Haq O, Utsumi T, *et al.* Intestinal and plasma VEGF levels in cirrhosis: the role of portal pressure. J Cell Mol Med 2012; 16(5): 1125-33.
[http://dx.doi.org/10.1111/j.1582-4934.2011.01399.x] [PMID: 21801303]

[67]   Garcia-Pras E, Gallego J, Coch L, *et al.* Role and therapeutic potential of vascular stem/progenitor cells in pathological neovascularisation during chronic portal hypertension. Gut 2017; 66(7): 1306-20.
[http://dx.doi.org/10.1136/gutjnl-2015-311157] [PMID: 26984852]

[68]   Gana JC, Serrano CA, Ling SC. Angiogenesis and portal-systemic collaterals in portal hypertension. Ann Hepatol 2016; 15(3): 303-13.
[http://dx.doi.org/10.5604/16652681.1198799] [PMID: 27049484]

[69]   Fernandez M, Vizzutti F, Garcia-Pagan JC, Rodes J, Bosch J. Anti-VEGF receptor-2 monoclonal antibody prevents portal-systemic collateral vessel formation in portal hypertensive mice. Gastroenterology 2004; 126(3): 886-94.
[http://dx.doi.org/10.1053/j.gastro.2003.12.012] [PMID: 14988842]

[70]   Fernandez M, Mejias M, Angermayr B, Garcia-Pagan JC, Rodés J, Bosch J. Inhibition of VEGF

receptor-2 decreases the development of hyperdynamic splanchnic circulation and portal-systemic collateral vessels in portal hypertensive rats. J Hepatol 2005; 43(1): 98-103.
[http://dx.doi.org/10.1016/j.jhep.2005.02.022] [PMID: 15893841]

[71] Angermayr B, Fernandez M, Mejias M, Gracia-Sancho J, Garcia-Pagan JC, Bosch J. NAD(P)H oxidase modulates angiogenesis and the development of portosystemic collaterals and splanchnic hyperaemia in portal hypertensive rats. Gut 2007; 56(4): 560-4.
[http://dx.doi.org/10.1136/gut.2005.088013] [PMID: 16854998]

[72] Gallego J, Garcia-Pras E, Mejias M, Pell N, Schaeper U, Fernandez M. Therapeutic siRNA targeting endothelial KDR decreases portosystemic collateralization in portal hypertension. Sci Rep 2017; 7(1): 14791.
[http://dx.doi.org/10.1038/s41598-017-14818-7] [PMID: 29093528]

[73] Chan CC. Portal-systemic collaterals and angiogenesis. J Chin Med Assoc 2009; 72(5): 223-4.
[http://dx.doi.org/10.1016/S1726-4901(09)70060-7] [PMID: 19467943]

[74] Albillos A, Bañares R, González M, *et al.* The extent of the collateral circulation influences the postprandial increase in portal pressure in patients with cirrhosis. Gut 2007; 56(2): 259-64.
[http://dx.doi.org/10.1136/gut.2006.095240] [PMID: 16837532]

[75] Arora A, Rajesh S, Meenakshi YS, Sureka B, Bansal K, Sarin SK. Spectrum of hepatofugal collateral pathways in portal hypertension: an illustrated radiological review. Insights Imaging 2015; 6(5): 559-72.
[http://dx.doi.org/10.1007/s13244-015-0419-8] [PMID: 26337049]

[76] Yang Z, Tian L, Peng L, Qiu F. Immunohistochemical analysis of growth factor expression and localization in gastric coronary vein of cirrhotic patients. J Tongji Med Univ 1996; 16(4): 229-33.
[http://dx.doi.org/10.1007/BF02888113] [PMID: 9389088]

[77] Hashizume M, Kitano S, Sugimachi K, Sueishi K. Three-dimensional view of the vascular structure of the lower esophagus in clinical portal hypertension. Hepatology 1988; 8(6): 1482-7.
[http://dx.doi.org/10.1002/hep.1840080603] [PMID: 3192160]

[78] Turmakhanov ST, Asadulaev ShM, Akhmetkaliev MN. Morpho-functional Changes of the Azygos Vein and Other Veins of the Gastroesophageal Zone in Portal Hypertension. Ann hir gepatol 2008; 13(2): 58-65.

[79] Vianna A, Hayes PC, Moscoso G, *et al.* Normal venous circulation of the gastroesophageal junction. A route to understanding varices. Gastroenterology 1987; 93(4): 876-89.
[http://dx.doi.org/10.1016/0016-5085(87)90453-7] [PMID: 3623028]

[80] Noda T. Angioarchitectural study of esophageal varices. With special reference to variceal rupture. Virchows Arch A Pathol Anat Histopathol 1984; 404(4): 381-92.
[http://dx.doi.org/10.1007/BF00695222] [PMID: 6437071]

[81] Gaba RC, Couture PM, Lakhoo J. Gastroesophageal Variceal Filling and Drainage Pathways: An Angiographic Description of Afferent and Efferent Venous Anatomic Patterns. J Clin Imaging Sci 2015; 5: 61.
[http://dx.doi.org/10.4103/2156-7514.170730] [PMID: 26713177]

[82] Gracia-Sancho J, Maeso-Díaz R, Bosch J. Pathophysiology and a Rational Basis of Therapy. Dig Dis 2015; 33(4): 508-14.
[http://dx.doi.org/10.1159/000374099] [PMID: 26159267]

[83] Libby P. Inflammatory mechanisms: the molecular basis of inflammation and disease. Nutr Rev 2007; 65(12 Pt 2): S140-6.
[http://dx.doi.org/10.1301/nr.2007.dec.S140-S146] [PMID: 18240538]

[84] de Las Heras N, Aller MA, Martín-Fernández B, *et al.* A wound-like inflammatory aortic response in chronic portal hypertensive rats. Mol Immunol 2012; 51(2): 177-87.
[http://dx.doi.org/10.1016/j.molimm.2012.03.016] [PMID: 22463791]

[85]   Fernández-Varo G, Ros J, Morales-Ruiz M, *et al.* Nitric oxide synthase 3-dependent vascular remodeling and circulatory dysfunction in cirrhosis. Am J Pathol 2003; 162(6): 1985-93.
[http://dx.doi.org/10.1016/S0002-9440(10)64331-3] [PMID: 12759254]

[86]   Kiyono S, Maruyama H, Kondo T, *et al.* Hemodynamic effect of the left gastric artery on esophageal varices in patients with cirrhosis. J Gastroenterol 2016; 51(9): 900-9.
[http://dx.doi.org/10.1007/s00535-015-1157-x] [PMID: 26781661]

[87]   Piva A, Zampieri F, Di Pascoli M, Gatta A, Sacerdoti D, Bolognesi M. Mesenteric arteries responsiveness to acute variations of wall shear stress is impaired in rats with liver cirrhosis. Scand J Gastroenterol 2012; 47(8-9): 1003-13.
[http://dx.doi.org/10.3109/00365521.2012.703231] [PMID: 22774919]

[88]   Resch M, Wiest R, Moleda L, *et al.* Alterations in mechanical properties of mesenteric resistance arteries in experimental portal hypertension. Am J Physiol Gastrointest Liver Physiol 2009; 297(4): G849-57.
[http://dx.doi.org/10.1152/ajpgi.00084.2009] [PMID: 19696142]

[89]   Geerts AM, De Vriese AS, Vanheule E, *et al.* Increased angiogenesis and permeability in the mesenteric microvasculature of rats with cirrhosis and portal hypertension: an *in vivo* study. Liver Int 2006; 26(7): 889-98.
[http://dx.doi.org/10.1111/j.1478-3231.2006.01308.x] [PMID: 16911473]

[90]   Bolognesi M, Di Pascoli M, Verardo A, Gatta A. Splanchnic vasodilation and hyperdynamic circulatory syndrome in cirrhosis. World J Gastroenterol 2014; 20(10): 2555-63.
[http://dx.doi.org/10.3748/wjg.v20.i10.2555] [PMID: 24627591]

[91]   Wei W, Pu YS, Wang XK, *et al.* Wall shear stress in portal vein of cirrhotic patients with portal hypertension. World J Gastroenterol 2017; 23(18): 3279-86.
[http://dx.doi.org/10.3748/wjg.v23.i18.3279] [PMID: 28566887]

[92]   Wen B, Liang J, Deng X, Chen R, Peng P. Effect of fluid shear stress on portal vein remodeling in a rat model of portal hypertension. Gastroenterol Res Pract 2015; 2015: 545018.
[http://dx.doi.org/10.1155/2015/545018] [PMID: 25892988]

[93]   Zeng X, Huang P, Chen M, *et al.* TMEM16A regulates portal vein smooth muscle cell proliferation in portal hypertension. Exp Ther Med 2019; 15(1): 1062-8.
[PMID: 29434696]

[94]   Lautt WW. Mechanism and role of intrinsic regulation of hepatic arterial blood flow: hepatic arterial buffer response. Am J Physiol 1985; 249(5 Pt 1): G549-56.
[PMID: 3904482]

[95]   Moeller M, Thonig A, Pohl S, Ripoll C, Zipprich A. Hepatic arterial vasodilation is independent of portal hypertension in early stages of cirrhosis. PLoS One 2015; 10(3): e0121229.
[http://dx.doi.org/10.1371/journal.pone.0121229] [PMID: 25793622]

[96]   Eipel C, Abshagen K, Vollmar B. Regulation of hepatic blood flow: the hepatic arterial buffer response revisited. World J Gastroenterol 2010; 16(48): 6046-57.
[http://dx.doi.org/10.3748/wjg.v16.i48.6046] [PMID: 21182219]

[97]   Li T, Ni JY, Qi YW, Li HY, Zhang T, Yang Z. Splenic vasculopathy in portal hypertension patients. World J Gastroenterol 2006; 12(17): 2737-41.
[http://dx.doi.org/10.3748/wjg.v12.i17.2737] [PMID: 16718761]

[98]   Yang Z, Zhang L, Li D, Qiu F. Pathological morphology alteration of the splanchnic vascular wall in portal hypertensive patients. Chin Med J (Engl) 2002; 115(4): 559-62.
[PMID: 12133298]

[99]   Garbuzenko DV. Experimental methods of portal hypertension studying. Ros zhurn gastrojenterol gepatol koloproktol 2010; 20(2): 4-12.

[100] McDonald DM, Choyke PL. Imaging of angiogenesis: from microscope to clinic. Nat Med 2003; 9(6): 713-25.
[http://dx.doi.org/10.1038/nm0603-713] [PMID: 12778170]

[101] Van Steenkiste C, Trachet B, Casteleyn C, *et al.* Vascular corrosion casting: analyzing wall shear stress in the portal vein and vascular abnormalities in portal hypertensive and cirrhotic rodents. Lab Invest 2010; 90(11): 1558-72.
[http://dx.doi.org/10.1038/labinvest.2010.138] [PMID: 20714322]

[102] Niggemann P, Murata S, Naito Z, Kumazaki T. A comparative study of the microcirculatory changes in the developing liver cirrhosis between the central and peripheral parts of the main lobe in mice. Hepatol Res 2004; 28(1): 41-8.
[http://dx.doi.org/10.1016/j.hepres.2003.08.004] [PMID: 14734150]

[103] Yang YY, Huang YT, Lin HC, *et al.* Thalidomide decreases intrahepatic resistance in cirrhotic rats. Biochem Biophys Res Commun 2009; 380(3): 666-72.
[http://dx.doi.org/10.1016/j.bbrc.2009.01.160] [PMID: 19285019]

[104] Boerckel JD, Mason DE, McDermott AM, Alsberg E. Microcomputed tomography: approaches and applications in bioengineering. Stem Cell Res Ther 2014; 5(6): 144.
[http://dx.doi.org/10.1186/scrt534] [PMID: 25689288]

[105] Ehling J, Bartneck M, Wei X, *et al.* CCL2-dependent infiltrating macrophages promote angiogenesis in progressive liver fibrosis. Gut 2014; 63(12): 1960-71.
[http://dx.doi.org/10.1136/gutjnl-2013-306294] [PMID: 24561613]

[106] Bartneck M, Fech V, Ehling J, *et al.* Histidine-rich glycoprotein promotes macrophage activation and inflammation in chronic liver disease. Hepatology 2016; 63(4): 1310-24.
[http://dx.doi.org/10.1002/hep.28418] [PMID: 26699087]

[107] Jorgensen SM, Demirkaya O, Ritman EL. Three-dimensional imaging of vasculature and parenchyma in intact rodent organs with X-ray micro-CT. Am J Physiol 1998; 275(3 Pt 2): H1103-14.
[PMID: 9724319]

[108] Thabut D, Routray C, Lomberk G, *et al.* Complementary vascular and matrix regulatory pathways underlie the beneficial mechanism of action of sorafenib in liver fibrosis. Hepatology 2011; 54(2): 573-85.
[http://dx.doi.org/10.1002/hep.24427] [PMID: 21567441]

[109] Lin HC, Huang YT, Yang YY, *et al.* Beneficial effects of dual vascular endothelial growth factor receptor/fibroblast growth factor receptor inhibitor brivanib alaninate in cirrhotic portal hypertensive rats. J Gastroenterol Hepatol 2014; 29(5): 1073-82.
[http://dx.doi.org/10.1111/jgh.12480] [PMID: 24325631]

[110] Kline TL, Knudsen BE, Anderson JL, Vercnocke AJ, Jorgensen SM, Ritman EL. Anatomy of hepatic arteriolo-portal venular shunts evaluated by 3D micro-CT imaging. J Anat 2014; 224(6): 724-31.
[http://dx.doi.org/10.1111/joa.12178] [PMID: 24684343]

[111] Peeters G, Debbaut C, Laleman W, *et al.* A multilevel framework to reconstruct anatomical 3D models of the hepatic vasculature in rat livers. J Anat 2017; 230(3): 471-83.
[http://dx.doi.org/10.1111/joa.12567] [PMID: 27995631]

[112] Peeters G, Debbaut C, Friebel A, *et al.* Quantitative analysis of hepatic macro- and microvascular alterations during cirrhogenesis in the rat. J Anat 2019; 232(3): 485-96.
[http://dx.doi.org/10.1111/joa.12760] [PMID: 29205328]

[113] Hsu SJ, Lee JY, Lin TY, *et al.* The beneficial effects of curcumin in cirrhotic rats with portal hypertension. Biosci Rep 2017; 37(6): 1-13.
[http://dx.doi.org/10.1042/BSR20171015] [PMID: 29162665]

[114] Renier N, Wu Z, Simon DJ, Yang J, Ariel P, Tessier-Lavigne M. iDISCO: a simple, rapid method to immunolabel large tissue samples for volume imaging. Cell 2014; 159(4): 896-910.

[http://dx.doi.org/10.1016/j.cell.2014.10.010] [PMID: 25417164]

[115] Susaki EA, Tainaka K, Perrin D, *et al.* Whole-brain imaging with single-cell resolution using chemical cocktails and computational analysis. Cell 2014; 157(3): 726-39.
[http://dx.doi.org/10.1016/j.cell.2014.03.042] [PMID: 24746791]

[116] Arefyev NO, Garbuzenko DV, Emelyanov IV, Khasanov LR, Mineeva LV. Changes in the microvasculature of small bowel mesentery in rats with prehepatic portal Hypertension: the preliminary study *in vivo.* Abdomen 2017; 4: e1580.

[117] Maksan SM, Ryschich E, Ulger Z, Gebhard MM, Schmidt J. Disturbance of hepatic and intestinal microcirculation in experimental liver cirrhosis. World J Gastroenterol 2005; 11(6): 846-9.
[http://dx.doi.org/10.3748/wjg.v11.i6.846] [PMID: 15682478]

[118] Yamaki K, Lindbom L, Thorlacius H, Hedqvist P, Raud J. An approach for studies of mediator-induced leukocyte rolling in the undisturbed microcirculation of the rat mesentery. Br J Pharmacol 1998; 123(3): 381-9.
[http://dx.doi.org/10.1038/sj.bjp.0701617] [PMID: 9504377]

[119] De Backer D, Hollenberg S, Boerma C, *et al.* How to evaluate the microcirculation: report of a round table conference. Crit Care 2007; 11(5): R101.
[http://dx.doi.org/10.1186/cc6118] [PMID: 17845716]

[120] De Backer D, Creteur J, Preiser JC, Dubois MJ, Vincent JL. Microvascular blood flow is altered in patients with sepsis. Am J Respir Crit Care Med 2002; 166(1): 98-104.
[http://dx.doi.org/10.1164/rccm.200109-016OC] [PMID: 12091178]

[121] Spronk PE, Ince C, Gardien MJ, Mathura KR, Oudemans-van Straaten HM, Zandstra DF. Nitroglycerin in septic shock after intravascular volume resuscitation. Lancet 2002; 360(9343): 1395-6.
[http://dx.doi.org/10.1016/S0140-6736(02)11393-6] [PMID: 12423989]

[122] Klyscz T, Jünger M, Jung F, Zeintl H. [Cap image--a new kind of computer-assisted video image analysis system for dynamic capillary microscopy]. Biomed Tech (Berl) 1997; 42(6): 168-75.
[http://dx.doi.org/10.1515/bmte.1997.42.6.168] [PMID: 9312307]

[123] Sumanovski LT, Battegay E, Stumm M, van der Kooij M, Sieber CC. Increased angiogenesis in portal hypertensive rats: role of nitric oxide. Hepatology 1999; 29(4): 1044-9.
[http://dx.doi.org/10.1002/hep.510290436] [PMID: 10094944]

[124] Anderson CR, Ponce AM, Price RJ. Immunohistochemical identification of an extracellular matrix scaffold that microguides capillary sprouting *in vivo.* J Histochem Cytochem 2004; 52(8): 1063-72.
[http://dx.doi.org/10.1369/jhc.4A6250.2004] [PMID: 15258182]

[125] Huang HC, Wang SS, Hsin IF, *et al.* Cannabinoid receptor 2 agonist ameliorates mesenteric angiogenesis and portosystemic collaterals in cirrhotic rats. Hepatology 2012; 56(1): 248-58.
[http://dx.doi.org/10.1002/hep.25625] [PMID: 22290687]

[126] Yang M, Stapor PC, Peirce SM, Betancourt AM, Murfee WL. Rat mesentery exteriorization: a model for investigating the cellular dynamics involved in angiogenesis. J Vis Exp 2012; 63(63): e3954.
[PMID: 22643964]

[127] McConnell M, Iwakiri Y. Biology of portal hypertension. Hepatol Int 2019; 12 (Suppl. 1): 11-23.
[http://dx.doi.org/10.1007/s12072-017-9826-x] [PMID: 29075990]

[128] Licks F, Hartmann RM, Marques C, *et al.* N-acetylcysteine modulates angiogenesis and vasodilation in stomach such as DNA damage in blood of portal hypertensive rats. World J Gastroenterol 2015; 21(43): 12351-60.
[http://dx.doi.org/10.3748/wjg.v21.i43.12351] [PMID: 26604642]

[129] Aperio Technologies I. Microvessel Analysis Algorithm, User'S Guide @ONLINE. 2008.

[130] Reyes-Aldasoro CC, Williams LJ, Akerman S, Kanthou C, Tozer GM. An automatic algorithm for the

segmentation and morphological analysis of microvessels in immunostained histological tumour sections. J Microsc 2011; 242(3): 262-78.
[http://dx.doi.org/10.1111/j.1365-2818.2010.03464.x] [PMID: 21118252]

[131] Fernández-Carrobles MM, Tadeo I, Bueno G, *et al.* TMA vessel segmentation based on color and morphological features: application to angiogenesis research. Sci World J 2013; 2013: 263190.
[http://dx.doi.org/10.1155/2013/263190] [PMID: 24489494]

[132] Chojkier M, Groszmann RJ. Measurement of portal-systemic shunting in the rat by using γ-labeled microspheres. Am J Physiol 1981; 240(5): G371-5.
[PMID: 7235023]

[133] Hodeige D, de Pauw M, Eechaute W, Weyne J, Heyndrickx GR. On the validity of blood flow measurement using colored microspheres. Am J Physiol 1999; 276(4): H1150-8.
[PMID: 10199837]

[134] Theodorakis N, Maluccio M, Skill N. Murine study of portal hypertension associated endothelin-1 hypo-response. World J Gastroenterol 2015; 21(16): 4817-28.
[http://dx.doi.org/10.3748/wjg.v21.i16.4817] [PMID: 25944995]

[135] Hsu SJ, Wang SS, Hsin IF, *et al.* Green tea polyphenol decreases the severity of portosystemic collaterals and mesenteric angiogenesis in rats with liver cirrhosis. Clin Sci (Lond) 2014; 126(9): 633-44.
[http://dx.doi.org/10.1042/CS20130215] [PMID: 24063570]

[136] Lee PC, Yang YY, Huang CS, *et al.* Concomitant inhibition of oxidative stress and angiogenesis by chronic hydrogen-rich saline and N-acetylcysteine treatments improves systemic, splanchnic and hepatic hemodynamics of cirrhotic rats. Hepatol Res 2015; 45(5): 578-88.
[http://dx.doi.org/10.1111/hepr.12379] [PMID: 24961937]

[137] Van Steenkiste C, Staelens S, Deleye S, *et al.* Measurement of porto-systemic shunting in mice by novel three-dimensional micro-single photon emission computed tomography imaging enabling longitudinal follow-up. Liver Int 2010; 30(8): 1211-20.
[http://dx.doi.org/10.1111/j.1478-3231.2010.02276.x] [PMID: 20497314]

[138] Dufour JF. Anti-angiogenic therapy for HCC. Minerva Gastroenterol Dietol 2012; 58(1): 81-6.
[PMID: 22419006]

[139] Llovet JM, Ricci S, Mazzaferro V, *et al.* Sorafenib in advanced hepatocellular carcinoma. N Engl J Med 2008; 359(4): 378-90.
[http://dx.doi.org/10.1056/NEJMoa0708857] [PMID: 18650514]

[140] Liu L, You Z, Yu H, *et al.* Mechanotransduction-modulated fibrotic microniches reveal the contribution of angiogenesis in liver fibrosis. Nat Mater 2017; 16(12): 1252-61.
[http://dx.doi.org/10.1038/nmat5024] [PMID: 29170554]

[141] Qu K, Huang Z, Lin T, *et al.* New Insight into the Anti-liver Fibrosis Effect of Multitargeted Tyrosine Kinase Inhibitors: From Molecular Target to Clinical Trials. Front Pharmacol 2016; 6: 300.
[http://dx.doi.org/10.3389/fphar.2015.00300] [PMID: 26834633]

[142] Garbuzenko DV, Arefyev NO, Kazachkov EL. Antiangiogenic therapy for portal hypertension in liver cirrhosis: Current progress and perspectives. World J Gastroenterol 2019; 24(33): 3738-48.
[http://dx.doi.org/10.3748/wjg.v24.i33.3738] [PMID: 30197479]

[143] Wang Y, Gao J, Zhang D, Zhang J, Ma J, Jiang H. New insights into the antifibrotic effects of sorafenib on hepatic stellate cells and liver fibrosis. J Hepatol 2010; 53(1): 132-44.
[http://dx.doi.org/10.1016/j.jhep.2010.02.027] [PMID: 20447716]

[144] Mejias M, Garcia-Pras E, Tiani C, Miquel R, Bosch J, Fernandez M. Beneficial effects of sorafenib on splanchnic, intrahepatic, and portocollateral circulations in portal hypertensive and cirrhotic rats. Hepatology 2009; 49(4): 1245-56.
[http://dx.doi.org/10.1002/hep.22758] [PMID: 19137587]

[145] Tugues S, Fernandez-Varo G, Muñoz-Luque J, *et al.* Antiangiogenic treatment with sunitinib ameliorates inflammatory infiltrate, fibrosis, and portal pressure in cirrhotic rats. Hepatology 2007; 46(6): 1919-26.
[http://dx.doi.org/10.1002/hep.21921] [PMID: 17935226]

[146] Majumder S, Piguet AC, Dufour JF, Chatterjee S. Study of the cellular mechanism of Sunitinib mediated inactivation of activated hepatic stellate cells and its implications in angiogenesis. Eur J Pharmacol 2013; 705(1-3): 86-95.
[http://dx.doi.org/10.1016/j.ejphar.2013.02.026] [PMID: 23454556]

[147] Yang YY, Liu RS, Lee PC, *et al.* Anti-VEGFR agents ameliorate hepatic venous dysregulation/microcirculatory dysfunction, splanchnic venous pooling and ascites of NASH-cirrhotic rat. Liver Int 2014; 34(4): 521-34.
[http://dx.doi.org/10.1111/liv.12299] [PMID: 23998651]

[148] Bieker JJ. Krüppel-like factors: three fingers in many pies. J Biol Chem 2001; 276(37): 34355-8.
[http://dx.doi.org/10.1074/jbc.R100043200] [PMID: 11443140]

[149] Taniguchi H, Jacinto FV, Villanueva A, *et al.* Silencing of Kruppel-like factor 2 by the histone methyltransferase EZH2 in human cancer. Oncogene 2012; 31(15): 1988-94.
[http://dx.doi.org/10.1038/onc.2011.387] [PMID: 21892211]

[150] Kawanami D, Mahabeleshwar GH, Lin Z, *et al.* Kruppel-like factor 2 inhibits hypoxia-inducible factor 1alpha expression and function in the endothelium. J Biol Chem 2009; 284(31): 20522-30.
[http://dx.doi.org/10.1074/jbc.M109.025346] [PMID: 19491109]

[151] Doddaballapur A, Michalik KM, Manavski Y, *et al.* Laminar shear stress inhibits endothelial cell metabolism *via* KLF2-mediated repression of PFKFB3. Arterioscler Thromb Vasc Biol 2015; 35(1): 137-45.
[http://dx.doi.org/10.1161/ATVBAHA.114.304277] [PMID: 25359860]

[152] Gracia-Sancho J, Russo L, García-Calderó H, García-Pagán JC, García-Cardeña G, Bosch J. Endothelial expression of transcription factor Kruppel-like factor 2 and its vasoprotective target genes in the normal and cirrhotic rat liver. Gut 2011; 60(4): 517-24.
[http://dx.doi.org/10.1136/gut.2010.220913] [PMID: 21112949]

[153] Das A, Shergill U, Thakur L, *et al.* Ephrin B2/EphB4 pathway in hepatic stellate cells stimulates Erk-dependent VEGF production and sinusoidal endothelial cell recruitment. Am J Physiol Gastrointest Liver Physiol 2010; 298(6): G908-15.
[http://dx.doi.org/10.1152/ajpgi.00510.2009] [PMID: 20338920]

[154] Zeng XQ, Li N, Pan DY, *et al.* Kruppel-like factor 2 inhibit the angiogenesis of cultured human liver sinusoidal endothelial cells through the ERK1/2 signaling pathway. Biochem Biophys Res Commun 2015; 464(4): 1241-7.
[http://dx.doi.org/10.1016/j.bbrc.2015.07.113] [PMID: 26212440]

[155] Miao Q, Zeng X, Ma G, *et al.* Simvastatin suppresses the proangiogenic microenvironment of human hepatic stellate cells *via* the Kruppel-like factor 2 pathway. Rev Esp Enferm Dig 2015; 107(2): 63-71.
[PMID: 25659387]

[156] Marrone G, Russo L, Rosado E, *et al.* The transcription factor KLF2 mediates hepatic endothelial protection and paracrine endothelial-stellate cell deactivation induced by statins. J Hepatol 2013; 58(1): 98-103.
[http://dx.doi.org/10.1016/j.jhep.2012.08.026] [PMID: 22989565]

[157] Garbuzenko DV, Mikurov AA, Smirnov DM. [Bacterial endotoxinemia and risk of hemorrhage from oesophageal varicose veins in patients with liver cirrhosis]. Klin Med (Mosk) 2012; 90(7): 48-51.
[PMID: 23019976]

[158] Zhu Q, Zou L, Jagavelu K, *et al.* Intestinal decontamination inhibits TLR4 dependent fibronectin-mediated cross-talk between stellate cells and endothelial cells in liver fibrosis in mice. J Hepatol

2012; 56(4): 893-9.
[http://dx.doi.org/10.1016/j.jhep.2011.11.013] [PMID: 22173161]

[159] DuPont HL. Biologic properties and clinical uses of rifaximin. Expert Opin Pharmacother 2011; 12(2): 293-302.
[http://dx.doi.org/10.1517/14656566.2011.546347] [PMID: 21226639]

[160] Liu Y, Salvador LA, Byeon S, *et al.* Anticolon cancer activity of largazole, a marine-derived tunable histone deacetylase inhibitor. J Pharmacol Exp Ther 2010; 335(2): 351-61.
[http://dx.doi.org/10.1124/jpet.110.172387] [PMID: 20739454]

[161] Liu Y, Wang Z, Wang J, *et al.* A histone deacetylase inhibitor, largazole, decreases liver fibrosis and angiogenesis by inhibiting transforming growth factor-β and vascular endothelial growth factor signalling. Liver Int 2013; 33(4): 504-15.
[http://dx.doi.org/10.1111/liv.12034] [PMID: 23279742]

[162] Fontaine H, Vallet-Pichard A, Equi-Andrade C, *et al.* Histopathologic efficacy of ribavirin monotherapy in kidney allograft recipients with chronic hepatitis C. Transplantation 2004; 78(6): 853-7.
[http://dx.doi.org/10.1097/01.TP.0000128911.87538.AA] [PMID: 15385804]

[163] Michaelis M, Michaelis R, Suhan T, *et al.* Ribavirin inhibits angiogenesis by tetrahydrobiopterin depletion. FASEB J 2007; 21(1): 81-7.
[http://dx.doi.org/10.1096/fj.06-6779com] [PMID: 17135367]

[164] Fernandez M, Mejias M, Garcia-Pras E, Mendez R, Garcia-Pagan JC, Bosch J. Reversal of portal hypertension and hyperdynamic splanchnic circulation by combined vascular endothelial growth factor and platelet-derived growth factor blockade in rats. Hepatology 2007; 46(4): 1208-17.
[http://dx.doi.org/10.1002/hep.21785] [PMID: 17654489]

[165] D'Amico M, Mejías M, García-Pras E, *et al.* Effects of the combined administration of propranolol plus sorafenib on portal hypertension in cirrhotic rats. Am J Physiol Gastrointest Liver Physiol 2012; 302(10): G1191-8.
[http://dx.doi.org/10.1152/ajpgi.00252.2011] [PMID: 22403792]

[166] Garbuzenko DV. Current approaches to the management of patients with liver cirrhosis who have acute esophageal variceal bleeding. Curr Med Res Opin 2016; 32(3): 467-75.
[http://dx.doi.org/10.1185/03007995.2015.1124846] [PMID: 26804426]

[167] Woltering EA. Development of targeted somatostatin-based antiangiogenic therapy: a review and future perspectives. Cancer Biother Radiopharm 2003; 18(4): 601-9.
[http://dx.doi.org/10.1089/108497803322287691] [PMID: 14503956]

[168] Mejias M, Garcia-Pras E, Tiani C, Bosch J, Fernandez M. The somatostatin analogue octreotide inhibits angiogenesis in the earliest, but not in advanced, stages of portal hypertension in rats. J Cell Mol Med 2008; 12(5A): 1690-9.
[http://dx.doi.org/10.1111/j.1582-4934.2008.00218.x] [PMID: 18194463]

[169] Garbuzenko DV. The principles of management of patients with liver cirrhosis complicated by ascites. Klin Med (Mosk) 2017; 95(9): 789-6.

[170] Michel F, Ambroisine ML, Duriez M, Delcayre C, Levy BI, Silvestre JS. Aldosterone enhances ischemia-induced neovascularization through angiotensin II-dependent pathway. Circulation 2004; 109(16): 1933-7.
[http://dx.doi.org/10.1161/01.CIR.0000127112.36796.9B] [PMID: 15078792]

[171] Wilkinson-Berka JL, Tan G, Jaworski K, Miller AG. Identification of a retinal aldosterone system and the protective effects of mineralocorticoid receptor antagonism on retinal vascular pathology. Circ Res 2009; 104(1): 124-33.
[http://dx.doi.org/10.1161/CIRCRESAHA.108.176008] [PMID: 19038868]

[172] Gravez B, Tarjus A, Pelloux V, *et al.* Aldosterone promotes cardiac endothelial cell proliferation *in*

vivo. J Am Heart Assoc 2015; 4(1): e001266.
[http://dx.doi.org/10.1161/JAHA.114.001266] [PMID: 25564371]

[173] Miternique-Grosse A, Griffon C, Siegel L, Neuville A, Weltin D, Stephan D. Antiangiogenic effects of spironolactone and other potassium-sparing diuretics in human umbilical vein endothelial cells and in fibrin gel chambers implanted in rats. J Hypertens 2006; 24(11): 2207-13.
[http://dx.doi.org/10.1097/01.hjh.0000249698.26983.4e] [PMID: 17053542]

[174] Hsu SJ, Wang SS, Huo TI, *et al.* The Impact of Spironolactone on the Severity of Portal-Systemic Collaterals and Hepatic Encephalopathy in Cirrhotic Rats. J Pharmacol Exp Ther 2015; 355(1): 117-24.
[http://dx.doi.org/10.1124/jpet.115.225516] [PMID: 26260462]

[175] Chikina SYu. Antioxidant effects of N-acetylcysteine in modern clinical practice. Jeffektivnaja farmakoterapija 2011; 32: 19-24.

[176] Garbuzenko DV. Pathophysiological mechanisms and new directions of therapy of portal hypertension at liver cirrhosis. Klin persp gastrojenterol gepatol 2010; 6: 11-20.

[177] Salani D, Taraboletti G, Rosanò L, *et al.* Endothelin-1 induces an angiogenic phenotype in cultured endothelial cells and stimulates neovascularization *in vivo.* Am J Pathol 2000; 157(5): 1703-11.
[http://dx.doi.org/10.1016/S0002-9440(10)64807-9] [PMID: 11073829]

[178] Hsu SJ, Lin TY, Wang SS, *et al.* Endothelin receptor blockers reduce shunting and angiogenesis in cirrhotic rats. Eur J Clin Invest 2016; 46(6): 572-80.
[http://dx.doi.org/10.1111/eci.12636] [PMID: 27091078]

[179] Gerasimenko ND, Degtyar NI, Racin MS. Systemic inflammation and aging: the role of nuclear transcription factors and therapeutic possibilities (Review of the literature). Probl starenija i dolgoletija 2016; 25: 554-61.

[180] Dana N, Javanmard SH, Rafiee L. Role of peroxisome proliferator-activated receptor alpha and gamma in antiangiogenic effect of pomegranate peel extract. Iran J Basic Med Sci 2016; 19(1): 106-10.
[PMID: 27096071]

[181] Schwabl P, Payer BA, Grahovac J, *et al.* Pioglitazone decreases portosystemic shunting by modulating inflammation and angiogenesis in cirrhotic and non-cirrhotic portal hypertensive rats. J Hepatol 2014; 60(6): 1135-42.
[http://dx.doi.org/10.1016/j.jhep.2014.01.025] [PMID: 24530596]

[182] Enomoto N, Takei Y, Hirose M, *et al.* Thalidomide prevents alcoholic liver injury in rats through suppression of Kupffer cell sensitization and TNF-α production. Gastroenterology 2002; 123(1): 291-300.
[http://dx.doi.org/10.1053/gast.2002.34161] [PMID: 12105857]

[183] Li TH, Huang CC, Yang YY, *et al.* Thalidomide Improves the Intestinal Mucosal Injury and Suppresses Mesenteric Angiogenesis and Vasodilatation by Down-Regulating Inflammasomes-Related Cascades in Cirrhotic Rats. PLoS One 2016; 11(1): e0147212.
[http://dx.doi.org/10.1371/journal.pone.0147212] [PMID: 26820153]

[184] Hsin IF, Lee JY, Huo TI, *et al.* 2'-Hydroxyflavanone ameliorates mesenteric angiogenesis and portal-systemic collaterals in rats with liver fibrosis. J Gastroenterol Hepatol 2016; 31(5): 1045-51.
[http://dx.doi.org/10.1111/jgh.13197] [PMID: 26474184]

[185] Coriat R, Gouya H, Mir O, *et al.* Reversible decrease of portal venous flow in cirrhotic patients: a positive side effect of sorafenib. PLoS One 2011; 6(2): e16978.
[http://dx.doi.org/10.1371/journal.pone.0016978] [PMID: 21340026]

[186] Pinter M, Sieghart W, Reiberger T, Rohr-Udilova N, Ferlitsch A, Peck-Radosavljevic M. The effects of sorafenib on the portal hypertensive syndrome in patients with liver cirrhosis and hepatocellular carcinoma--a pilot study. Aliment Pharmacol Ther 2012; 35(1): 83-91.

[http://dx.doi.org/10.1111/j.1365-2036.2011.04896.x] [PMID: 22032637]

[187] Garcia-Tsao G, Fallon M, Reddy K, *et al.* Placebo-controlled, randomized, pilot study of the effect of sorafenib on portal pressure in patients with cirrhosis, portal hypertension and ablated hepatocellular carcinoma (HCC). Hepatology 2015; 62 (Suppl. S1): 580A.

[188] D'Amico G. Stages classification of cirrhosis: Where do we stand? In: de Franchis R, Ed. Portal Hypertension V Proceedings of the Fifth Baveno International Consensus Workshop. 132-9.

[189] Vorobioff JD, Groszmann RJ. Hepatic venous pressure gradient measurement in pre-primary and primary prophylaxis of variceal hemorrhage. Ann Hepatol 2013; 12(1): 22-9.
[PMID: 23293190]

[190] Villanueva C, Albillos A, Genescà J, *et al.* Development of hyperdynamic circulation and response to β-blockers in compensated cirrhosis with portal hypertension. Hepatology 2016; 63(1): 197-206.
[http://dx.doi.org/10.1002/hep.28264] [PMID: 26422126]

[191] Vorobioff JD, Groszmann RJ. Prevention of portal hypertension: from variceal development to clinical decompensation. Hepatology 2015; 61(1): 375-81.
[http://dx.doi.org/10.1002/hep.27249] [PMID: 24913395]

[192] Jaurigue MM, Cappell MS. Therapy for alcoholic liver disease. World J Gastroenterol 2014; 20(9): 2143-58.
[http://dx.doi.org/10.3748/wjg.v20.i9.2143] [PMID: 24605013]

[193] Chung GE, Lee JH, Kim YJ. Does antiviral therapy reduce complications of cirrhosis? World J Gastroenterol 2014; 20(23): 7306-11.
[http://dx.doi.org/10.3748/wjg.v20.i23.7306] [PMID: 24966601]

[194] Libânio D, Marinho RT. Impact of hepatitis C oral therapy in portal hypertension. World J Gastroenterol 2017; 23(26): 4669-74.
[http://dx.doi.org/10.3748/wjg.v23.i26.4669] [PMID: 28765688]

SUBJECT INDEX

A

Abdominal aorta 178, 184, 199
Activated HSC 164, 165, 166, 170, 172, 173, 182, 193, 194
Activation 1, 8, 9, 11, 12, 42, 43, 45, 58, 65, 69, 114, 139, 141, 142, 145, 146, 148, 149, 164, 165, 166, 167, 168, 191, 196
  endothelial cell 167
  ligand-induced receptor 58, 69
Active neovascularization 119
Adenoid 71, 72
Advanced RCC 57, 61, 63
Adventitial veins 175, 176, 177
Agents 34, 49, 50, 52, 54, 55, 57, 61, 64, 66, 68, 74, 97, 99, 102, 103, 104, 108, 143
  anti-cancer 54, 55
  cytotoxic 49, 50
  negatively-acting 97, 99, 104
  positively-acting 97, 99, 104
  vascular disrupting 103
Age-related Macular Degeneration (AMD) 1, 4, 6, 9, 12, 13, 111, 112, 114, 115, 119, 120, 128, 131, 133
Akt signaling 197, 198, 201
Alanine transaminase (ALT) 70, 75
Aldose reductase (AR) 1, 10
Aldosterone 164, 196, 201
Alpha lipoic acid 148
Alzheimer's disease 72, 73
Anemia 59, 70, 72
Angioblasts 37, 109
Angiogenesis 1, 2, 3, 4, 5, 7, 9, 11, 12, 13, 19, 20, 21, 26, 27, 29, 30, 34, 35, 36, 37, 38, 39, 40, 41, 42, 43, 44, 45, 46, 47, 48, 49, 52, 53, 54, 55, 56, 64, 65, 69, 71, 74, 75, 97, 98, 99, 104, 108, 109, 110, 111, 112, 113, 137, 138, 139, 140, 141, 143, 144, 145, 146, 147, 148, 149, 162, 163, 164, 167, 168, 169, 170, 171, 172, 173, 180, 183, 185, 186, 188, 189, 190, 191, 192, 193, 194, 195, 196, 198, 199, 201, 203
  antagonize 56, 71

cascade 140
choroidal 4, 7, 12
fibrosis-associated 170, 194
inhibiting pathologic 97, 99, 104
intussusceptive 189
postnatal 109
splanchnic 185
stimulate 36, 111, 169, 172
superfluous 48
suppress 74
suppressing 146
sustained 35
targeting 19, 47, 49, 56
tumoral 110
tumour 98
tumoural 98
Angiogenesis inhibitors 37, 48, 49, 50, 51, 52, 53, 54, 55, 97, 98, 99, 104, 111, 112, 115, 162, 169, 190, 196
  administration of 49, 50
  endogenous 48
Angiogenesis processes 34, 35, 37, 38, 47, 51, 98, 109, 138, 139, 143, 144, 145, 146, 148, 149
  perplex 34, 35
Angiogenic 1, 2, 7, 9, 12, 128, 129, 130, 137, 139, 142, 144, 146, 147, 167, 170, 172, 173, 179
  factors 128, 129, 130, 139, 170, 172, 173
  processes 1, 2, 7, 9, 12, 137, 142, 144, 146, 147, 167, 170, 172, 179
Angiopoietins 43, 109, 110, 140, 169
Angiostatin 48, 97, 99, 169
Angiotensin 12, 13, 164
Anti-angiogenic 19, 39, 40, 48, 50, 51, 52, 53, 55, 56, 60, 61, 74, 75, 76, 112, 162, 163, 190, 191, 198, 199
  activity 60, 61, 74
  agents 48, 50, 51, 52, 55, 56, 74, 76
  effects 75, 76
  factors 39
    family 40
  therapy 19, 53, 112, 162, 163, 190, 191, 198, 199